Comorbidity in Affective Disorders

Medical Psychiatry

Series Editor

William A. Frosch, M.D.

Cornell University Medical College
New York, New York

1. Handbook of Depression and Anxiety: A Biological Approach, *edited by Johan A. den Boer and J. M. Ad Sitsen*
2. Anticonvulsants in Mood Disorders, *edited by Russell T. Joffe and Joseph R. Calabrese*
3. Serotonin in Antipsychotic Treatment: Mechanisms and Clinical Practice, *edited by John M. Kane, H.-J. Möller, and Frans Awouters*
4. Handbook of Functional Gastrointestinal Disorders, *edited by Kevin W. Olden*
5. Clinical Management of Anxiety, *edited by Johan A. den Boer*
6. Obsessive-Compulsive Disorders: Diagnosis • Etiology • Treatment, *edited by Eric Hollander and Dan J. Stein*
7. Bipolar Disorder: Biological Models and Their Clinical Application, *edited by L. Trevor Young and Russell T. Joffe*
8. Dual Diagnosis and Treatment: Substance Abuse and Comorbid Medical and Psychiatric Disorders, *edited by Henry R. Kranzler and Bruce J. Rounsaville*
9. Geriatric Psychopharmacology, *edited by J. Craig Nelson*
10. Panic Disorder and Its Treatment, *edited by Jerrold F. Rosenbaum and Mark H. Pollack*
11. Comorbidity in Affective Disorders, *edited by Mauricio Tohen*
12. Practical Management of the Side Effects of Psychotropic Drugs, *edited by Richard Balon*

ADDITIONAL VOLUMES IN PREPARATION

Psychiatric Treatment of the Medically Ill, *edited by Robert G. Robinson and William R. Yates*

Comorbidity in Affective Disorders

edited by

Mauricio Tohen

Lilly Research Laboratories
Indianapolis, Indiana and
McLean Hospital, Harvard Medical School
Boston, Massachusetts

MARCEL DEKKER, INC. NEW YORK • BASEL

ISBN: 0-8247-0212-3

This book is printed on acid-free paper.

Headquarters
Marcel Dekker, Inc.
270 Madison Avenue, New York, NY 10016
tel: 212-696-9000; fax: 212-685-4540

Eastern Hemisphere Distribution
Marcel Dekker AG
Hutgasse 4, Postfach 812, CH-4001 Basel, Switzerland
tel: 44-61-261-8482; fax: 44-61-261-8896

World Wide Web
http://www.dekker.com

The publisher offers discounts on this book when ordered in bulk quantities. For more information, write to Special Sales/Professional Marketing at the headquarters address above.

Current printing (last digit):
10 9 8 7 6 5 4 3 2 1

PRINTED IN THE UNITED STATES OF AMERICA

About the Series

Welcome to the world of multiple diagnoses.

When dinosaurs roamed the earth and all we had for psychiatric nosologic guidance was DSM-2, a single diagnosis was commonly considered adequate for each patient. The classification was usually thought of as hierarchical: when the patient was diagnosed as having schizophrenia, the presence of obsessive-compulsive symptoms was thought of as a manifestation of the underlying illness rather than as an additional syndrome. The patient's avoidant behavior was merely symptomatic of schizophrenia and not seen as indicative of a personality or personality disorder. The development of multiple diagnostic axes of Spitzer and the DSM-3 taskforce was powerfully shaped by a number of forces. Important among these were the development of research criteria for diagnosis of potential subjects (patients) for controlled study of uncomplicated illness, and the realization that most patients had personalities as well as illnesses. I believe that the introduction of the personality axis was also, unconsciously, an atonement for the deinstitutionalization of the previously beloved term "neurosis." In addition, and also probably outside of awareness, was Dr. Spitzer's experience as a medical student with the New York Heart Association's multi-axial diagnostic scheme for heart disease. In that system, every patient received an etiological, anatomical, physiological, and functional diagnosis.

DSM-3R and DSM-4 have further eroded the hierarchic structure of our diagnostic scheme. This, along with the use of criteria sets, has resulted in many, and perhaps most, patients receiving several diagnoses. In the absence of known etiologies and clear pathophysiologic and/or psychopathologic pathways, this may be the sensible system to use until we deepen our understanding of underlying processes. Certainly, for example, the presence of substance abuse appears to complicate the course and response to treatment of other psychiatric illnesses. Similarly, at least some substance abuse is precipitated or reinforced by psychiatric illness. Our ability to make the necessary multiple diagnoses will help us refine prognoses and shape our treatments to the real needs of patients.

Dr. Tohen has gathered a distinguished group of contributors for this volume which summarizes our current knowledge of comorbidity in affective illness. Careful reading and application will help us to help those in need.

William A. Frosch

Preface

Considering that half of all psychiatric patients have more than one diagnosis, comorbidity can be considered the rule rather than the exception. Individuals with affective disorders are especially susceptible to comorbid conditions in both treatment- and population-based samples. Two large population-based studies conducted in the United States estimated the lifetime rate of comorbidity in affective disorders as high as 75%. Not only is comorbidity in affective disorders highly prevalent, but in addition it has major implications for complicating treatment and worsening patient outcome. Comorbidity also has tremendous impact on the design of clinical trials and outcome research.

This textbook was conceptualized as a tool for both clinicians and researchers. For clinicians, it offers assistance in the diagnosis and treatment of patients with affective disorders. Knowledge of the epidemiological and diagnostic challenges presented by comorbidity in affective disorders aids the clinician in treatment planning by taking into account the impact of comorbidity on both treatment and outcome. For the researcher, knowledge of comorbidity in affective disorders is essential for the proper design of clinical trials and outcome studies. In the design of clinical trials, the investigator needs to consider if the exclusion of patients with comorbidity will affect the generalizability of the findings or if inclusion of these patients will affect the validity of the results. For outcome studies, the presence of comorbidity may need to be considered as a separate factor and analyzed as such.

Contributors of this textbook were carefully selected and are leading experts in their respective fields. The book is divided into two major parts: Depression (Chapters 2–6) and Bipolar Disorder (Chapters 7–11). Both sections have "parallel" development with respect to the comorbid conditions or issues which are presented in separate chapters. The first chapter, by Ronald C. Kessler, presents the major findings from the National Comorbidity Survey on Comorbidity in Depression and in Bipolar Disorder. This chapter provides an excellent foundation for subsequent chapters by highlighting the importance of recognizing and addressing comorbid conditions in affective disorders.

The first comorbid disorder that is addressed in the book is substance abuse, a highly prevalent condition in affective disorder patients. Chapter 2, written by

Douglas M. Ziedonis, Conor K. Farren, and Tony P. George, is entitled "Depression and Substance Abuse" and describes the epidemiological risk and treatment factors associated with the use of alcohol and illicit drugs by patients with major depression. A parallel chapter in the bipolar disorder section entitled "Bipolar Disorder and Substance Abuse" (Chapter 7) is by Susan C. Sonne and Kathleen T. Brady.

"Depression in the Medically Ill" (Chapter 3), by Jeffrey Newport and Charles B. Nemeroff, and "The Co-occurrence of Bipolar Disorder with Medical Illness" (Chapter 8), authored by Kenji W. Sax and Stephen M. Strakowski, emphasize the challenges of pharmacological treatment in the respective patient populations.

The comorbidity of personality disorders in depression and bipolar disorder are areas of research that are sparse in both outcome and treatment-response data. Patients with these conditions represent major challenges for clinicians due to psychosocial and pharmacological considerations. "Comorbidity of Depressive Illnesses and Personality Disorders" (Chapter 4), contributed by Thomas J. Doyle, Ming T. Tsuang, and Michael J. Lyons, along with "Bipolar Disorder and Comorbid Axis I Disorders" (Chapter 9) and "Bipolar Disorder and Comorbid Axis II Disorders" (Chapter 10), both authored by Carlos A. Zarate, Jr., and Mauricio Tohen, provide important clinical insight into personality disorder comorbidity.

Comorbidity in mood disorders is present throughout the lifespan but has different diagnostic and treatment challenges in children, adults, and the elderly. Chapter 5, "The Comorbidity of Depression and Medical Illness in the Elderly," written by Andrew Satlin, and Chapter 11, "Comorbidity and Bipolar Disorder in Old Age," by Kenneth Israel Shulman and Anu Singh, focus on comorbidity in the elderly and address the major issues in comorbid medical conditions with an emphasis on both pharmacological and psychosocial treatments. "Comorbidity with Depression in Children and Adolescents," by Elizabeth Jane Costello, Adrian Angold, and Mark E. Sweeney, emphasizes the aspects of comorbid conditions that one encounters in children and adolescents.

The objective of this textbook has been to produce a comprehensive yet succinct overview of comorbidity in affective disorders. Not all possible psychiatric comorbidities have been included. The textbook is limited to the major conditions that are comorbid with mood disorders.

As editor of this textbook, I would like to acknowledge the efforts of the contributing authors, all of whom have made a major contribution to the field of psychiatry. I would also like to acknowledge the support of our publisher, Marcel Dekker, Inc.

Mauricio Tohen

Contents

About the Series *iii*
Preface *v*
Contributors *ix*

1. Comorbidity of Unipolar and Bipolar Depression with Other Psychiatric Disorders in a General Population Survey 1
Ronald C. Kessler

2. Depression and Substance Abuse 27
Douglas M. Ziedonis, Conor K. Farren, and Tony P. George

3. Depression in the Medically Ill 57
D. Jeffrey Newport and Charles B. Nemeroff

4. Comorbidity of Depressive Illnesses and Personality Disorders 105
Thomas J. Doyle, Ming T. Tsuang, and Michael J. Lyons

5. The Comorbidity of Depression and Medical Illness in the Elderly 157
Andrew Satlin

6. Comorbidity with Depression in Children and Adolescents 179
Elizabeth Jane Costello, Adrian Angold, and Mark E. Sweeney

7. Bipolar Disorder and Substance Abuse 197
Susan C. Sonne and Kathleen T. Brady

8. The Co-occurrence of Bipolar Disorder with Medical Illness 213
Kenji W. Sax and Stephen M. Strakowski

9. Bipolar Disorder and Comorbid Axis I Disorders 229
Carlos A. Zarate, Jr., and Mauricio Tohen

10. Bipolar Disorder and Comorbid Axis II Disorders 241
Carlos A. Zarate, Jr., and Mauricio Tohen

11. Comorbidity and Bipolar Disorder in Old Age 249
Kenneth Israel Shulman and Anu Singh

12. Developmental Aspects of Comorbidity in Mania 263
Gabrielle A. Carlson

Index *281*

Contributors

Adrian Angold, M.R.C.Psych. Department of Psychiatry and Behavioral Sciences, Duke University Medical Center, Durham, North Carolina

Kathleen T. Brady, M.D., Ph.D. Institute of Psychiatry and Behavioral Sciences, Medical University of South Carolina, Charleston, South Carolina

Gabrielle A. Carlson, M.D. Department of Psychiatry and Behavioral Sciences, State University of New York University of Stony Brook, Stony Brook, New York

Elizabeth Jane Costello, Ph.D. Department of Psychiatry and Behavioral Sciences, Duke University Medical Center, Durham, North Carolina

Thomas J. Doyle Department of Psychiatry, Institute of Psychiatric Epidemiology and Genetics, Harvard Medical School, Boston, Massachusetts

Conor K. Farren, M.D., Ph.D. Department of Psychiatry, Yale University School of Medicine, New Haven, Connecticut

Tony P. George, M.D. Department of Psychiatry, Yale University School of Medicine, New Haven, Connecticut

Ronald C. Kessler, Ph.D. Department of Health Care Policy, Harvard Medical School, Boston, Massachusetts

Michael J. Lyons, Ph.D. Department of Psychology, Boston University, Boston, Massachusetts

Charles B. Nemeroff, M.D., Ph.D. Department of Psychiatry and Behavioral Sciences, Emory University School of Medicine, Atlanta, Georgia

D. Jeffrey Newport, M.D., M.Div. Department of Psychiatry and Behavioral Sciences, Emory University School of Medicine, Atlanta, Georgia

Andrew Satlin, M.D. Department of Psychiatry, Harvard Medical School, Boston, Massachusetts

Kenji W. Sax, Ph.D. Department of Psychiatry, University of Cincinnati, Cincinnati, Ohio

Kenneth Israel Shulman, M.D. Department of Psychiatry, Sunnybrook Health Science Center, University of Toronto, Toronto, Ontario, Canada

Anu Singh, M.D., F.R.C.P.(C) Department of Psychiatry, Sunnybrook Health Science Center, University of Toronto, Toronto, Ontario, Canada

Susan C. Sonne, Pharm.D. Institute of Psychiatry and Behavioral Sciences, Medical University of South Carolina, Charleston, South Carolina

Stephen M. Strakowski, M.D. Department of Psychiatry, University of Cincinnati, Cincinnati, Ohio

Mark E. Sweeney Department of Psychiatry and Behavioral Sciences, Duke University Medical Center, Durham, North Carolina

Mauricio Tohen, M.D., Dr.P.H. Lilly Research Laboratories, Indianapolis, Indiana, and McLean Hospital, Harvard Medical School, Boston, Massachusetts

Ming T. Tsuang, M.D., Ph.D., D.Sc. Department of Psychiatry, Institute of Psychiatric Epidemiology and Genetics, Harvard Medical School, Boston, Massachusetts

Carlos A. Zarate, Jr., M.D. Bipolar and Psychotic Disorders Program, University of Massachusetts Medical School, Worcester, Massachusetts

Douglas M. Ziedonis, M.D., M.P.H. Department of Psychiatry, Robert Wood Johnson Medical School, Piscataway, New Jersey

Comorbidity in Affective Disorders

1

Comorbidity of Unipolar and Bipolar Depression with Other Psychiatric Disorders in a General Population Survey

RONALD C. KESSLER
Harvard Medical School
Boston, Massachusetts

I. INTRODUCTION

Studies of diagnostic patterns in both treatment samples (1–4) and community samples (5–8) show that mood disorders often co-occur with other psychiatric disorders. Indeed, comorbidity appears to be the norm, with up to two-thirds of those with a lifetime major depressive episode also having a history of at least one other psychiatric disorder and an even higher proportion of those with lifetime mania having other lifetime disorders (7). Furthermore, the majority of people in an episode of either depression or mania meet criteria for at least one other current psychiatric disorder if diagnostic hierarchy rules are relaxed (9).

There is controversy about these results relating to the possibility that they are, at least in part, artifacts of changes in the DSM diagnostic system used in most recent studies of comorbidity (10–12). Beginning with DSM-III (13) and continuing with DSM-III-R (14) and DSM-IV (15), these changes included a dramatic increase in the number of diagnostic categories and a reduction in the number of exclusion criteria. These changes were made in an effort to retain potentially important differentiating information (10). As a result of these changes, many patients who would previously have received only a single diagnosis received multiple diagnoses.

Critics have argued that these changes in the DSM system had the undesirable consequence of artificially increasing the estimated prevalence of comorbidity and introducing distinctions among cases that are not clinically useful (11). However, it is impossible to judge this without making the distinctions and investigating whether they are useful. The disaggregation successively introduced into recent versions of the DSM system allows this to be done using established criteria for determining the validity of diagnostic distinctions (16, 17). Although this work is still in progress, it is likely to result in the conclusion that some of the diagnostic distinctions currently in vogue are useful, whereas others are not.

The bulk of work in this area is being done in treatment studies and is aimed at determining whether a target symptom approach to treatment can be enhanced by introducing evidence about comorbidity. Longitudinal family genetic studies and biological studies are also being carried out to improve our understanding of the underlying pathogenesis of pure and comorbid disorders. It is important that these results be interpreted against the backdrop of descriptive general population data on the distributions and associations among sets of diagnostic criteria. General population data of this sort provide a context in which clinical results can be interpreted, as well as an external validity check to guard against the selection biases that exist in clinical samples.

The present chapter presents an overview of recent general population epidemiological research of this sort from the U.S. National Comorbidity Survey (NCS), a large ($n = 8098$), nationally representative, face-to-face survey of people in the age range 15–54 in the U.S. household population designed explicitly to study the epidemiology of comorbid psychiatric disorders. For a more complete description of the NCS design and methods, see Kessler et al. (18). We begin by examining comorbidities of depression and mania with other psychiatric disorders. We next consider temporal priorities in the predictive relationships between comorbid disorders. We then close with a presentation of data on the consequences of comorbidity for course and severity.

II. THE PREVALENCES OF UNIPOLAR AND BIPOLAR DEPRESSION

Epidemiological studies consistently find that mood disorders are highly prevalent (8,19–24). In the NCS, for example, we estimated that 17.1% of the 8098 respondents met lifetime DSM-III-R criteria for a major depressive episode (MDE), 14.9% for a nonbipolar major depressive disorder (MDD), and 1.6% for bipolar I disorder (BPI) (18).

The vast majority of community epidemiological studies, including the NCS, use fully structured interviews administered by interviewers who are not clinicians to make diagnoses. In the case of the NCS, the World Health Organization (WHO) Composite International Diagnostic Interview (CIDI) (25) was utilized. A clinical reappraisal study of the CIDI diagnoses in the NCS found that the vast majority of people classified as having a depressive episode were independently confirmed by blind clinical reinterviews as having a history of depression (26). However, only a minority of the people classified as having a history of mania were confirmed in the clinical reappraisal study (27).

It was possible to develop a revised CIDI mania diagnostic algorithm based on post hoc comparisons of the clinical reappraisal data that had an acceptable positive predictive value. This revised algorithm classified 0.4% of respondents as having a lifetime history of BPI, approximately half of the clinically confirmed manics evaluated in the reappraisal study. The algorithm required euphoria (either a period of abnormally elevated mood or a period of being unusually active to a degree that friends and family members were concerned) and associated symptoms of inflated self-esteem or grandiosity and a decreased need for sleep. It is this subset of manics who are the focus of subsequent data on the epidemiology of bipolar disorder in the NCS.

III. COMORBIDITIES OF MDD AND BPI WITH OTHER DSM-III-R DISORDERS

As shown in Table 1, the majority of the NCS respondents with a lifetime history of MDD (61.8%) can be characterized as secondary in the sense that they had at least one of the other DSM-III-R disorders assessed in the NCS before or in the same year as their first onset of depression. Only about one-quarter (26.0%) of lifetime cases reported that MDD was their only lifetime

Table 1 Prevalences of Lifetime Pure, Primary, and Secondary Major Depressive Disorder and Bipolar I Disorder, with Standard Errors

	Pure[a]		Primary		Secondary	
	%	(s.e.)	%	(s.e.)	%	(s.e.)
I. Major Depressive disorder						
Total	26.0	(2.5)	12.2	(1.2)	61.8	(2.6)
Women	30.1*	(3.0)	12.2	(1.6)	57.7*	(2.9)
Men	18.6	(2.7)	12.1	(2.2)	69.3	(3.4)
II. Bipolar I disorder						
Total	0.0	—	20.5	16.3	79.5	16.3
Women	0.0	—	38.1	27.0	61.9	27.0
Men	0.0	—	0.0	—	100.0	—

[a]Respondents with lifetime MDD and lifetime dysthymia only were coded as pure.
*$p < 0.05$, women versus men.
Source: Reproduced, in part, by permission of the *British Journal of Psychiatry*.

DSM-III-R disorder. The final 12.2% reported that MDD was their first lifetime disorder followed by the later onset of one or more other disorders. MDD is significantly more likely to be secondary among men than women (69.3% vs. 57.7%, $t = 2.6$, $p < .05$) and significantly more likely to be pure among women than men (30.1% vs. 18.6%, $t = 2.8$, $p < .05$).

Parallel analyses for BPI showed that the majority of the NCS respondents with a lifetime history of bipolar disorder (79.5%) can be characterized as secondary in the sense that they had at least one other DSM-III-R disorder before or in the same year as their first onset of either depression or mania. The other 20.5% reported that either depression or mania was their first lifetime disorder followed by the later onset of one or more other disorders. None reported that BPI was their only lifetime DSM-III-R disorder. No significant sex difference was found in the temporal priority of BPI compared to other disorders.

Table 2 presents more detailed data concerning lifetime and 12-month comorbidity between MDD and the other DSM-III-R disorders assessed in the NCS. The results in the first three columns concern lifetime comorbidity. As shown there, 58.0% of the NCS respondents with lifetime MDD also had a lifetime anxiety disorder and 38.6% a lifetime substance use disorder. More than one-third (31.9%) of people with lifetime MDD also had three or more other lifetime disorders. The odds ratios (ORs) reported in the second column are all significant at the .05 level and greater than 1.0, with the exception of an insignificant OR associated with alcohol abuse without dependence.

The results in the last three columns concern 12-month comorbidity. As shown there, 58.9% of the respondents with 12-month MDD also experienced at least one other DSM-III-R disorder during this same period of time, including 51.2% who had a 12-month anxiety disorder and 18.5% who had a 12-month substance use disorder. The ORs in the next column show that nine of the 11 NCS disorders assessed for 12-month prevalence have significant ORs with 12-month MDD, the exceptions being alcohol and drug abuse without dependence.

A comparison of lifetime and 12-month results in Table 2 shows that the ORs associated with lifetime comorbidity are generally smaller than those associated with 12-month comorbidity, indicating that the tendency for 12-month episodes of MDD to co-occur with episodes of other disorders is more powerful than the tendency for lifetime depression to be more prevalent among people with a lifetime history of other disorders. Inspection of the results in the last three rows of the table shows that episodes of MDD have much higher odds of co-occurring with two or three or more other recent disorders than with only a single other disorder, a pattern that is considerably more pronounced than the tendency for lifetime MDD to be comorbid with two or three or more other lifetime disorders. A final observation is that MDD is more strongly comorbid with the anxiety disorders than with the other NCS disorders. Among the anxi-

Table 2 Comorbidities of Major Depressive Disorder (zero-order odds ratios, ORs) with Other DSM-III-R Disorders

	Lifetime MDD			12-month MDD		
Other disorders	%	OR	(95% CI)	%	OR	(95% CI)
I. Anxiety disorders						
Generalized anxiety disorder	17.2	6.0*	(4.2–8.6)	15.4	8.2*	(5.0–13.5)
Agoraphobia	16.3	3.4*	(2.5–4.6)	12.6	4.4*	(2.8–6.9)
Simple phobia	24.3	3.1*	(2.5–3.8)	23.7	3.7*	(2.8–4.8)
Social phobia	27.1	2.9*	(2.3–3.6)	20.0	3.3*	(2.4–4.5)
Panic disorder	9.9	4.0*	(2.7–6.1)	8.6	5.0*	(3.1–8.0)
Posttraumatic stress disorder	19.5	4.0*	(3.1–5.2)	15.2	6.0*	(4.1–8.6)
Any	58.0	4.2*	(3.4–5.2)	51.2	5.1*	(4.3–6.0)
II. Substance use disorders						
Alcohol dependence	23.5	2.0*	(1.6–2.6)	13.0	2.0*	(1.3–3.0)
Drug dependence	13.3	2.0*	(1.5–2.6)	7.5	3.1*	(2.0–4.6)
Alcohol abuse without dependence	4.1	0.9	(0.7–1.2)	1.4	1.1	(0.6–1.9)
Drug abuse without dependence	6.5	1.6*	(1.1–2.2)	1.1	1.4	(0.3–6.1)
Any	38.6	1.8*	(1.4–2.2)	18.5	1.9*	(1.4–2.8)
III. Other disorders						
Dysthymia	6.7	2.8*	(1.8–4.4)	4.0	5.2*	(2.4–11.2)
Conduct disorder[a]	16.2	1.3*	(1.0–1.6)	—	—	—
IV. Aggregate number of disorders[b]						
One+	74.0	4.1*	(3.2–5.4)	58.9	4.7*	(3.8–5.7)
One	24.7	1.3*	(1.1–1.5)	26.9	2.0*	(1.6–2.5)
Two	17.4	1.9*	(1.6–2.2)	15.4	3.3*	(2.4–4.5)
Three+	31.9	4.0*	(3.1–5.1)	16.5	7.1*	(5.0–10.0)

[a]This disorder was only assessed on a lifetime basis.
[b]Dysthymia was excluded from aggregate categories.
*$p < 0.05$.
Source: Reproduced by permission of the *British Journal of Psychiatry*.

ety disorders, furthermore, MDD is most strongly comorbid with generalized anxiety disorder.

The results in the first column of Table 3 show lifetime prevalence estimates of individual NCS/DSM-III-R disorders among respondents with BPI. Virtually all respondents with a history of BPI (93.0%) reported at least one lifetime anxiety disorder, while 71.1% reported at least one lifetime substance use disorder, 59.5% reported a history of conduct disorder (CD), and 85.7% reported having three or more of the above disorders in their lifetime. The ORs range between insignificant values for alcohol and drug abuse without dependence and

Table 3 Comorbidities of Bipolar I Disorder (zero-order odds ratios, ORs) with Other DSM-III-R Disorders

	Lifetime bipolar I disorder			12-month bipolar I disorder		
Other disorders	%	OR	(95% CI)	%	OR	(95% CI)
I. Anxiety disorders						
Generalized anxiety disorder	42.4	14.0*	(5.3–36.7)	26.6	11.5	(0.7–200.0)
Agoraphobia	62.1	23.9*	(13.2–43.0)	61.5	42.7*	(24.7–73.7)
Simple phobia	66.6	16.1*	(6.6–39.3)	59.4	15.4*	(3.0–78.7)
Social phobia	47.1	5.9*	(1.8–19.6)	32.8	5.8*	(3.0–11.2)
Panic disorder	32.9	14.0*	(1.9–101.7)	31.0	20.1*	(1.9–208.4)
Posttraumatic stress disorder	38.7	8.9*	(2.7–29.5)	27.8	10.9*	(2.3–52.2)
Any	93.0	34.8*	(11.0–110.8)	95.0	82.4*	(23.2–293.0)
II. Substance use disorders						
Alcohol dependence	61.2	9.8*	(6.0–16.0)	27.6	5.0*	(2.7–9.2)
Drug dependence	40.6	8.6*	(3.5–21.2)	15.0	6.1	(0.9–39.7)
Alcohol abuse without dependence	3.1	0.3	(0.04–2.2)	1.8	0.7	(0.4–1.4)
Drug abuse without dependence	5.4	1.2	(0.4–4.1)	1.8	2.4*	(1.1–5.1)
Any	71.1	6.9*	(3.6–13.1)	42.2	5.8*	(1.6–21.7)
III. Other disorders						
Dysthymia	49.7	14.9*	(10.2–21.7)	44.3	32.6*	(7.2–148.4)
Conduct disorder[a]	59.5	10.0*	(2.8–36.3)	—	—	—
IV. Aggregate number of disorders[b]						
One+	100.0	—	—	100.0	—	—
One	4.8	0.2	(0.05–0.7)	13.6	0.8	(0.3–2.5)
Two	9.5	0.8	(0.3–2.0)	20.4	3.8*	(1.6–8.9)
Three+	85.7	40.1*	(16.6–97.0)	66.0	49.7*	(27.2–90.7)

[a]This disorder was only assessed on a lifetime basis.
[b]Dysthymia was excluded from aggregate categories.
*$p < 0.05$.

23.9 for agoraphobia. The OR for any lifetime anxiety disorder (34.8) is especially high. It is noteworthy that the ORs of BPI with other disorders are consistently much higher than those associated with MDD.

IV. THE EFFECTS OF EARLIER DISORDERS ON SECONDARY MDD AND BPI

Virtually all previous research on temporal priorities in comorbid disorders has focused exclusively on age-of-onset comparisons. But this is a limited approach because it fails to consider information on the relative sizes and age-of-onset distributions of pure versus comorbid cases (28). The problem can be illustrated with a simple example (29). Imagine two disorders, A and B, with a lifetime OR of 2.3, having equal lifetime prevalences and equal temporal priorities (i.e., 50% A before B and 50% B before A). This does not mean that the two disorders are equally powerful in predicting each other. Indeed, it is a simple matter to generate these observed results from an underlying process in which disorder A has no effect in predicting B but B has a strong effect in predicting A. One such process is as follows: 80% of lifetime cases of A have onsets at birth; 100% of lifetime cases of B have onsets at age 10 for reasons that are totally unrelated to prior A; and the remaining 20% of lifetime cases of A have onsets of age 20 that are powerfully influenced by prior history of B (OR of 20). This set of processes will yield a cross-sectional OR of 2.3 between the two lifetime disorders among people older than 20 years.

This example shows that rigorous evaluation of temporal priority requires the researcher to go beyond a simple comparison of onset ages to examine reciprocal conditional risks in a way that takes into consideration the relative prevalences and age-of-onset distributions of both pure and comorbid cases. Such an analysis can more accurately be carried out in a general population sample than a clinical sample. This is true because age-of-onset distributions are biased in clinical samples due to the significant association between age of onset and probability of seeking treatment (30).

The most elegant way to examine temporal priority is by means of reciprocal survival analysis in which each disorder in a comorbid pair is treated as a time-varying covariate to predict the first onset of the other disorder in the pair. This was done in the NCS by estimating a series of survival models to study the extent to which temporally primary disorders predict the subsequent first onset of MDD and BPI and vice versa. Results showed that these reciprocal effects are generally quite similar in magnitude in bivariate models that assume constant effects. Indeed, the differences between the reciprocal effects were found to be less than their standard errors in almost all cases.

Results of the analyses in which earlier disorders were used to predict first onset of MDD are presented in Table 4. The ORs in this table are exponentiated discrete-time survival coefficients with the year as the unit of analysis. Two models were specified and each was estimated in a series of univariate prediction equations. Model 1 stipulated that the onset of MDD within a given year is a function of the respondent s prior history of one of the other NCS disorders. As shown in the first column in Table 4, the ORs based on this model are all greater than 1.0 and all but three of 12 are statistically significant at the 0.5 level. This means that most of the disorders considered here predict the subsequent onset of secondary depression.

Model 2 was designed to study time trends in the significant time-lagged effects documented in Model 1. Model 2 stipulated that the onset of MDD within a given year is a function of first onset of another disorder in the same

Table 4 The Effects (exponentiated discrete-time survival coefficients) of Prior Disorders on First Onset of MDD

	Model 1[a]		Model 2[b]					
	Time-lagged effect		Same-year effect		Time-lagged effect		Time-trend effect	
Prior disorders	OR	(95% Cl)	OR	(95% Cl)	OR	(95% Cl)	OR	(95% Cl)
I. Anxiety disorders								
Generalized anxiety disorder	2.9*	(1.1–5.50)	62.0*	(37.06–103.87)	7.6*	(3.56–16.29)	0.85*	(0.77–0.94)
Agoraphobia	2.8*	(1.97–4.08)	15.7*	(9.67–25.63)	2.5*	(1.02–6.10)	1.02	(0.92–1.12)
Simple phobia	2.7*	(2.13–3.41)	9.1*	(5.76–14.39)	4.2*	(2.25–7.68)	0.95	(0.89–1.01)
Social phobia	2.6*	(2.10–3.26)	6.5*	(3.71–11.39)	3.0*	(1.91–4.76)	0.98	(0.94–1.03)
Panic disorder	1.3	(0.73–2.32)	28.0*	(15.69–49.81)	2.4*	(1.07–5.54)	0.91	(0.77–1.08)
Posttraumatic stress disorder	2.4*	(1.84–3.10)	9.2*	(4.74–17.80)	3.0*	(1.67–5.37)	0.97	(0.90–1.05)
Any	2.6*	(2.06–3.19)	12.0*	(8.93–16.05)	2.7*	(1.70–4.42)	0.99	(0.94–1.04)
II. Substance use disorders								
Alcohol dependence	2.5*	(2.19–2.87)	6.0*	(4.38–8.16)	2.9*	(2.27–3.68)	0.99	(0.96–1.02)
Drug dependence	2.1*	(1.77–2.49)	7.5*	(5.62–10.05)	1.8*	(1.38–2.37)	1.03	(0.99–1.07)
Alcohol abuse without dependence	1.1	(0.86–1.36)	1.7*	(1.09–2.57)	1.3	(0.77–2.13)	0.97	(0.91–1.04)
Drug abuse without dependence	1.5*	(1.14–1.88)	2.5*	(1.86–3.27)	1.3	(0.86–1.97)	1.02	(0.96–1.08)
Any	2.0*	(1.78–2.30)	4.5*	(3.70–5.51)	2.1*	(1.72–2.48)	0.99	(0.97–1.02)

III. Other disorders								
Dysthymia[c]	1.5	(0.77–3.00)	4.5	(2.03–10.08)	2.1	(0.85–5.36)	0.94	(0.81–1.10)
Conduct disorder	1.6*	(1.12–2.32)	3.1*	(1.34–6.94)	1.7	(0.99–2.97)	0.99	(0.93–1.05)
IV. Aggregate number of disorders								
One+	2.4*	(1.83–3.10)	10.5*	(8.22–13.44)	1.9*	(1.32–2.81)	1.03	(0.99–1.07)
One	2.0*	(1.49–2.73)	8.8*	(6.42–12.07)	2.0*	(1.19–3.23)	1.00	(0.96–1.06)
Two	2.9*	(2.03–4.10)	17.3*	(10.82–27.68)	1.9	(0.88–3.91)	1.05	(0.98–1.13)
Three+	2.8*	(1.81–4.20)	51.6	NC	2.4	(0.70–8.34)	1.01	(0.91–1.13)

[a]Model 1 is a discrete-time survival mode in which first onset of MDD is predicted from prior history of one other DSM-III-R disorder. To be defined as "time-lagged" a disorder must have an age of onset of least 1 year earlier than that of MDD (at least 2 years earlier in the case of dysthymia).

[b]Model 2 is a discrete-time survival model in which first onset of MDD is predicted from the onset of one other disorder in the same year as MDD, prior onset of this disorder, and a time-trend for number of years since the onset of the prior disorder.

[c]Consistent with DSM-III-R diagnostic hierarchy rules, dysthymia was not diagnosed if it began within 2 years of the onset of MDD.

NC = standard error estimate did not converge in the design-based model estimation.

$*p \leq 0.05$.

Source: Reproduced by permission of the *British Journal of Psychiatry*.

year as MDD (same-year effect), first onset of the other disorder in the years prior to the onset of MDD (time-lagged effect), and a linear term for change in the time-lagged effect depending on the number of years since the onset of the earlier disorder (time-trend effect). As shown in Table 4, same-year effects are generally quite large, especially those associated with the anxiety disorders where the ORs range between 6.5 (social phobia) and 62.0 (generalized anxiety disorder). Consistent with the results of Model 1, there are also significant time-lagged ORs for all disorders other than alcohol and drug abuse without dependence. The time-lagged effects are consistently smaller than the same-year effects.

The results concerning time trends show that the effects of earlier disorders on secondary depression are generally quite persistent. Twelve disorders have significant time-lagged effects on MDD. The time trends are insignificant for all but one, which means that the elevated risk of MDD associated with an earlier onset of these disorders persists for many years without any significant change in magnitude. The situation is different for the one disorder with significant time trends in its lagged effects on risk of depression—generalized anxiety disorder (GAD), whose effects decay with time. The decline in the time-lagged effects of GAD is linear and fairly gradual after the first year. It is noteworthy that despite the decline, the estimated effect of GAD remains greater than zero for more than a decade after onset.

The small number of respondents with BPI in the NCS made it impossible to have the power needed to study time trends of the type reported in Table 4. However, a series of linear discrete-time survival models was nonetheless estimated in each of which prior history of one other NCS/DSM-III-R disorder was used as a time-varying predictor of the subsequent onset of BPI. The ORs were found to be consistently greater than 1.0 and four were significant at the .05 level, indicating that they predict an increased probability of first onset of bipolar disorder. Three of the four significant coefficients were associated with anxiety disorders [GAD, posttraumatic stress disorder (PTSD), any anxiety], while the fourth was associated with prior history of either conduct disorder or adult antisocial behavior. It is noteworthy that the ORs were all found to be smaller than the comparable cross-sectional ORs in Table 3, especially for the anxiety disorders, indicating that only part of these comorbidities are due to other disorders predicting the onset of temporally secondary BPI.

Although the aggregate measures of substance use disorders in the discrete-time survival analyses were not significant predictors of the subsequent onset of BPI, more detailed disaggregated analyses showed that there are effects of specific substances. Cocaine was the only drug for which prior use had a meaningfully elevated OR (4.2; 95% CI: 0.3–57.2) in predicting subsequent onset of BPI, a result consistent with a prospective epidemiological investigation by Anthony and Petronis (31) based on the ECA data. Stimulant abuse (OR + 3.1,

95% CI: 1.0–9.9) and dependence (OR = 5.7, 95% CI: 1.8–18.4) were the only illicit drug use disorders with estimable ORs that meaningfully predicted subsequent onset of BPI.

V. THE DISTRIBUTIONS OF SECONDARY MDD AND BPI

A classification scheme was constructed to describe secondary MDD and BPI in terms of their associated primary disorder. Results are reported in Table 5. As shown in the first column, 67.9% of the cases of secondary MDD are associated with a primary anxiety disorder, 19.2% with a primary substance use disorder, 1.8% with primary dysthymia, and 12.6% with primary conduct disorder. The average difference between the age of onset of the primary disorder and secondary MDD is reported in the second column. Very short time lags are involved when the primary disorder is either GAD (1.5 year) or panic disorder (1.5 years), consistent with hierarchy rules in earlier diagnostic schemes. In other cases of primary anxiety and secondary depression, however, the average time lag is between 10.6 (primary agoraphobia) and 13.6 (primary simple phobia) years. The average time lag for primary conduct disorder is within this range (11.8 years), whereas the time lags for substance use disorders are shorter (4.3–6.5 years).

Results for secondary BPI, shown in the remainder of Table 5, are quite different from those for MDD. As shown in the third column, a much smaller proportion of cases of secondary BPI (31.2%) than secondary MDD (67.9%) are associated with a primary anxiety disorder, while roughly equal proportions are associated with primary substance use disorder (18.5% of secondary BPI vs. 19.2% of secondary MDD), and a much higher proportion of cases of secondary BPI (50.2%) than MDD (12.3%) are associated with primary conduct disorder. The average difference between the age of onset of the primary disorder and secondary BPI is 8.1 years compared to 4.2 years for primary substance disorders and 10.3 for primary conduct disorder.

VI. THE EFFECTS OF COMORBIDITY ON COURSE AND SEVERITY OF MDD AND BPI

A series of logistic regression equations was estimated to study the associations between prior lifetime disorders and the subsequent course and severity of MDD and BPI. Results are reported for MDD in Table 6. The ORs represent contrasts between respondents with various types of secondary MDD versus those with pure and primary MDD. These ORs have been adjusted for the effects of demographic variables (age, gender, and race/ethnicity), age of onset of depression, and time since onset of depression.

The results in the first column show that comorbidity of MDD with a primary

Table 5 The Primary Disorders Associated with Secondary Major Depressive Disorder and Bipolar I Disorder

	Major depressive disorder				Bipolar I disorder			
	Percentage of secondary MDD[a]		Mean difference of primary vs. secondary onset ages (years)		Percentage of secondary BPI[a]		Mean difference of primary vs. secondary onset ages (years)	
Primary disorders	%	(s.e.)	$\bar{x}$	(s.e.)	%	(s.e.)	$\bar{x}$	(s.e.)
I. Anxiety disorders								
Generalized anxiety disorder	9.4	(1.6)	1.5	(0.8)	0.0	—	—	—
Agoraphobia	9.4	(1.4)	10.6	(1.5)	2.3	2.3	25.0	0.0
Simple phobia	21.9	(2.1)	13.6	(0.7)	11.3	7.5	3.6	3.2
Social phobia	22.4	(2.3)	11.9	(1.1)	15.1	8.4	11.9	2.5
Panic disorder	2.3	(0.5)	1.5	(0.7)	2.3	2.3	25.0	0.0
Posttraumatic stress disorder	11.2	(1.5)	11.6	(1.5)	4.7	4.6	7.0	0.0
Any	67.9	(2.5)	11.2	(0.5)	31.2	11.8	8.1	2.7
II. Substance use disorders								
Alcohol dependence	4.0	(0.6)	4.3	(1.1)	18.5	12.0	4.2	0.6
Drug dependence	1.6	(0.4)	5.3	(1.0)	0.0	—	—	—
Alcohol abuse without dependence	15.2	(1.8)	6.5	(0.7)	0.0	—	—	—
Drug abuse without dependence	4.8	(0.8)	5.5	(0.8)	0.0	—	—	—
Any	19.2	(2.1)	6.6	(0.6)	18.5	12.0	4.2	0.6
III. Other disorders								
Dysthymia	1.8	(0.8)	3.4	(1.3)	0.0	—	—	—
Conduct disorder	12.3	(1.5)	11.8	(1.0)	50.2	16.5	10.3	1.8

[a]In cases where the respondent had two or more disorders prior to the onset of MDD or BPI, the one with the earliest age of onset is considered primary. In cases where two disorders had the same earliest onset, both are considered primary. As a result of his decision, the column totals are greater than 100%.

Source: Reproduced in part by permission of the *British Journal of Psychiatry*.

Table 6 The Effects (exponentiated logistic regression coefficients) of Prior Disorders on the Persistence and Severity of Major Depressive Disorder[a]

	30-day prevalence		LT chronic MDD		MDD interferes a lot		Hospitalization for MDD		LT suicide attempt	
Prior disorders	OR	(95% Cl)	OR	(95% Cl)	OR	(95% Cl)	OR	(95% Cl)	OR	(95% Cl)
I. Anxiety disorders										
Generalized anxiety disorder	1.6	(0.69–3.47)	2.1	(0.83–5.28)	2.4*	(1.12–4.99)	3.1*	(1.22–7.75)	1.1	(0.58–2.28)
Agoraphobia	1.9	(0.97–3.53)	1.0	(0.46–2.07)	1.3	(0.69–2.40	1.9	(0.92–3.98)	1.2	(0.64–2.45)
Simple phobia	1.8*	(1.07–2.87)	1.0	(0.68–1.49)	1.2	(0.91–1.72)	1.6	(0.82–3.15)	1.4	(0.80–2.39)
Social phobia	1.4	(0.88–2.32)	1.0	(0.64–1.72)	1.4	(0.92–2.16)	1.8*	(1.08–3.03)	0.9	(0.53–1.42)
Panic disorder	0.3	(0.04–2.56)	0.5	(0.15–2.03)	1.9	(0.56–6.39)	3.2	(0.79–13.16)	0.9	(0.15–6.03)
Posttraumatic stress disorder	1.5	(0.86–2.56)	1.3	(0.80–2.27)	1.2	(0.73–1.93)	2.3*	(1.34–4.10)	3.4*	(1.88–6.25)
Any	1.6*	(1.11–2.35)	1.2	(0.89–1.72)	1.5*	(1.13–1.88)	2.5*	(1.61–4.00)	1.8*	(1.13–2.83)
II. Substance use disorders										
Alcohol dependence	0.8	(0.46–1.45)	1.0	(0.54–1.78)	1.5	(0.83–2.73)	1.1	(0.47–2.44)	1.5	(0.76–2.94)
Drug dependence	0.7	(0.26–1.72)	1.1	(0.53–2.48)	2.3*	(1.18–4.48)	0.9	(0.35–2.46)	2.4	(0.98–5.66)
Alcohol abuse without dependence	0.9	(0.50–1.48)	1.2	(0.69–2.03)	1.5	(0.90–2.43)	2.2*	(1.07–4.69)	1.7	(0.92–3.07)
Drug abuse without dependence	0.6	(0.30–1.31)	1.1	(0.63–1.97)	1.7*	(1.08–2.73)	1.2	(0.52–2.59)	1.8	(0.84–4.07)
Any	0.8	(0.50–1.40)	1.2	(0.72–1.97)	1.6*	(1.00–2.46)	2.1*	(1.08–4.06)	1.6	(0.87–3.10)
III. Other disorders										
Dysthymia[b]	1.2	(0.67–2.30)	3.5*	(1.89–6.33)	1.4	(0.66–2.88)	1.5	(0.48–4.51)	1.4	(0.52–3.51)
Conduct disorder	1.0	(0.59–1.56)	0.9	(0.51–1.56)	0.7	(0.42–1.11)	0.5	(0.19–1.30)	1.3	(0.74–2.26)
IV. Aggregate number of disorders										
One+	1.5*	(1.05–2.05)	1.1	(0.78–1.52)	1.3*	(1.03–1.75)	2.3*	(1.48–3.49)	1.9*	(1.25–2.95)
One	1.5	(0.95–2.23)	1.0	(0.68–1.51)	1.3	(0.91–1.83)	1.8*	(1.12–2.97)	1.9*	(1.09–3.39)
Two	1.5	(0.87–2.50)	1.1	(0.58–2.03)	1.3	(0.88–1.96)	2.6*	(1.18–5.68)	1.7	(0.90–3.39)
Three+	1.5	(0.90–2.42)	1.2	(0.79–1.94)	1.5	(0.99–2.27)	2.9*	(1.55–5.38)	2.2*	(1.17–4.07)

[a]The analysis is based on a series of logit equations estimated in the subsample of all NCS respondents with a lifetime history of MDD. Each equation controlled for age at onset of MDD, years since first onset of MDD, and sex, and estimated the effect (OR) of prior history of one other disorder on various indicators of the persistence of lifetime severity of MDD. [b]Consistent with DSM-III-R diagnostic hierarchy rules, dysthymia was not diagnosed if it began within 2 years of the onset of MDD. $^{*}p \leq 0.05$. *Source*: Reproduced by permission of the *British Journal of Psychiatry*.

anxiety disorder but not with any other primary disorder is associated with significantly increased odds of a more persistent course, as indicated by 30-day prevalence adjusted for variation in age of onset and time since onset. The results in the second column show that primary dysthymia is associated with lifetime chronicity of MDD. The results in the next three columns show that primary anxiety disorders are associated with self-perceived interference with life and activities, suicide attempts, and hospitalization for depression, whereas primary substance use disorders are associated with interference and hospitalization, but not attempted suicide. The results in the last three rows show that there is not much of a dose-response relationship between the number of prior disorders and the subsequent persistence and severity of MDD. For the most part, the distinction between having any prior disorder (secondary MDD) versus none (pure or primary MDD) is the more important distinction.

Parallel models were estimated for BPI, but none of the ORs was significant. This is due, at least in part, to low statistical power because of the small number of respondents with BPI and the high comorbidity of BPI with other disorders. However, the magnitudes of the ORs were generally not greatly different from zero, suggesting that even if the sample had been larger we would not have found meaningfully elevated risks of persistence and severity of BPI associated with comorbidity.

VII. DISCUSSION

The results presented above have two important limitations. One is that they provide no way of assessing the extent to which failure to report lifetime disorders distorts the results concerning patterns and correlates of comorbidity. We know very little about the cognitive processes involved in forgetting, but we do know from a number of prospective studies that it occurs with alarmingly high frequency in this population (32–34). A complicating factor is that there are now two separate studies that have documented that forgetting depression is more common among men than women (34–36). This factor could lead to an artificial increase in the estimated comorbidity between depression and anxiety and a related decrease in the estimated comorbidity between depression and substance use disorders due to the fact that anxiety disorders are much more common among women and substance disorders among men (18). Based on this evidence, caution is needed in interpreting any results concerning comorbidity based on cross-sectional lifetime recall data such as those generated in most general population epidemiological studies.

A related limitation is that the distinction between primary and secondary disorders is based on retrospective reports concerning age of onset that are subject to memory error. This is true not only in epidemiological samples but also in clinical samples. There is some evidence in the cognitive psychological literature that first experiences have a special place in autobiographical memory (37,38), but the extent to which this is true varies as a function of a number of factors. Our analysis of responses to the question "Can you remember your *exact* age the *very* first time [emphasis in the original] disorders of particular types occurred?" documented clearly that vivid memories are much more likely to exist for acute-onset disorders such as panic and mania than for disorders with insidious onsets such as depression (39). This difference could lead to incorrect recall of the temporal priority of MDD and BPI compared to other disorders in retrospective studies. Long-term longitudinal studies of representative community samples beginning in childhood are needed to resolve this problem of recall bias and arrive at a clear description of the natural history and correlates of pure, primary, and secondary comorbid depression and mania.

Within the context of these limitations, the results reported above show that MDD is a prevalent and highly comorbid disorder in the general population, whereas BPI is an uncommon and extremely highly comorbid disorder. Most lifetime cases of comorbid MDD and BPI are temporally secondary. However, the increased relative odds of the subsequent onset of other disorders associated with prior MDD and BPI are for the most part as large as the relative odds of subsequent MDD and BPI associated with prior disorders. The time-lagged effects for MDD generally persist for many years without change. Our sample of cases with BPI is too small to know whether the same is true for mania. Some forms of comorbid MDD and BPI are more severe and persistent than pure MDD or other types of BPI.

The finding that MDD and BPI are highly comorbid with other NCS/DSM-III-R disorders is consistent with evidence of high comorbidity of major depression and bipolar disorder from both treatment samples (2–4,41,42) and general population samples (5–8). While alcohol and drug disorders are usually found to be the most prevalent comorbid disorders in treatment samples, comorbid anxiety disorders were found to be much more common on our analysis. This difference could reflect an impact of comorbid substance use disorders on increased probability of seeking help. The evaluation of this possibility would be of particular interest in light of evidence that high comorbidity with anxiety disorders is associated with poor treatment response and worse outcome in patients having both unipolar and bipolar disorders (43–45).

In making sense of the finding that the majority of cases of lifetime MDD and BPI are comorbid, it is important to keep in mind that this finding is based on DSM-III-R, a diagnostic system that encourages multiple diagnoses. For example, while DSM-III did not allow the diagnosis of panic disorder in the presence of MDD, DSM-III-R does. As noted at the beginning of this chapter, there is currently a good deal of controversy concerning whether cases of this sort should be conceived of as multiple comorbid disorders or a single disorder with a complex phenomenological expression. It is too early to know how this controversy will be resolved. Until we do, it is important to continue carrying out research with a diagnostic scheme that encourages multiple diagnoses while avoiding the reification of the notion of comorbidity in favor of an empirical approach that allows us to learn more abut which clusters of narrowly defined comorbid disorders do and do not matter (11).

Putting aside the importance of the diagnostic system, the high comorbidities documented above could be due to a number of causal processes, including the possibility of an impact of earlier disorders on subsequent mood disorders, possibly by precipitating mood disorder in genetically predisposed individuals, an effect of MDD and BPI on the subsequent onset of other disorders, an effect of some underlying vulnerability shared by MDD, BPI, and other conditions, or some combination of these processes. In the case of comorbidities involving substance use, it is also possible that substance-related problems could represent attempts to modulate the distress and mood lability associated with MDD and BPI or that they could be symptoms of mood disturbance. Although the NCS design does not allow us to sort out these various possibilities, we were able to examine temporal priority between mood disorders and comorbid disorders. The results showed that first onset of both manic and depressive episodes usually occurred after the prior onset of some other comorbid disorder. Consistent with this finding, our survival analysis showed that prior disorders are associated with an increased risk of the subsequent onset of both MDD and BPI.

The analysis of same-year and time-lagged associations between MDD and prior disorders was motivated by the results of an earlier investigation of comorbid PTSD in the NCS, where we found that many of the people who experienced a traumatic event such as rape or assault responded not only by developing PTSD but also by experiencing their first episodes of depression, panic, agoraphobia, or substance abuse (46,47). This result led us to speculate that a similar sort of within-year clustering or one-year lagged effect of other disorders on MDD might exist. Consistent with our earlier PTSD work, the time trend analysis documented a tendency for the ORs associated with comorbidity to be much higher for same-year onsets of MDD and other disorders than for time-lagged onsets.

We suspect that this finding is, at least in part, due to the effects of precipitating life experiences. Not only is this interpretation consistent with our own findings concerning same-year onset of PTSD and other disorders in the wake of a traumatic life experience, but it is also consistent with Monroe's (48) review of the literature on stressful life experiences and episode onset of depression and anxiety. The latter documented a number of common precipitating stresses associated with the two types of disorders. Furthermore, a small number of epidemiological studies have shown that there is specificity in the stresses associated with episodes of pure and comorbid depression. For example, stresses that involved interpersonal conflict and a mixture of danger and loss appear to be more powerfully predictors of mixed anxiety-depression than pure depression (49–52).

It is relevant in this regard to note that clinical researchers have suggested that certain primary psychiatric disorders, if they are sufficiently impairing, can also operate as stressors that promote secondary depression (53,54). The NCS results concerning same-year comorbidities of depression and other DSM-III-R disorders are consistent with this thinking.

The finding that cocaine use and stimulant use disorders predict subsequent bipolar disorder is consistent with the related suggestion of several authors that drugs can precipitate bipolar illness (55,56) as well as with the finding of Post et al. (57) that cocaine is a powerful inducer of kindling, a sensitization-like process that may be a model for the development of bipolar illness. The findings that conduct disorder (CD) and adult antisocial behavior (AAB) are associated with a significantly increased risk of subsequent mania are, at least superficially consistent with the findings regarding the effects of drug use disorders. However, it is also important to recognize that the antisocial behaviors giving rise to diagnoses of CD and AAB could be early expressions of bipolar disorder. This sort of symptom overlap is one of a number of diagnostic complexities that make it difficult to distinguish temporal order of early-onset disorders with subsequent mania in the absence of detailed longitudinal investigation (58).

Also important is the evidence that at least some forms of comorbidity may be due to genetic influences rather than to precipitating life experiences (52,59–62). This is most clear in the case of comorbidity between depression and GAD (59,63). This raises the possibility that an underlaying genetic vulnerability might interact with stressful experiences of various sorts to determine whether high-risk people manifest exclusively with depression or with a comorbid disorder.

This kind of underlying genetic diathesis could explain the finding reported above that the time-lagged effects of earlier disorders on temporally secondary MDD persist for many years without change. This could be because the earlier disorder represents a marker for an enduring genetic vulnerability. This result appears at first glance to be inconsistent with the observations of clinical investigators that secondary depression often occurs only many years after a chronic primary psychiatric disorder (54) or in the context of a chronic and seriously impairing physical illness (64), an observation that has been the basis of an argument that secondary depression is often a response to the exhaustion and demoralization created by chronic intractable stress (53,65).

This inconsistency, however, is more apparent than real because a constant time-lagged effect will lead to a preponderance of cases where the secondary depression does not occur until many years after the primary disorder. Furthermore, as noted by Akiskal (65), the response of exhaustion or demoralization can occur as quickly as several months after the onset of the primary disorder, rather than invariably requiring years of unremitting prior exposure to the primary disorder. More detailed analysis is likely to show that the speed of onset of the secondary disorder is a joint function of the persistence and impairment caused by the primary disorder and the coping resources that characterize the person confronting the challenges imposed by the primary disorder.

Although our current understanding of these processes is only partial, one clear conclusion is that same-year and time-lagged comorbidities are quite different in the sense that the ORs for same-year comorbidities are much larger than those for time-lagged comorbidities. Each of these two types is quite common in the general population. It would be informative to know whether the same-year and time-lagged forms differ in other important ways such as age of onset and course. These issues have not yet been investigated comprehensively, although there is preliminary evidence that comorbid panic-depression with same-year onsets has a stronger pattern of family aggregation than comorbid panic-depression with time-lagged onsets (66). It would be informative, in light of the above results, to determine whether same-year comorbidities are more likely than time-lagged comorbidities invariably to co-occur in recurring episodes of disorder. For example, in cases where the first onset of MDD occurs a few months after the first onset of panic, is the invariable co-occurrence of subsequent episodes of panic and depression throughout the life course more likely than in cases where the first onset of MDD occurred many years after the onset of a persistent panic disorder? This question cannot be answered with the baseline NCS data because information was not obtained about either the consistency of syndrome co-occurrence throughout the life course or the chronicity of primary disorders. A second wave of the NCS is planned, however, in which this additional information will be collected along with prospective data that can help resolve some of the current uncertainties in the cross-sectional data.

Most previous research on the consequences of comorbidity has focused on the predictors of episode recovery and relapse in treatment samples (e.g., 67–69) and has generally found that patients with comorbidity have a poorer prognosis than those with pure disorders (e.g., 69–71). In contrast, the focus of our analysis was on lifetime consequences. We found that comobidity is consistently associated with the persistence of depression and mania. It is noteworthy that we have elsewhere found that comorbid depression and mania are not consistently associated with the persistence of any of the anxiety disorders (9,72). This asymmetry is inconsistent with a purely genetic hypothesis, but is consistent with the notion, mentioned earlier, that secondary depression might be a severity marker of chronic anxiety linked to exhaustion and demoralization (53,65). This observation raises the possibility that genetic influences are more important in accounting for lifetime comorbidity than episode co-occurrence among people with a history of comorbidity, while the opposite is true for environmental influences.

It is unclear from these results whether comorbidity has implications for treatment. A good deal of evidence suggests that the treatment of MDD and BPI with modern medications is equally effective whether or not the patient presents with co-occurring disorders (9,73). Epidemiological data of the sort presented here are not able to shed much light on this matter.

Epidemiological data are more useful, however, in raising questions about the implications of comorbidity for prevention. It is clear from the results reviewed in this chapter that comorbid disorders are more severe than pure disorders. Furthermore, it is clear from studies of service use that most people with comorbid MDD and BPI do not come into contact with the treatment system until after they have had onsets of comorbidity (9). The question could be raised, then, whether more aggressive early outreach and treatment of people with pure temporally primary disorders could be successful in preventing the onset of temporally secondary comorbid disorders and, if so, whether success in this secondary prevention could help reduce the severity and persistence of the primary disorders.

The science of prevention is too underdeveloped to provide answers to these questions. Furthermore, clinical research on comorbidity is not yet advanced enough to tell us much about the etiology of comorbidity. If MDD and BPI and their comorbid disorders are manifestations of a common underlying genetic vulnerability, then there is no reason to think that the successful treatment of primary disorders will prevent the subsequent onset of secondary MDD or BPI. If, on the other hand, primary disorders are either causal or in a casual pathway linked to risk of secondary MDD and BPI, early interventions aimed at treatment of primary disorders could well be effective in preventing secondary disorders. Furthermore, if primary disorders are early warnings of risk that are amenable to environmental intervention, early inerventions aimed at preventing secondary disorders among people who already have primary disorders might prove to be effective. Given the enormous complexities involved in sorting out contending causal hypotheses about the reasons for comorbidity with nonexperimental data, experimental interventions of these types might be the most promising way to study the etiology of comorbidity as well as to deal with it implications (29).

ACKNOWLEDGMENTS

Preparation of this report was supported by a Research Scientist Award from the U.S. National Institute of Mental Health (NIMH; K05 MH00507). The data reported here were collected and analyzed with the support of NIMH Grants

R01 MH46376, R01 MH49098, and RO1 MH52861, with supplemental support from the National Institute of Drug Abuse (through a supplement to MH46376) and the W. T. Grant Foundation (Grant 90135190). Parts of this chapter appeared previously in the *British Journal of Psychiatry* (1996; 168 (suppl 30): 17–30) and *Psychological Medicine* (1997; 27:1079–1089) and are reproduced here with permission. A complete list of all NCS publications along with abstracts, study documentation, interview schedules, and the raw NCS public-use data files can be obtained directly from the NCS Homepage by using the URL http://www.hcp.med.harvard.edu/ncs/.

REFERENCES

1. Ross HE, Glaser FB, Germanson T. The prevalence of psychiatric disorders in patients with alcohol and other drug problems. Arch Gen Psychiatry 1988; 45: 1023–1031.
2. Wolf AW, Schubert DSP, Patterson MB, Grande TP, Brocco KJ, Pendleton L. Associations among major psychiatric diagnoses. J Consult Clin Psychol 1988; 56: 292–294.
3. Mezzich JE, Ahn CW, Fabrega H Jr. Pilkonis PA. Patterns of psychiatric comorbidity in a large population presenting for care. In: Maser JD, Cloninger CR, eds. Comorbidity of Mood and Anxiety Disorders. Washington, DC: American Psychiatric Press, 1990:189–204.
4. Rounsaville BJ, Anton SF, Carroll K, Budde D, Prusoff BA, Gawin F. Psychiatric diagnosis of treatment-seeking cocaine abusers. Arch Gen Psychiatry 1991; 48: 43–51.
5. Angst J, Vollrath M, Merikangas KR, Ernst C. Comorbidity of anxiety and depression in the Zurich Cohort Study of young adults. In: Maser JD, Cloninger CR, eds. Comorbidity of Mood and Anxiety Disorders. Washington, DC: American Psychiatric Press, 1990:123–137.
6. Hagnell O, Grasbeck A. Comorbidity of anxiety and depression in the Lundby 25-Year prospective study: the pattern of subsequent episodes. In: Maser JD, Cloninger CR, eds. Comorbidity of Mood and Anxiety Disorders. Washington, DC: American Psychiatric Press, 1990:139–152.
7. Robins LN, Locke BZ, Regier DA. An overview of psychiatric disorders in America. In: Robins LN, Regier DA, eds. Psychiatric Disorders in America: The Epidemiologic Catchment Area Study. New York: The Free Press, 1991:328–366.
8. Wittchen H-U, Essau CA, Von Zersen D, Krieg J-C, Zaudig M. Lifetime and six-month prevalence of mental disorders in the Munich Follow-up Study. Eur Arch Psychiatry Clin Neurosci 1992; 241:247–258.
9. Kessler RC. The prevalence of psychiatric comorbidity. In: Wetzler S, Sanderson WD, eds. Treatment Strategies for Patients with Psychiatric Comorbidity. New York: Wiley, 1997:23–48.
10. First MB, Spitzer, RL, Williams JBW. Exclusionary principles and the comorbidity of psychiatric diagnoses: historical review and implications for the future. In: Maser

JD, Cloninger CR, eds. Comorbidity of Mood and Anxiety Disorders. Washington, DC: American Psychiatric Press, 1990:83–109.
11. Frances A, Widiger T, Fyer MR. The influence of classification methods on comorbidity. In: Maser JD, Cloninger CR, eds. Comorbidity of Mood and Anxiety Disorders. Washington, DC: American Psychiatric Press, 1990:41–59.
12. Frances A, Manning D, Marin D, Kocsis J, McKinney K, Hall W, Kline M. Relationship of anxiety and depression. Psychopharmacology 1992; 106:S82–S86.
13. American Psychiatric Association. Diagnostic and Statistical Manual of Mental Disorders, 3rd ed. Washington, DC: American Psychiatric Press, 1980.
14. American Psychiatric Association. Diagnostic and Statistical Manual of Mental Disorders, revised 3rd ed. Washington, DC: American Psychiatric Press, 1987.
15. American Psychiatric Association. Diagnostic and Statistical Manual of Mental Disorders, 4th ed. Washington, DC: American Psychiatric Press, 1994.
16. Robins LN, Guze SB. Establishment of diagnostic validity in psychiatric illness: its application to schizophrenia. Am J Psychiatry 1970; 126:983–987.
17. Cloninger CR. Establishment of diagnostic validity in psychiatric illness: Robins and Guze's method revised. In: Robins LN, Barrett J, eds. Validity of Psychiatric Diagnosis. New York: Raven Press, 1989:9–18.
18. Kessler RC, McGonagle KA, Zhao S, Nelson CB, Hughes M, Eshleman S, Wittchen H-U, Kendler KS. Lifetime and 12-month prevalence of DSM-III-R psychiatric disorders in the United States: results from the National Comorbidity Survey. Arch Gen Psychiatry 1994; 51:8–19.
19. Bland RC, Orn H, Newman SC. Lifetime prevalence of psychiatric disorders in Edmonton. Acta Psychiatr Scand 1988; 338:24–32.
20. Canino GJ, Bird HR, Shrout PE, Rubio-Stipec M, Bravo M, Martinez R, Sesman M, Guevara LM. The prevalence of specific psychiatric disorders in Puerto Rico. Arch Gen Psychiatry 1987; 44:727–735.
21. Hwu HG, Yeh EK, Chang LY. Prevalence of psychiatric disorders in Taiwan defined by Chinese diagnostic interview schedule. Acta Psychiatr Scan 1989; 79: 136–147.
22. Lee CK, Kwak YS, Yamamoto J, Rhee H, Kim YS, Han JH, Choi JO, Lee YH. Psychiatric epidemiology in Korea. Part I. Gender and age differences in Seoul. J Nerv Ment Dis 1990; 178:242–246.
23. Wells JE, Bushnell JA, Hornblow AR, Joyce PR, Oakley-Browne MA. Christchurch psychiatric epidemiology study. Part I. Methodology and lifetime prevalence for specific psychiatric disorders. Aust NZ J Psychiatry 1989; 23:315–326.
24. Oakley-Browne MA, Joyce PR, Wells JE, Bushnell JA, Hornblow AR. Christchurch psychiatric epidemiology study. Part II. Six month and other period prevalences for specific psychiatric disorders Aust NZ J Psychiatry 1989; 23:327–340.
25. World Health Organization. Composite International Diagnostic Interview (CIDI, Version 1.0) Geneva, Switzerland: World Health Organization, 1990.
26. Blazer DG, Kessler RC, McGonogle KA, Swartz MS. The prevalence and ditribution of major depression in a national community sample: The National Comorbidity Survey. Am J Psychiatry 1994; 151:979–986.
27. Kessler RC, Rubinow DR, Holmes C, Abelson JM, Zhao S. The epidemiology of

DSM-III-R bipolar I disorder in a general population survey. Psychol Med 1997; 27:1079–1089.
28. Lavori PW. Double diagnosis: the role of the prior odds on each disorder. In: Maser JD, Cloninger CR, eds. Comorbidity of Mood and Anxiety Disorders. Washington, DC: American Psychiatric Press, 1990: 681–692.
29. Kessler RC, Price RH. Primary prevention of secondary disorders: a proposal and agenda. Am J Commun Psychol 1993; 21:607–634.
30. Kessler RC, Olfson M, Berglund P. Patterns and predictors of treatment contact after first onset of a psychiatric disorder. Am J Psychiatry 1998; 155:62–69.
31. Anthony JC, Petronis KR. Epidemiologic evidence on suspected associations between cocaine use and psychiatric disturbances. NIDA Res Monogr 1991; 110: 71–94.
32. Bromet EJ, Dunn LO, Connell MM, Dew MA, Schulberg HC. Long-term reliability of diagnosing lifetime major depression in a community sample. Arch Gen Psychiatry 1986; 43:435–440.
33. McLeod JD, Turnbull JE, Kessler RC, Abelson JM. Sources of discrepancy in the comparison of a lay-administered diagnostic instrument with clinical diagnosis. Psychiatry Res 1990; 31:145–159.
34. Wilhelm K, Parker G. Sex differences in lifetime depression rates: fact or artefact? Psychol Med 1994; 24:97 111.
35. Angst J, Dobler-Mikola A. Do the diagnostic criteria determine the sex ratio in depression? J Affect Disord 1984; 7:189–198.
36. Angst J, Dobler-Mikola A. The definition of depression. Psychiatry Res 1984; 18: 401–406.
37. Pillemer DB, Goldsmith LR, Panter AT, White SH. Very long-term memories of the first year in college. J Exp Psychol Learn Mem Cogn 1988; 14:709–714.
38. Robinson JA. First experience memories: contexts and functions in personal histories. In: Conway MA, Rubin DC, Spinnler H, Wagennar WA, eds. Theoretical Perspectives on Autobiographical Memory. Boston: Kluwer Academic, 1992:223–239.
39. Kessler RC, Mroczek DK, Belli RF. Retrospective adult assessment of childhood psychopathology. In: Shaffer D, Richters J, eds. Assessment in Child Psychopathology. New York: Guilford Press (in press).
40. Black DW, Winokur G, Bell S, Nasrallah A, Hulbert J. Complicated mania: comorbidity and immediate outcome in the treatment of mania. Arch Gen Psychiatry 1988; 45:232–236.
41. Kutcher SP, Marton P, Korenblum M. Relationship between psychiatric illness and conduct disorder in adolescents. Can J Psychiatry 1989; 34:526–529.
42. Brady K, Lydiard RB. Bipolar affective disorder and substance abuse. J Clin Psychopharmacol 1992; 12:17S–22S.
43. Murphy JM. Continuities in community-based psychiatric epidemiology. Arch Gen Psychiatry 1980; 37:1215–1223.
44. Roth M. Problems in the classification of affective disorders. Acta Psychiatr Scand 1981; 290:42–57.
45. Van Valkenburg CH, Akiskal HS, Puzantian V, Rosenthal T. Anxious depression—

clinical family history and naturalistic outcome—comparisons with panic and major depressive disorders. J Affect Disord 1984; 6:67–82.
46. Kessler RC, Sonnega A, Bromet E, Hughes M, Nelson CB. Post-traumatic stress disorder in the National Comorbidity Survey. Arch Gen Psychiatry 1995; 52:1048–1060.
47. Kessler RC, Sonnega A, Bromet E, Hughes M, Nelson CB, Breslau N. Epidemiologic risk factors for trauma and PTSD. In: Yehuda R, ed. Risk Factors for Post Traumatic Stress Disorder. Washington, DC: American Psychiatric Press (in press).
48. Monroe SM. Psychosocial factors in anxiety and depression. In: Maser JD, Cloninger CR, eds. Comorbidity of Mood and Anxiety Disorders. Washington, DC: American Psychiatric Press, 1990:463–497.
49. Cooke DJ. Life events and syndrome of depression in the general population. Soc Psychiatry 1981; 16:181–186.
50. Finlay-Jones R, Brown GW. Types of stressful life events and the onset of anxiety and depressive disorders. Psychol Med 1981; 11:803–815.
51. Prudo R, Harris T, Brown GW. Psychiatric disorder in a rural and an urban population. 3. Social integration and the morphology of affective disorder. Psychol Med 1984; 14:327–345.
52. Torgersen S. A twin-study perspective of the comorbidity of anxiety and depression. In: Maser JD, Cloninger CR, eds. Comorbidity of Mood and Anxiety Disorders. Washington, DC: American Psychiatric Press, 1990: 367–378.
53. Akiskal HS. Anxiety: Definition, relationship to depression, and proposal for an integrative model. In: Tuma AH, Maser JD. Anxiety and the Anxiety Disorders. Hillsdale, NJ: Lawrence Erlbaum Associates, 1985:787–797.
54. Cloninger CR, Martin RL, Guze SB, Clayton PJ. The empirical structure of psychiatric comorbidity and its theoretical significance. In: Maser JD, Cloninger CR, eds. Comorbidity of Mood and Anxiety Disorders. Washington, DC: American Psychiatric Press, 1990:439–462.
55. El-Guebaly N. Manic-depressive psychosis and drug abuse. Can Psychiatr Assoc 1975; 20:595–598.
56. Weller MPI, Ang PC, Latimer-Sayer DT, Zachary A. Drug abuse and mental illness. Lancet 1988; 1:997.
57. Post RM, Rubinow DR, Ballenger JC. Conditioning and sensitization in the longitudinal course of affective illness. Br J Psychiatry 1986; 149:191–201.
58. Bukstein OG, Brent DA, Kaminer Y. Comorbidity of substance abuse and other psychiatric disorders in adolescents. Am J. Psychiatry 1989; 146:1131–1141.
59. Kendler KS. Major depression and generalized anxiety disorder: same genes (partly) different environments—revisited. Br J Psychiatry 1996; 168:68–75.
60. Kendler KS, Neale MC, Kessler RC, Heath AC, Eaves LJ. Major depression and phobias: the genetic and environmental sources of comorbidity. Psychol Med 1993; 23:361–371.
61. Merikangas KR. Comorbidity for anxiety and depression: review of family and genetic studies. In: Maser JD, Cloninger CR, eds. Comorbidity of Mood and Anxiety Disorders. Washington, DC: American Psychiatric Press, 1990:331–348.
62. Weissman MM. Evidence for comorbidity of anxiety and depression: family and

genetic studies of children. In: Maser JD, Cloninger CR, eds. Comorbidity of Mood and Anxiety Disorders. Washington, DC: American Psychiatric Press, 1990:349–365.

63. Kendler KS, Neale MC, Kessler RC, Heath AC, Eaves LJ. Major depression and generalized anxiety disorder: same genes (partly) different environments? Arch Gen Psychiatry 1992; 49:716–722.
64. Hong B, Smith MD, Robson AM, Wetzel RD. Depressive symptomatology and treatment in patients with end-stage renal disease. Psychol Med 1987; 17:185–190.
65. Akiskal HS. Toward a clinical understanding of the relationship of anxiety and depressive disorders. In: Maser JD, Cloninger CR, eds. Comorbidity of Mood and Anxiety Disorders. Washington, DC: American Psychiatric Press, 1990:597–607.
66. Kessler RC, Stang P, Wittchen H-U, Ustun B, Roy-Byrne PP, Walters EE. Patterns, predictors, and consequences of lifetime panic-depression comorbidity in the National Comorbidity Survey Arch Gen Psychiatry (in press).
67. Bronisch T, Hecht H. Major depression with and without a coexisting anxiety disorders: social dysfunction, social integration, and personality features. J Affect Disord 1990; 20:151–157.
68. Joffe RT, Babgy RM, Levitt A. Anxious and nonanxious depression. Am J Psychiatry 1993; 150:1257–1258.
69. Keitner GI, Ryan CE, Miller IW, Kohn R, Epstein NB. 12-month outcome of patients with major depression and comorbid psychiatric or medical illness (compound depression). Am J Psychiatry 1991; 148:345–350.
70. Coryell W, Endicott J, Andreasen NC, Keller MB, Clayton PJ, Hirschfeld RMA, Scheftner WA, Winokur G. Depression and panic attacks: the significance of overlap is reflected in follow-up and family study data. Am J Psychiatry 1988; 145: 293–300.
71. Fawcett J, Kravitz HM. Anxiety syndromes and their relationship to depressive illness. J Clin Psychiatry 1983; 44:8–11.
72. Kessler RC, Nelson CB, McGonagle KA, Liu J, Swartz M, Blazer DG. Comorbidity of DSM-III-R major depressive disorder in the general population: results from the US National Comorbidity of DSM-III-R major depressive disorder in the general population: results from the US National Comorbidity Survey. Br J Psychiatry 1996; 168:17–30.
73. Montgomery S, den Boer JA, eds. SSRIs in Depression and Anxiety. London: Wiley (in press).

APPENDIX The Effects (exponentiated logistic regression coefficients) of Prior Disorders on the Persistence and Severity of Biopolar I Disorder[a]

	30-day prevalence		Hospitalization for bipolar I disorder		LT suicide attempt		High number of LT episodes	
Prior disorders	OR	(95% Cl)	OR	(95% Cl)	OR	(95% Cl)	OR	(95% Cl)
I. Anxiety disorders								
Generalized anxiety disorder	NC	—	NC	—	NC	—	NC	—
Agoraphobia	NC	—	NC	—	NC	—	NC	—
Simple phobia	0.2	(0.02–1.1)	60.8	(0.5–7027.1)	0.4	(0.0–172.5)	NC	—
Social phobia	0.2	(0.0–106.0)	0.03	(0.0–0.2)	0.7	(0.1–5.9)	0.1	(0.01–1.1)
Panic disorder	NC	—	NC	—	NC	—	2.0	(0.03–113.2)
Posttraumatic stress disorder	1.0	(0.01–81.2)	67.0*	(1.0–4457.1)	0.2	(0.02–1.7)	0.1	(0.01–1.8)
Any	0.3	(0.01–21.3)	18.3	(0.5–616.4)	0.4	(0.02–8.7)	0.3	(0.1–1.6)
II. Substance use disorders								
Alcohol dependence	2.6	(0.1–86.2)	0.3	(0.2–5.6)	0.1	(0.0–4.0)	514.1	(0.6–423784)
Drug dependence	NC	—	NC	—	NC	—	NC	—
Alcohol abuse without dependence	NC	—	NC	—	NC	—	NC	—
Drug abuse without dependence	NC	—	NC	—	NC	—	NC	—
Any	1.7	(0.03–99.5)	0.2	(0.01–4.3)	0.9	(0.1–17.0)	3.9	(0.1–99.2)
III. Other disorders								
Dysthymia[b]	57.0*	(1.1–2825.9)	0.6	(0.03–14.8)	14.8	(0.1–1916.9)	82.2*	(4.6–1468.1)
Conduct disorder	0.03	(0.0–0.7)	56.2	(0.0–2221716.1)	2.1	(0.3–16.0)	0.7	(0.1–6.1)
IV. Aggregate number of disorders								
One+	0.3	(0.0–30.7)	57.4*	(2.7–1203.8)	0.4	(0.01–23.7)	77.5	(0.1–95007.3)
One	0.04	(0.0–15.5)	1.5	(0.04–56.0)	0.3	(0.0–57.0)	8.3	(0.5–137.8)
Two	0.9	(0.1–12.1)	14.5*	(1.5–141.1)	0.8	(0.1–7.2)	1.0	(0.1–6.5)
Three+	7.7	(0.1–902.4)	0.02	(0.0–0.7)	2.5	(0.03–180.0)	2.0	(0.1–57.9)

[a]The analysis is based on a series of logit equations estimated in the subsample of all NCS respondents with a lifetime history of BPI. Each equation controlled for age at onset of BPI, years since first onset of BPI, and sex, and estimated the effect (OR) of prior history of one other disorder on various indicators of the persistence of lifetime severity of BPI.

[b]Consistent with DSM-III-R diagnostic hierarchy rules, dysthymia was not diagnosed if it began within 2 years of the onset of BPI.

NC = parameter estimate did not converge in the design-based model estimation.

$^{*}p \leq 0.05$.

2

Depression and Substance Abuse

DOUGLAS M. ZIEDONIS
Robert Wood Johnson Medical School
Piscataway, New Jersey

CONOR K. FARREN and TONY P. GEORGE
Yale University School of Medicine
New Haven, Connecticut

I. INTRODUCTION

Substance abuse is common among individuals with depression. High current and lifetime rates of this comorbidity are found in the community and in both the mental health and addiction systems. The relationship between the depression and substance abuse is complex, and each disorder modifies the clinical course and treatment of the other disorder. The relative age of onset of depression and substance abuse varies in general and according to gender. Of course, the age of onset of substance use precedes both the onset of the substance use disorder and the depressive disorder.

Individuals with both depression and substance abuse tend to have a poor prognosis and poor response to traditional treatment approaches. There are numerous subtypes based on the type and severity of depression and the type(s) of substance use disorders, including alcohol, tobacco, and other drugs. Severity of disorder is reflected by the intensity of symptoms as well as how broadly the illness affects other psychiatric, medical, legal, social, family, and employment problems. Another important factor is a patient's motivation to stop the substance abuse and motivation to acknowledge and treat the depression. Motivation is a state that changes during progression of the disorders and recovery. When either disorder is untreated and/or undetected, the overall course of treatment is impacted. This chapter focuses on assessing and treating coexisting depression and substance use disorders.

II. EPIDEMIOLOGY

In the Epidemiological Catchment Area study (ECA; Regier et al., 1990), a lifetime history of either an alcohol or illicit drug use disorder was found in 32% of individuals with a mood disorder, and alcohol or drug use disorders were nearly equal in frequency (about 20%). The National Comorbidity Study (NCS; Kessler et al., 1997) study also demonstrated high rates of comorbidity; however, it also provided evidence that the depression comorbidity rates varied according to diagnosis of alcohol abuse versus alcohol dependence and being male versus female. For example, alcohol abuse was more often associated with depression among women (30%) compared to men (9%). Alcohol dependence was also more often associated with depression among women (49%) versus men (24%). Men with alcohol abuse or dependence had lower rates of depression comorbidity and alcohol use disorder was temporally primary. In contrast, women reported the onset of an alcohol use disorder in the same year or after the onset of the depression.

Lifetime and current comorbidity rates are higher among individuals in addiction and mental health treatment settings. In mental health treatment settings, about 25–60% of individuals with depression have a current alcohol use disorder, and these rates vary according to specific treatment setting (higher rates in emergency rooms, inpatient settings, and outreach programs). In addiction treatment programs, about 5–70% of individuals with an alcohol use disorder have coexisting depression (Davidson et al., 1995). The temporal pathway of the depressive symptoms is individually variable, with a large proportion being relieved within a few days or weeks of abstinence from alcohol (Dachis et al., 1986; Pottenger et al., 1978; O'Sullivan et al., 1983). Dachis et al. (1986) found that depression diagnosed in a current episode of alcohol dependence remitted after 2 weeks of abstinence and detoxification from alcohol. Brown and Schuckit (1988) found depressive symptoms decreasing most rapidly between the first and second weeks of abstinence with only about 6% of the alcoholics continuing to have depression after 4 weeks of abstinence. This finding contrasts with depressed patients without substance abuse who often continue to have some symptoms for about 3–4 months (Coryell et al., 1989). In contrast, Pottenger et al. (1978) found a significant persistence of depressive symptoms in a group of alcoholics who were found to be depressed while drinking at baseline, but a high percentage (72%) of those depressed alcoholics were still drinking at follow-up after 1 year of treatment for alcohol dependence. Prospective follow-up data for the collaborative Study on the Psychobiology of Depression also showed that 28% of alcohol-dependent patients without depression at intake developed major depression within 6 years compared with 12% of never-ill subjects (Coryell et al., 1992).

The ECA study found that about 35% of cocaine addicts had an affective disorder during their lifetime. About 10–30% of depressed psychiatric patients have a current cocaine use disorder. About 30% of substance-abuse-treatment-seeking cocaine addicts have a current affective disorder, and about 62% have had an affective disorder during their life (Rounsaville et al., 1991). Compared to the rates found in the general population, the cocaine addicts had higher rates of *current* major depression (5%), alcohol dependence (29%), minor bipolar disorders (e.g., hypomania 2% and cyclothymic personality 20%), and anxiety disorders (phobia 12% and generalized anxiety 4%). Compared to non-treatment-seeking cocaine abusers, treatment seekers use cocaine in a higher intensity manner, have longer periods of depression, and have more adverse consequences associated with cocaine use including drug overdoses and losses of jobs and relationships (Rounsaville et al., 1991).

Although lifetime and current affective disorders are very common in cocaine addicts, most patients presenting for treatment have depressive symptoms and do not meet diagnostic criteria for depression after an initial abstinence period. The intensity of the acute cocaine withdrawal depressive symptoms appears to be independent of other cocaine withdrawal symptoms such as the intensity of cocaine craving (Ho et al., 1991). For many cocaine addicts there is an initial improvement in depressive symptoms during the first month of treatment, with some patients maintaining this improved mood state. Unfortunately, many patients experience a reemergence of the depressive symptoms including difficulty concentrating, anxiety, fatigue, boredom, anhedonia, loss of sex drive, irritability, and insomnia. These symptoms often develop after about 6 weeks of abstinence and can last for months during a stage of recovery labeled "the wall" (Rawson et al., 1990). Relapse to cocaine is common during this period.

Cigarette smoking and severity of nicotine dependence are strongly associated with major depression and depressive symptoms. For the general population, smokers are twice as likely to have had a major depressive episode in their lifetime compared to nonsmokers (Glassman et al., 1990). The association with smoking is even stronger with recurrent major depression than with a single episode (Glassman, 1993). The risk for major depression increases with the severity of nicotine dependence and average number of cigarettes consumed. There may be an increased risk of suicide in smokers versus nonsmokers (Hemenway et al., 1993), but whether the presence of depression of smoking per se is responsible for this association is not currently resolved.

At least 50% of psychiatric patients with depression meet criteria for nicotine dependence, and the heavy smokers (>25 cigarettes per day) are three times more likely to have a current substance use disorder (Ziedonis et al., 1994). About 25–40% of smokers who enter smoking cessation programs have a history of major depression and many have dysthymic symptoms (Glassman, 1993b; Hall, 1993). Smokers with a depression history are twice as likely not to succeed at smoking cessation compared to those without a depression history

(14% vs. 28%, Glassman, 1990). The poorer prognosis is most likely secondary to the fact that depressed smokers have more severe nicotine withdrawal symptoms (especially depressive symptoms) and are at risk for a depressive episode relapse (Hall et al., 1993). Barriers to implementing nicotine dependence treatment in mental health settings include clinician fears of exacerbating the psychiatric disorder, lack of training in smoking cessation, the belief that psychiatric patients are not interested and cannot quit (i.e., low patient motivation), the perceived need to use smoking as a positive behavioral reinforcement in treatment, and the lack of provider reimbursement for smoking cessation treatment services and medications.

The development of a substance use disorder results in adverse medical, legal, vocational, social, family, and psychological consequences. Substance use has a deleterious impact on the course of depression, but studies report that effects vary according to the type of substance used and the severity of the problem. The impact of substances varies according to the route of administration and the state of use. Chronic abuse of alcohol can result in substantial cognitive difficulties, especially on complex tasks that require simultaneous consideration of several elements. The severity of these deficits relates to the quantity of alcohol intake and the duration of the drinking problem (Grant and Reed, 1985). The effect of stimulants on neuropsychological functioning is a pattern of mild impairment with specific deficits noted in the areas of concentration, memory, nonverbal problem solving, and abstracting ability (Cocores et al., 1987). But other studies have suggested that stimulant use enhances attention. Chronic cocaine use, however, may impair attention and motor function through overstimulation of the brain reward areas and through a rebound hypoexcitability of these regions when the drug is discontinued (Gawin et al., 1986).

III. ETIOLOGY OF SUBSTANCE ABUSE AND DEPRESSION

Why is there such a strong association between depression and alcohol, tobacco, and other drug use disorders? Biopsychosocial factors appear to influence the onset of both disorders and the likelihood that both disorders will coexist. These factors may also cause an individual in recovery to relapse and have a recurrence of depressive symptoms and/or substance use/abuse.

A. Psychosocial Factors

Despite all the negative consequences associated with substance abuse, some individuals with depression report that using substances helps them cope with their symptoms of depression. They report using substances for pleasure, to alleviate boredom, to relieve feelings of anxiety, sadness, or distress, and to share the excitement of "getting high" with friends who are also using. Some individuals report that substance use reduces their social inhibitions. The "self-medication theory" suggests that people self-select a particular type of drug (cocaine, opiates, or alcohol) based on particular psychological characteristics or psychiatric diagnoses. For some people, the energizing properties of cocaine are thought to help overcome boredom, emptiness, and fatigue related to depression, personality disorder, or alcohol dependence. Also, some people develop severe depressive symptoms during cocaine withdrawal and are caught in a cycle of trying to medicate these withdrawal feelings. For other people, the usage of cocaine leads to increased assertiveness, self-esteem, and frustration tolerance, which has been speculated to relate to an addict's disturbances in "self-regulation," including an inability to recognize, tolerate, and regulate affect. Some people chose cocaine because it helps them augment a hyperactive lifestyle and an exaggerated need for self-sufficiency (Khantzian, 1985). The self-medication theory suggests that individuals may use chemicals to alleviate the symptoms of depression; however, the research data supporting this clinical perception are mixed. First, from study to study patients with depression do not appear to preferentially select specific substances. Second, although some patients report feeling less depressed when using substances, this phenomenon appears to be only a temporary effect with some substances, and many individuals develop increased depression, anxiety, and insomnia during the acute and protracted abstinence periods.

Alcohol is a central nervous system depressant that some individuals state they use to forget their problems, reduce their anxiety, or improve their ability to sleep. However, alcohol has the potential to cause depressive symptoms. The idea of self-medicating a primary depression with alcohol has not been supported in the literature (Schuckit and Monteiro, 1988). Serious depression can follow prolonged drinking. As many as 70–80% of severely depressed people do not increase their alcohol use; they either decrease or maintain a similar pattern of use (Anthenelli and Schuckit, 1993). Only 5–10% of those with a major depressive episode develop secondary alcohol dependence. In one survey almost all of the newly admitted alcohol-dependent inpatients reported some degree of depressive symptoms (Brady and Roberts, 1995). The quality of the depression is equal in primary versus secondary depression; however, secondary depression is transient and disappears with several days or weeks of abstinence (Gibson and Becker, 1973; Brown and Schuckit, 1988; Davidson, 1993).

Social factors can be important in initiating and maintaining depression and/or substance abuse. Some specific factors include family-of-origin issues, early loss of a parent, peer group pressure, and community. Recently, the role of the entitlement system in maintaining substance abuse has been suggested.

B. Biological Factors

There appear to be common neurobiological underpinnings and genetic factors underlying the comorbidity between depression and alcohol and other drugs (Merikangas and Gelernter, 1990). Among individuals with a primary depression disorder, close relatives have been reported to have a greater incidence of depression, but not alcohol dependence (Hesselbrock et al., 1983; Hasegawa et al., 1991). There may be a higher incidence of depression in female alcoholics relative to the general female population, and that depression may be primary in the majority of cases (66%), whereas alcohol abuse may be primary in depressed alcoholic men (Helzer and Pryzbeck, 1988). With regard to comorbid nicotine dependence, twin studies appear to demonstrate that smoking does not cause depression and depression does not cause smoking, but that shared genetic factors may predispose individuals to both smoking and depression (Kendler et al., 1993).

From a biological perspective, the mesolimbic dopamine pathway appears to play an important role in drug reinforcement and reward (Koob, 1992). Increasing evidence suggests that increased mesolimbic dopamine release results in increased pleasure and reward. However, multiple pathways influence mesolimbic dopamine release, including the endogenous opioid peptide system. Each specific substance has a unique pharmacological effect that modifies cognition, thought, and mood. Even relatively small amounts of substances over a shorter period may result in substantial consequences. Individuals with depression appear to progress rapidly from substance use to abuse or dependence. In addition, substances of abuse can have pharmacokinetic and pharmacodynamic interactions with psychiatric medications used to treat the depression. This typically reduces the medications' effectiveness.

Like cigarettes, caffeinated beverages, such as coffee and tea, are known to interfere with the absorption and metabolism of psychiatric medication. Cigarette smoking increases the metabolism of psychiatric medication and typically decreases plasma drug levels, which can reduce medication effectiveness and side effects. The "tar" (polynuclear aromatic hydrocarbons), not nicotine, in cigarettes causes this effect. Abstinence from smoking increases medication blood levels, and smokers are usually prescribed higher dosages of medication as compared to nonsmokers (Ziedonis et al., 1994).

IV. BIOLOGICAL MARKERS

Biological markers of depression and specific substances may help to clarify the neurobiological linkage between the disorders. Each substance has a specific pharmacology and potential interaction with the neurobiology of depression. These findings can help us to better understand the etiology of the disorders and lead to innovative ways to identify individuals at risk for the disorders and ways to implement prevention strategies and pharmacotherapy treatments.

A. Alcohol Dependence

Whether the comorbidity of alcohol dependence and depression represents a significant neurobiological correlation remains to be fully explored. A study of the cerebrospinal fluid variables in nondepressed versus depressed alcoholics 3 weeks postdetoxification revealed lower cerebrospinal fluid (CSF) levels of the dopamine metabolite homovanillic acid (HVA) and of γ-aminobutyric acid (GABA) in the depressed alcoholics (Roy et al., 1991). Petty et al. (1996) have recently shown decreased serum GABA levels in abstinent alcoholics. Interestingly, several investigators have found a reduced CSF HVA in depressed subjects without alcoholism (Roy et al., 1985). Other dopamine abnormalities, including a reduced growth hormone response to the dopamine agonists apomorphine (Balldin et al., 1992; Dettling et al., 1995), and bromocriptine (Farren et al., 1995a) in alcoholics, have been found. While dopamine has been implicated in the etiology of depression (Manki et al., 1996), and dopamine receptor abnormalities have been implicated in a subset of depressed patients (Ebert et al., 1996), most theories of depression emphasize other neurotransmitters (i.e., serotonin and norepinephrine), which may indirectly interact with dopamine to contribute to depression (Brown and Gershon, 1993).

Abnormalities of serotonin (5-HT) metabolism have frequently been found in alcoholism (for review see LeMarquand et al., 1994) as well as in depression (Heninger et al., 1984). Indeed, neuroendocrine investigations using the same serotonergic probes have found similar abnormalities in alcoholics (Farren et al., 1995b), and in depressives (O'Keane and Dinan, 1992). CSF measurement of 5-hydroxyindolacetic acid (5-HIAA), a 5-HT metabolite, were nonsignificantly reduced in the alcoholics with depression relative to the nondepressed (Roy et al., 1991). Unfortunately, these abnormalities are not specific for either disorder, as these and similar serotonergic abnormalities have also been documented in obsessive-compulsive disorder (Lucey et al., 1992) and autism (McDougle et al., 1996).

Abnormalities of hypothalamic-pituitary axis activation using the dexamethasone suppression test (DST) have been found in alcohol dependence (Swartz and Dunner, 1982) and in depression (Carroll et al., 1981). DST abnormalities in alcohol dependence have been found to return to baseline after 4 weeks of abstinence (Brizer et al., 1988). Low basal levels of cortisol were found to distinguish alcoholics without major depression from those with a current depression in the postwithdrawal period (Halbreich et al., 1989), but alcoholics have also been found to have high levels of basal cortisol (Farren et al., 1995c), also in the postwithdrawal period. Other neuroendocrine abnormalities in depression include a blunted TSH response to TRH infusion (Staner et al., 1994) and a blunted growth hormone response to dexamethasone (Thakore and Dinan, 1996), but they are nonspecific to this disorder.

Other biochemical abnormalities found in alcohol dependence include diminished response to alcohol in the sons of alcoholics (Schuckit et al., 1994), lowered platelet adenylyl cyclase activity in alcoholics (Katamura et al., 1996), and lowered serum β-endorphin levels. This latter abnormality may be of relevance as the μ-opioid receptor antagonist naltrexone has been found to be helpful in treatment of nondepressed alcoholics (O'Malley et al., 1992; Volpicelli et al., 1992).

B. Cocaine Dependence

The effects of cocaine administration on HPA axis function have been extensively reviewed by Mello and Mendelson (1997). Through monoamine reuptake blockade, cocaine stimulates ACTH and cortisol secretion (or corticosterone in rodents) and decreases secretion of prolactin (since dopamine inhibits prolactin release). Since there are abnormalities in HPA function in depressives, cocaine may modulate the course of primary major depressive illness through its effects on pituitary secretion, and secondary depression induced by cocaine withdrawal may similarly relate to altered neuroendocrine function.

C. Opiate Dependence

Few studies have investigated biological correlates between depression and opiate dependence. However, opiates such as heroin and morphine had been used until the 1950s to treat depressive symptoms, and evidence for learned helplessness models in animals (an animal model of depression) suggests that opiates can have antidepressant effects. Antidepressant actions of opiates are practically limited by dose-dependent side effects such as respiratory depression. Bodkin et al. (1995) investigated the efficacy of the partial μ-opiate receptor antagonist buprenorphine in an open-label study of 10 treatment-refractory unipolar depressed subjects for 4–6 weeks and found that this agent had substantial antidepressant properties, particularly within the first week of treatment.

D. Nicotine Dependence

Although there have not been any biological studies to date that link depression and nicotine dependence, there is evidence from preclinical and clinical studies that nicotine dependence and withdrawal can alter monoamine function. Several preclinical studies in rodents suggest that nicotine can stimulate dopamine (catecholamine) turnover and release in mesolimbic dopamine systems (Nisell et al., 1995) and nicotine withdrawal produces reduced dopamine function in nucleus accumbens and dorsolateral striatum, but not the prefrontal cortex (Fung et al., 1996; Hildebrand et al., 1997; George et al., 1998).

Nicotine withdrawal effects on adrenergic function have been well characterized in human subjects, and smoking cessation is associated with decreased plasma levels and urinary excretion of epinephrine and norepinephrine (Myrsten et al., 1977; Elgerot, 1978; West et al., 1984; Ward et al., 1991), and elevated leukocyte β-2 adrenergic binding (Laustiola et al., 1991). Since reduced catecholamine function has been implicated in depression and smoking cessation can precipitate depressive relapse in smokers with a history of depression (Glassman et al., 1990), it is obvious that depression and nicotine dependence may have common biological substrates. The antidepressant bupropion, a catecholamine reuptake blocker, has recently been showed to have efficacy in smoking cessation (Hurt et al., 1997), which further substantiates the common role of catecholamines in depression and smoking.

Effects of serotonin systems are not significant, though there may be selective changes in hippocampus (Benwell and Balfour, 1979) and the SSRI sertraline can attenuate nicotine withdrawal-induced weight gain and food/water consumption in rodents (Levin et al., 1993). Furthermore, nicotine and smoking can stimulate HPA axis function, but the effects of smoking cessation on HPA function (ACTH and cortisol levels) are equivocal (Pickworth et al., 1996) and require further study.

V. ASSESSMENT AND DIFFERENTIAL DIAGNOSIS

An initial evaluation of every patient should include a mental status examination and an assessment of medical conditions, prescribed medications, and use of alcohol, tobacco, and other drugs. The diagnostic assessment should consider other psychiatric disorders associated with depression, including personality and anxiety disorders (generalized anxiety, agoraphobia, and panic disorders). A bipolar disorder should be ruled out. Patients should be asked about their previous substance abuse and psychiatric treatment, including previous diagnoses, severity of illness, type(s) of treatment, intensity of treatment, and length of treatment.

Patients with depressive symptoms should be assessed for suicidal ideation. Compared to the general population, the incidence of suicide among substance abusers is about 20 times higher (Blumental, 1988). The risk for suicidal behavior increases with a history of previous attempts, family history of suicide, having a plan, lack of support system, recent losses, and feelings of hopelessness and helplessness.

Individuals treated for depression in mental health settings often have not been carefully screened for substance use and problem usage. Mental health staff have often had limited training in identifying and treating the dually diagnosed client. A number of studies have demonstrated that many mental health clinicians have had difficulties detecting current substance abuse among psychiatric patients. One problem can be that depressed patients abusing substances may attempt to protect their drug supply, deny usage, and minimize the consequences of their usage. Information from the patient's family or friends can help in the assessment of process and help engage these individuals in the treatment process. Patients should be asked questions about their family history for mental illness or addiction. Addicts with a strong family history for affective disorders are at higher risk for an underlying affective disorder (Weiss et al., 1988). Urine toxicology and breathalizer tests are important in the diagnostic process. In evaluating a positive or negative test result, the clinician should be aware of the day of last use and the time required for a specific drug to be metabolized and not detected in the urine test.

Establishing a DSM-IV diagnosis helps the clinician to focus on the differences between symptoms versus syndromes, such as drinking and alcoholism, sadness and major depression, and nervousness and panic disorder. Establishing a substance use disorder in psychiatric patients can be complicated, especially if the patient minimizes his or her substance-related problems and attributes those problems to other causes. Psychiatric patients tend to have more severe consequences from smaller amounts of substance use than nonpsychiatric patients, and clinicians may be lulled into a false sense of security by focusing only on the amount of substance use reported. A patient's smoking status can be a clue to a hidden substance use disorder. As with the general population, cigarette smoking is associated with other substance use among individuals with depression. Heavy smokers (more than 25 cigarettes per day) have rates of substance abuse three to four times that of nonsmokers. Other screening clues for a substance use disorder include the occurrence of the common consequences of substance abuse. These consequences include episodes of homelessness, legal problems, verbal threats, violence, treatment noncompliance, need for higher-dose medications, multiple medical problems, frequent emergency room visits or hospitalizations, and suicidal ideation/attempts.

A substance abuse assessment should include asking about the patterns of usage (specific amounts, frequency, last use, route of administration), consequences of use, past treatment history, severity of the symptoms, family history for both mental illness and substance abuse, the perception of the benefits for continued use as well as reasons to quit using the substance, and the motivational level to quit using each substance.

One method to evaluate motivation is the five-stage scale by Prochaska and DiClemente (precontemplation, contemplation, preparation, action, and maintenance). Using these Prochaska and DiClemente stages to evaluate a sample of 105 individuals with both depression and a substance use disorder, about 77% were assessed as having low motivation (precontemplation or contemplation), with the motivation varying according to the individual substance and the presence or absence of polysubstance abuse. Low motivation was assessed in 53% who abused alcohol, 65% who abused cocaine, and 73% who abused marijuana (Ziedonis D and Trudeau K, personal communication).

Recent substance use can cause a variety of psychiatric symptoms, and these symptoms can vary depending on whether they are associated with chronic usage, intoxication, acute withdrawal, and protracted withdrawal states. For example, cocaine use can cause paranoia/psychosis, mood lability, euphoria, sleep disturbances, appetite disturbance, grandiosity, depression, agitation, irritability, anhedonia, suicidal ideation, and anxiety (Post et al., 1974; Gawin and Kleber, 1986).

The DSM-IV criteria for substance-related disorders and substance-induced mood disorders include 11 classes of substances: alcohol; amphetamines; caffeine; cannabis; cocaine; hallucinogens; inhalants; nicotine; opioids; phencyclidine (PCP); and sedatives, hypnotics, and anxiolytics. These diagnoses differ from a substance-induced mood disorder in that the latter identifies the cause of the depressive symptoms to be the direct result of the use of a substance. Substance-induced mood disorders occur only in association with intoxication and withdrawal, as opposed to primary mood disorders, which may precede substance use or remain during extended periods of abstinence (at least 1 month) from substances (APA, 1994).

DSM-IV substance use disorders for each substance include substance dependence, abuse, intoxication, and withdrawal. Substance intoxication is a reversible state that develops secondary to the recent ingestion or exposure to a substance. Substance withdrawal is the development of maladaptive behavioral, physiological, and cognitive changes secondary to the cessation of, or reduction in, heavy substance use. Substance abuse is a maladaptive pattern of substance use leading to clinically significant impairment in one or more of the following over a 12-month period: (1) recurrent use resulting in failure to fulfill major role obligations; (2) recurrent use of substances in situations that may be hazardous; and (3) continued use despite persistent social or interpersonal problems. Substance dependence refers to a cluster of behavioral, physiological, and cognitive symptoms indicating that an individual continues to use a substance despite significant negative consequences. To meet criteria for dependence, a person must manifest three or more of the following symptoms within a 12-month period of time: (1) tolerance, a marked need for increased amounts of a substance or a diminished effect of the same amount over time; (2) withdrawal symptoms upon discontinuing the substance or taking another substance to relieve/avoid withdrawal; (3) taking larger amounts than intended; (4) desire to quit or failed attempts at quitting; (5) spending a great deal of time obtaining, using, or recovering from the substance; (6) interference in social/occupational functioning due to use; and (7) continued use despite knowledge of detrimental physical or psychological consequences. Physiological dependence requires the presence of symptom (1) and/or (2) (APA, 1994).

Some clinicians use structured instruments to help in the diagnostic assessment. Several studies comparing different instruments suggest that the special nature of the dual diagnosis population favors a clinician-administered, structured interview, such as the Structured Clinical Interview for DSM (SCID). The combination of a clinical assessment and a structured interview can lead to a more reliable and valid diagnosis than either approach alone (Ford, 1989).

Establishing a definitive diagnosis of depression in the context of a substance use can be difficult because of the patient's continued substance usage and the difficulty in remembering details of the clinical history. Creating a time line of the patient's life and establishing when an individual first met diagnostic criteria for either disorder can sometimes be helpful. A primary depression disorder is established if the criteria for a depression disorder occurred either prior to the substance use disorder or after an extended period of abstinence from substances (this period varies in the literature between 2 weeks and 6 months). Otherwise, the depressive symptoms are thought to be a secondary depression. Some practical problems in organizing the time line include the patient's ability to recall information, the fact that many patients have few protracted drug-free periods, and the fact that the typical onset of mental illness occurs after the time in which many patients already have developed a substance abuse disorder. Without a clear history of a primary psychiatric disorder, the diagnosis of a primary or coexisting psychiatric disorder in the context of recent drug usage is difficult. The accuracy of a diagnosis should improve by continuing to observe a patient's condition over time (Schuckit and Monteiro, 1988).

Another method for subgrouping individuals with both substance abuse and depression is the substance-induced versus independent depressive episodes division (Schuckit et al., 1996). Analysis of the large Collaborative Study on the Genetics of Alcoholism (COGA) data set using semistructured interviews given to 2945 alcoholics gave an incidence of independent depressions of 15.2%, and an incidence of substance-induced depressions of 26/4%. This data set represents by far the largest number of alcoholic subjects ever studied for comorbidity. Those subjects with independent major depressive episodes were more likely to be married, Caucasian, and female, to have experience with fewer drugs and less treatment for alcoholism, to have attempted suicide and have a close relative with a mood disorder relative to those alcoholics with a substance-abuse-induced depressive episode (Schuckit et al., 1996). Consistent with the hypothesis that independent major depression might reflect a family history of affective disorder and not alcohol dependence are the 8-year follow-up data on 450 sons of alcoholics and controls that revealed a higher incidence of alcohol dependence among the sons of alcoholics but no increase in incidence of affective disorder (Schuckit and Smith, 1996). Indeed irrespective of the primary/

secondary dichotomy, a large number of alcoholics with histories of depression report a substance-induced depressive episode (Schuckit et al., 1996).

Although the primary-secondary distinction can help in the diagnostic process, this concept has polarized the way clinicians think about treatment, especially the use of antidepressants (Ziedonis and Kosten, 1991). Another method to describe the dually diagnosed is whether the depression is "transient" or "persistent." Psychiatrists working in both mental health and substance abuse settings often have different thresholds to establish a depression disorder. Patients often have the opportunity to chose which treatment setting, and this selection bias may help in assessment of both motivation and severity/priority of symptoms.

VI. TREATMENT OF DEPRESSION AND COMORBID SUBSTANCE USE DISORDERS

Treatment of comorbid substance abuse and depression can be effective; however, treatment must address both of the problems in an integrated manner that includes blending traditional psychiatric and substance abuse treatment approaches and blending psychotherapy and pharmacotherapy (Ziedonis and Fisher, 1996; Beitman and Klerman, 1991; Carroll et al. 1991). The primary substance abuse psychosocial treatments that appear fundamental to dual-diagnosis treatment are motivation enhancement therapy, relapse prevention, and 12-step facilitation. However, clinical experience suggests that these three treatment approaches need modification due to the vulnerabilities associated with depression. Substance abuse relapse prevention (Marlatt and Gordon, 1985; Carroll et al., 1991) integrates easily with traditional psychiatric treatment modalities such as cognitive therapy (Beck et al., 1979) and interpersonal therapy (IPT) (Klerman et al., 1984). Both cognitive therapy and IPT are specific psychotherapy approaches effective in treating depression, and these approaches can be adapted easily to fit the structure of traditional substance abuse treatment therapies and programs. Assertiveness training, problem solving therapy, and mood management can also be helpful (Hall et al., 1991).

Treatment of the dually diagnosed should be specific to the type and severity of depression and substance use disorder. Based on the specific substance abused, specific medications are used for detoxification and maintenance treatments.

Treatment should target the individual's motivational level and stage of recovery. Several models of dual-diagnosis treatment and recovery have been described. Treatment is described in a phase-specific manner that considers individual needs. In general, these models can be described as having three phases: (1) an initial engagement phase; (2) an action/changing behaviors phase; and (3) maintenance—a long-term life-style/paradigm shift phase.

Several models of care have developed to attempt to blend the traditional mental health and addiction systems. In the mental health system, Drake and colleagues have successfully improved the coordination of substance abuse services for the dually diagnosed by developing the *assertive community treatment team model*. This approach relies on multidisciplinary teams that serve as the primary clinician for a relatively small number of patients and are involved in a patient's treatment in all settings. The teams are outpatient-oriented; they execute intensive case management within the patient's natural environment. The treatment model is a stage-wise, cognitive-behavioral substance abuse treatment, and provides comprehensive community mental health services that include outreach, case management, and medications. The stage-wise treatment phases are based on Osher and Kofoed's five stages of dual-diagnosis treatment, i.e., engagement, persuasion, coercion, relapse prevention, and action. In the addiction treatment setting, dual-diagnosis treatment often is organized in a "consultation model." In this approach, a dual-diagnosis expert is hired to evaluate addicts with depression and suggest/manage the psychiatric component of treatment. Since most individuals in early recovery complain of depression, anxiety, and anger, the traditional group therapy provides a forum to address psychiatric symptoms. The addiction model of dual recovery begins with abstinence: (1) achieving sobriety, (2) maintaining abstinence and early recovery, and (3) advanced recovery (Kaufman, 1989). The addiction treatment system usually has an "abstinence only" treatment philosophy, except in methadone maintenance treatment programs. In this model, therapy is initially supportive, directive, and focused on achieving abstinence from all substances. In treating the depressed addict, the clinician should provide the patient with opportunities to ventilate depressive feelings with an emphasis on the here and now. In early recovery, the patient's psychological defenses are recognized, but only redirected and used to maintain abstinence. Therapy is also directed toward decreasing the acute depressive feelings through understanding of psychosocial stressors, facilitating medication compliance, developing coping skills, and reframing ways of perceiving the patient's situation. Only in the advanced recovery phase may the patient be able to handle the feelings that would surface from a more psychodynamic therapy approach. In the advanced phase, the patient's defenses can be confronted more directly, but new and more mature defenses should be substituted in the place of the old defenses. Also, clinicians should recognize that the old defenses might have developed as a protective manner by the patient to resist an unhealthy, adverse situation.

Minkoff has proposed an *integrated treatment model* based on the parallels between the disorders of depression and substance abuse. Both are conceptualized as chronic relapsing conditions with a biological underpinning and social stigma. Individuals affected with depression or substance abuse often deny or minimize the presence or impact of the disorder. This approach emphasizes case management in which both problems are addressed simultaneously, and the patient is educated about the parallels between the two disorders.

The *motivation-based dual-diagnosis treatment approach* was developed to integrate mental health and addiction treatment (Ziedonis and Fisher, 1996; Ziedonis and D'Avanso, 1998). Motivation-based treatment incorporates the values underpinning the other models and articulates specific goals and treatment approaches for patients based on their motivation to address the addiction problem, the type of substance(s) abused, and the severity of both disorders. This model takes into consideration issues related to motivation, self-efficacy, interpersonal limitations, and the establishment of the therapeutic alliance. Motivation-based treatment incorporates the primary substance abuse psychosocial interventions with the necessary modifications needed for individuals with depression and substance abuse. The five motivational stages of Prochaska and DiClemente (precontemplation, contemplation, preparation, action, and maintenance) are incorporated into the assessment of all patients. Each motivational stage is matched with specific treatment approaches. The transtheoretical model articulated by Prochaska and DiClemente organizes a conceptualization of process underlying change, acknowledging that individuals vary in their readiness for change. Treatment approaches and treatment goals (abstinence or reduction, medication compliance, etc.) should be matched with the patient's level of motivation.

In motivation-based treatment, the clinician is encouraged to develop realistic and appropriate treatment goals. While the overall approach is eclectic, specific treatment approaches are suggested during the different motivational stages. Clinicians should have skills and knowledge in integrating different therapy approaches: motivational enhancement therapy, psychoeducation, relapse prevention, 12-step, pharmacotherapies (for both psychiatric and substance use disorders, including detoxification and maintenance), behavioral contracting, ongoing assessments including urine and breath toxicology monitoring, social skills training, peer support/counseling, vocational/educational counseling, and family/network therapies.

Usually psychiatric patients must be engaged in treatment to address the comorbid substance use disorder. Most patients enter treatment at a low level of motivation for substance use treatment, but are often motivated to stabilize and decrease their depression. This situation lends itself to the initiation of motivational enhancement therapy (MET) techniques around the engagement of psychiatric issues, eventually branching out to possible concerns and issues related to substance use. Treatment of the lower-motivated clients can be a lengthy process. The addition of multiple supports, external motivators, and monitors can help quicken the process through the stages of treatment.

Traditional motivational enhancement therapy and techniques are described in *Motivational Interviewing* (Miller and Rollnick, 1991). MET is based on the recognition that substance-abusing individuals vary in their readiness for change, and it attempts to build motivation for change and strengthen the commitment to change through "empathic exploration." MET emphasizes the fundamental role of ambivalence in change processes and the role of vacillation between levels of readiness. The concept of relapse is an integral part of a continuous change process. MET is especially helpful for the lower-motivated dually diagnosed clients who do not perceive their substance use as a problem; they do not perceive a need for change, nor do they seek treatment for themselves. The low-motivation client minimizes the physical risks or complications of substance use on mood or its impact on thought processes, or even its impact on significant others. The therapist attempts to engage the client in a discussion about his/her substance use in an open and nonjudgmental approach using "empathic exploration." The therapist attempts to elicit self-motivational statements from the patient regarding issues or problems related to substance use. A useful MET technique is to ask patients to discuss or write a "decisional balance" of the pros and cons of their continued substance use and of stopping their substance use. The low-motivation client is more likely to discuss reasons for continued use and the perceived benefits of use. Some may disclose their sense of hopelessness or their fears of quitting. General discussions about their life, their goals and hopes, may lead them to take a different look at their substance use and their feelings of ambivalence about substance use. The most difficult part of MET for the clinician is to refrain from providing advice, agreement/disagreement, interpretation, lecturing, or judgment.

The vulnerabilities inherent to depression (biological, cognitive, affective, and interpersonal) underlie the need to modify traditional psychosocial treatments for substance use disorders. MET for dual diagnosis must be modified to include ongoing contacts using a MET approach; using MET tools (i.e., the decisional balance tool can help the clinician explore the subjective experience of using drugs and having depression); intensive case management to facilitate possible alternatives that may improve the immediate quality of life for patients; more active participation by the clinician in making direct suggestions to help reduce substance use; and the reinforcement of other positive behaviors in patients' lives. MET is an ongoing part of treatment rather than a four-session treatment as originally developed for nondepressed substance abusers. Finally, individuals with a dual diagnosis may fluctuate with their acceptance of their diagnosis of depression and their motivation to maintain medication for depression. The clinician's efforts at increasing motivation to address the substance use disorder must not deny or minimize the depression problem and the need for medications to manage the depression.

The community reinforcement approach (CRA) offers a way to develop external motivation for a dually diagnosed population with few external motivators. CRA uses behavioral therapy principles of contingencies, rewards, and consequences. Disability income, probation, and family can provide external motivation to engage in treatment and progress to abstinence. As the patient's motivation for substance use treatment unfolds, the second phase of motivation-based treatment begins with the integration of relapse prevention and 12-step interventions.

Relapse prevention therapy is based on a cognitive/behavioral perspective, and change is believed to occur when the therapist helps the patient to unlearn "bad habits." It is based on the principles of classic and operant conditioning. It assumes that within a teacher-student model of treatment, using cognitive learning strategies, individuals can identify high-risk situations and develop alternative behaviors to either avoid or escape situations that induce craving or that have been associated with using. Traditional relapse prevention interventions were designed to facilitate and heighten the sense of self-efficacy by building skills that help reduce the probability of using.

Relapse prevention and 12-step recovery interventions have been successful in reducing and eliminating substance use in motivated people. Both relapse prevention and 12-step treatment revolve around social skills, which consist of the ability to interact with others, i.e., to communicate, and the ability to solve problems. The 12-step recovery program should be integrated into general substance abuse relapse prevention, psychotherapy approaches for depression (Evans and Sullivan, 1990), and methadone maintenance programs (Obuchowsky and Zweben, 1987). The spiritual aspect of the 12-step recovery program broadens the traditional psychiatric "biopsychosocial" model to the "biopsychosocial-spiritual" model. In the "social" component of this model, the clinician must include an awareness of the patient's family, sociocultural, and ethnic background and how these factors influence the patient's psychological state and ability to interact with a therapist (Acosta et al., 1982).

Clinical experience in referring individuals with depression to 12-step programs has been helpful except when some individuals are told to stop their antidepressant medication. Not all self-help groups are right for all individuals. The individual with depression should be encouraged to find the 12-step meeting in which he or she is most comfortable.

Further in the recovery process, the client develops extended periods of abstinence and is in the maintenance stage. The transition from action to maintenance can be difficult. During the maintenance phase, the goal shifts from an exclusive focus on abstinence to improving core areas of one's life. For the nondepressed substance abuser, this stage has been labeled stage II recovery (Larsen, 1985). The focus is on reducing dysfunctional relationships and increasing healthy relationships. Clients are attempting to pursue alternative highs, including employment, better relationships with significant others, and other social outlets with nonusers. This stage in treatment can be more difficult for the individual with depression. Encouraging involvement in self-help at this time may be very appropriate, particularly 12-step meetings. The 12 steps guide individuals through the recovery process. Sustaining change can be difficult, and positive patterns may need to be learned and relearned until they are fully integrated into patients' lives.

Individuals may cycle through the motivational levels at various times in their lives. Both the patient and the clinician must remember that the change process is ongoing, not finite. Relapse is always a possibility. Old patterns may reemerge, and new stressors may bring on cravings and ineffective coping strategies. However, dual recovery can be very rewarding and healthy. Individuals develop new ways to deal with life and self-actualize. Some individuals may have a lifetime of recovery from addiction and yet still have recurrent depression episodes.

VII. PHARMACOLOGICAL TREATMENT OF DEPRESSION AND COMORBID SUBSTANCE ABUSE

The treatment of primary depression often includes pharmacotherapy. Primary depressive disorders are heterogeneous, and a variety of antidepressants are available based on the side effect profile and specific neurotransmitters affected. Like substance abuse disorders, primary depression can also be a relapsing condition. To prevent depression relapses, medications are used as maintenance treatment for 6 months to as long as several years (Charney et al., 1981). From our clinical experience, having several first-line antidepressants allows flexibility to adapt to the individual's needs. With the depressed substance abuser we have found bupropion (activating), sertraline (neutral), and nefazadone (sedating) to be excellent first-line options.

Medications that specifically target specific substance use disorders are used for detoxification, craving reduction, relief of protracted abstinence withdrawal symptoms, and as agonist maintenance agents. These medications vary according to the specific chemical(s) involved in the substance use disorder(s) (i.e., alcohol, cocaine, opiates, nicotine, etc.). Some of these medications may also help to further reduce and stabilize the symptoms of depression. Unfortunately there have been limited pharmacotherapy trials for the substance-abusing individual with depression. There is, however, a growing clinical experience in using these medications safely and effectively.

A. Depression and Alcohol

Adjunctive medications that are approved by the Food and Drug Administration (FDA) for use in the treatment of alcohol use disorders include disulfiram (Antabuse) and naltrexone (Revia). Clinical experience with disulfiram is mixed in this population, but randomized control trials are lacking. Because of the potential alcohol-disulfiram reaction, the patient must be able to fully understand the risks of the medication and have the judgment to not drink because of the risk. At high doses of disulfiram (1000 mg), some clinicians have reported psychotic symptoms in non-dual-diagnosis patients. At the lower dose of 125–250 mg, the medication is well tolerated.

Naltrexone's record is more consistent. It has been used as an effective pharmacological agent in the treatment of alcohol dependence in nonpsychiatric patients, and has been shown to reduce alcohol consumption and lower rates of relapse when compared to placebo. Specifically, naltrexone-treated patients reported fewer drinking days, fewer drinks consumed per occasion, and lower rates of relapse to heavy alcohol use. Clinical experience suggests that naltrexone may help treat the individual with depression and alcohol dependence, especially in patients for whom the use of disulfiram is a concern. Opioid antagonists may have a role in improving psychiatric symptoms, and these data suggest that the medication is well tolerated by this population and does not increase their psychiatric symptoms. Research studies to date have not found any serious negative interactions with naltrexone and other psychiatric medications (including neuroleptics, lithium, and antidepressants). No drug interaction was noted between naltrexone and several antidepressants in a study with over 500 subjects.

Acamprosate is currently only available and approved in Europe; however, clinical trials are being completed in the United States. This drug's efficacy in alcohol dependence (Whitworth et al., 1996) probably relates to its actions on central glutamatergic systems. No studies with acamprosate in depressed alcoholics have been published.

Some studies have addressed the issue of serotonergic agents and other antidepressants in alcoholics. Older trials of antidepressants did not generally support efficacy, but these studies may have used doses that were too low and for too short a duration of treatment. There is evidence, however, that desipramine reduces depressive symptoms in both secondarily depressed and nondepressed alcoholics. There was an improvement in depressive scores on desipramine, a significant benefit in maintenance of abstinence, and a trend for the depressed desipramine subjects to have a longer time to relapse. A recent large trial of nortriptyline and bromocriptine in 216 subjects divided into alcoholics alone, depressed/anxious alcoholics, and nondepressed alcoholics with antisocial personality disorder (ASPD) proved that the only benefit was in those subjects with ASPD taking nortriptyline, both in depression scores and in overall drinking outcome. Other trials included the use of imipramine in 69 primarily depressed alcoholics, which showed a significant benefit in decreased alcohol consumption in those whose mood improved, without an increase in attainment of full sobriety. An open-label trial of fluoxetine showed an improvement in mood and a modest improvement in drinking measures in severely depressed alcoholics on antidepressant treatment. A double-blind, placebo-controlled trial of fluoxetine in alcoholics without major depression revealed a significant reduction in drinking and in depressive symptoms in the fluoxetine group of subjects with some depressive symptoms (Kranzler et al., 1995). Thus, there is some evidence that some serotonergic compounds and other antidepressants help relative depression but have only modest effects upon drinking in the population of depressed alcoholics.

There is modest evidence that sertraline may help relieve depression and have a modest effect upon drinking behavior in depressed alcoholics. Sertraline has also been used in an open trial in depressed alcoholic patients over a 12-week period (Anton et al. 1996). Nine subjects with alcohol abuse or dependence with an admission diagnosis of major depression or dysthymia were treated with sertraline in variable doses from 200 mg daily to between 25 and 50 mg/day. Overall alcohol use, obsessive thoughts about alcohol, and depression scores were all reduced during the study. In another open clinical trial, sertraline has been shown to help reduce alcohol consumption in seven nondepressed subjects with alcohol abuse or dependence (George et al., 1994). This serotonin-selective reuptake inhibitor (SSRI) has also been successfully used in an open-label study of posttraumatic stress disorder and alcoholism, with encouraging results (Brady et al., 1995).

B. Depression and Cocaine

Pharmacotherapeutic strategies for non–dually diagnosed cocaine addicts have focused on medications with monoaminergic activity that might reverse or compensate for the neurophysiological changes that result from chronic cocaine administration. Cocaine is a dopamine (and to a lesser extent NE and 5-HT) reuptake blocker that acutely increases activity in dopamine (monoamine) pathways. Chronic cocaine administration results in up-regulation of presynaptic impulse-modulating dopamine (DA) autoreceptors, which reduces activity in the (mesolimbic) DA system, which might cause the dysphoria and other affective changes. Numerous studies have evaluated the non–dually diagnosed cocaine addict using dopamine reuptake blockers and dopamine agonists. Most of these studies did not find clinically significant improvements in outcomes.

Cocaine addicts who are diagnosed with a secondary depressive disorder (i.e., duration of more than 2 weeks) should be considered for pharmacotherapy. Dopamine agonists and tricyclic antidepressants (TCAs) have been helpful in stabilizing depressive symptoms and decreasing cocaine craving and usage in cocaine addicts with secondary depression (Ziedonis and Kosten, 1991). However, studies with desipramine and cocaine use outcome measures have generally been disappointing. One study compared desipramine and placebo in cocaine addicts with depressed mood, who did not meet criteria for a current or lifetime diagnosis of depression. Results suggested that desipramine was more effective in improving depressed mood than placebo; cocaine abuse outcome measures were not reported (Giannini et al., 1986). In a study of the effectiveness of imipramine (Nunes et al., 1995) for 12 weeks in 113 cocaine-abusing subjects, imipramine was more effective compared to placebo in producing cocaine abstinence, particularly in intranasal versus intravenous and freebase users, and in subjects with a depressive history.

C. Depression and Opiates

Methadone, L-alpha-acetylmethadol (LAAM), naltrexone, and buprenorphine are medications used in the treatment of opiate dependence. There does not appear to be strong antidepressant qualities to these medication options, and adjunctive medications should be considered. Ziedonis and Kosten (1991) found that adjunctive desipramine or amantadine improved substance abuse outcomes for depressed methadone-maintained cocaine subjects compared to placebo. Previous studies have demonstrated effective results for depression alone (Rounsaville et al., 1985) and mixed results in cocaine abuse treatment (Kosten, 1989) in methadone-maintained subjects. Margolin et al. (1995) studied the efficacy of bupropion (300 mg/day) versus placebo for 12 weeks in 149 cocaine-dependent methadone patients. No significant differences between drug and placebo groups were reported for cocaine use, depression, or psychosocial functioning. Finally, Petrakis et al. (1994) examined the effectiveness of open-label fluoxetine in 22 methadone-maintained subjects with mixed depression and cocaine dependence. They found that although fluoxetine decreased depressive symptoms, there were no significant effects on substance abuse outcomes in this heterogeneous group of subjects.

D. Depression and Nicotine

As in all areas of psychiatry, combining pharmacotherapies and psychotherapies is important and leads to improved outcomes. This seems especially important when considering smoking cessation in a depressed smoker. The FDA-approved pharmacological approaches to smoking cessation include (1) nicotine replacement therapies (NRTs; i.e., patch, gum, spray, and inhaler), and (2) bupropion (Zyban). These products aim to reduce withdrawal symptoms and nicotine craving. Patient preference is an important factor in considering the medication options. Some patients will prefer a particular route of administration, and others may not want to receive nicotine replacement at all. Brief advice should include reviewing all FDA-approved options, and affirming hope that multiple combinations might also be considered if the first effort does not succeed. The use of NRTs for smoking cessation has been thoroughly reviewed elsewhere (Balfour and Fagerstrom, 1996; Ziedonis et al., 1998).

Bupropion is the only nonnicotine replacement medication that is FDA-approved for treating nicotine dependence. This heterocyclic, atypical antidepressant likely works by blocking reuptake of both dopamine and norepinephrine. The efficacy of this drug in smoking cessation was demonstrated in three double-blind, placebo-controlled trials in nondepressed chronic smokers (Hurt et al., 1997), and appears to further improve smoking cessation rates when combined with the nicotine patch (Glaxo Wellcome, unpublished data). Early studies demonstrated that bupropion (300 mg/day) could enhance smoking cessation rates in depressed male smokers compared to placebo (59% vs. 20% 1 week postquit date). Recently, Hurt et al. (1997) reported that in a multicenter study of 615 smokers, bupropion SR (sustained-release formulation) significantly enhanced smoking cessation rates after 7 weeks of treatment. The study also demonstrated that bupropion's effects were dose-dependent: abstinence rates were 19.0%, 28.8%, 38.6%, and 44.2% for placebo, 100 mg/day, 150 mg/day, and 300 mg/day groups, respectively. These effects are independent of bupropion's antidepressant effects.

Other promising antidepressants for smoking cessation are nortriptyline and doxepin (Humfleet et al., 1996). The SSRIs do not appear to have similar efficacy even though they may reduce dysphoria (Dalack et al., 1995) and the weight gain associated with nicotine withdrawal. However, one study is depressed alcoholic smokers found that fluoxetine concurrently reduced smoking and alcohol consumption.

Moclobemide is a reversible inhibitor of monoamine oxidase A (RIMA), which has been approved for the treatment of major depression in Canada and Europe. Since it increases synaptic availability of monoamines (DA, NE, 5-HT), it may have benefit in smoking cessation. Further, since a component in cigarette smoke other than nicotine inhibits both MAO-A (Fowler et al., 1996) and MAO-B (Fowler et al., 1996) activity, such agents may have a further effect on smoking cessation. Moclobemide has been shown to be effective in smoking cessation in highly dependent smokers at 6 and 12 months after quit date (Berlin et al., 1995), and this finding deserves further evaluation.

VIII. THE USE OF MEDICATIONS IN ADDICTION TREATMENT PROGRAMS

Other than during detoxification, substance abuse treatment programs often make limited use of pharmacotherapies. This can impact the treatment of the dually diagnosed. The limited use of pharmacotherapy often occurs because of a "drug-free" mentality that does not distinguish between addictive and nonaddictive medications and is often based on limited experience, knowledge, or skills in this area and remains unchallenged by a lack of medically trained staff. Pharmacotherapies for depression may increase the cost-effectiveness of treatment by improving treatment outcome, allowing for shorter inpatient treatments, decreasing the need for some inpatient treatments, and facilitating the transition from inpatient to outpatient services. However, pharmacotherapy is not a "magic bullet" and must be viewed realistically as one of several treatment approaches that can improve treatment outcome. As with any pharmacotherapy, practical issues include monitoring the side effects, medication blood levels, compliance, and target symptoms for treatment response. As with any medication, the patient should be explained the risks and benefits, including the risk of using alcohol or cocaine while on medications. Addicts can take nonaddictive medication in an addictive manner, such as doubling the prescribed dosage or taking the medication when they feel a certain way instead of the prescribed manner. Therefore, the clinician should encourage a patient to adhere closely to the prescribed dosage and manner of taking the medication. Staff education is important in the process of introducing the use of medication to a addiction treatment program. Providing staff and patients with Alcoholics Anonymous (AA) literature such as "The AA Member—Medications and Other Drugs" can help focus a discussion to correct misunderstandings of the differences between addictive and nonaddictive medications and to increase an appreciation for the official 12-step writings, which suggest leaving medical decisions to treatment providers (Alcoholics Anonymous, 1984).

IX. SUMMARY

The assessment and treatment of coexisting depression and substance abuse is challenging, but can be successful if one integrates a combination of traditional psychiatric and substance abuse approaches, including psychotherapy and pharmacotherapy. Advances in the neurobiology and treatment of both depression and specific drug dependencies will lead to more effective overall treatment outcomes in individuals with depression with comorbid substance abuse.

ACKNOWLEDGMENTS

This work was supported by NIDA Grants R01-DA09127 and K20-DA00193 (DMZ), K12 DA-00167 (CKF), and the Lucille P. Markey Foundation and a Young Investigator Award from NARSAD (TPG).

REFERENCES

Acosta FX, Yamamoto J, Evans LA. Effective psychotherapy for low-income and minority patients. New York: Plenum Press, 1982.

Alcoholics Anonymous. The A.A. Member-Medications and Other Drugs. New York: Alcoholics Anonymous World Services, Inc., 1984.

American Psychiatric Association: Diagnostic and statistical manual of mental disorders (4th ed). Washington DC, American Psychiatric Association, 1994.

Anthenelli RM, Schuckit MA. Affective and anxiety disorders and alcohol and drug dependence: diagnosis and treatment. In: Miller NS and Stimmel B (eds), Comorbidity of Addictive and Psychiatric Disorders. New York: Haworth Medical Press, 1993:73–87.

Anton RF, Moak DH, Latham PK. The obsessive compulsive drinking scale: A new method of assessing outcome in alcoholism treatment studies. Archives of General Psychiatry, 1996; 53(3):225–231.

Balfour DJK, Fagerstrom KO. Pharmacology of nicotine and its therapeutic use in smoking cessation and neurodegenerative disorders. Pharmacol Ther, 1996; 72:51–81.

Balldin J, Berggren UC, Lindstedt G. Neuroendocrine evidence for reduced dopamine receptor sensitivity in alcoholism. Alcoholism: Clin Exp Res 1992; 16:71–74.

Beck AT, Rush AJ, Shaw BG, Emoy G. Cognitive Therapy of Depression. New York: Guilford Press, 1979.

Beitman BD, Klerman GL (eds). Integrating Pharmacotherapy and Psychotherapy. Washington, DC: American Psychiatric Press Inc., 1991.

Benwell MEM, Balfour DJK. Effects of nicotine administration and its withdrawal on plasma corticosterone and brain 5-hydroxyindoles. Psychopharmacology 1979; 63: 7–11.

Berlin I, et al. A reversible monoamine oxidase A inhibitor (moclobemide) facilitates smoking cessation and abstinence in heavy, dependent smokers. Clin Pharmacol Ther 1995; 58:444–452.

Blumenthal SJ. A guide to risk factors, assessment, and treatment of suicidal patients. Medical Clinics of North America, 1988; 72:937–971.

Bodkin, JA, Zornberg GL, Lukas SE, Cole JO. Buprenorphine Treatment of Refractory Depression. J Clin PsychoPharmacol 1995; 15(1):49–57.

Brady KT, Roberts JM. The pharmacotherapy of dual diagnosis. Psychiatric Annals, 1995; 25(6):344–352.

Brady, K, Sonne SC, Roberts JM. Sertraline treatment of comorbid post traumatic stress disorder and alcohol dependence. J Clin Psychiatry 1995; 56:502–505.

Brizer D, Castaneda R, Weintraub A, Sperber J. Assessment and management of protracted abstinence symptoms in alcoholics. Course given at the 19th Annual Medical Scientific conference, American Medical Society on Alcoholism and Other Drug Dependencies, April 1988.

Brown AS, Gershon S. Dopamine and depression. J Neural Transm 1993; 91:75–109.

Brown SZ, Schukit MA. Changes in depression among abstinent alcoholics. J Studies on Alcohol 1988; 49:412–417.

Carroll BJ, Feinberg M, Greden J, Tarika J, Albala AA, Huskett RF, James WM, Kronfot A, Lohr N, Steiner M, de Vigue JP, Young E. A specific laboratory test for the diagnosis of melancholia: standardization, validation and clinical utility. Arch Gen Psychiatry 1981; 38:15–22.

Carroll KM, Rounsaville BJ, Keller DS. Relapse prevention strategies for the treatment of cocaine abuse. Am J Drug and Alcohol Abuse 1991; 17(3):249–265.

Charney DS, Menkes DB, Heninger, GR. Receptor sensitivity and the mechanism of action of antidepressant treatment. Implications for the etiology and therapy of depression. Arch Gen Psychiatry, 1981; 38:1160–1180.

Cocores JA, Patel MD, Gold MS, Pottash AC. Cocaine abuse, attention deficit disorder, and bipolar disorder. J Nerv Men Disease 1987; 175(7):431–432.

Coryell W, Keller M, Endicott J, et al. Bipolar II illness. Course and outcome over a five year period. Psychol Med 1989; 19:129–141.

Coryell W, Endicott J, Keller M. Major depression in a nonclinical sample. Arch Gen Psychiatry 1992; 49:117–125.

Covey LS, et al. Major depression following smoking cessation. Am J Psychiatry 1997; 154:263–265.

Dachis CA, Gold MS, Pottash ALC. Evaluating depression in alcoholics. Psychiatry Res 1986; 17:105–109.

Dalack GW, et al. Mood, major depression, and fluoxetine response in cigarette smokers. Am J Psychiatry 1995; 152:398–403.

Davidson L, Simsarian J, Marcus K. Providing services to persons dually diagnosed with prolonged mental illness and substance abuse. White paper prepared for the Connecticut Department of Mental Health, 1993.

Dettling M, Heinz A, Dufeu P, Rommelspacher H, Graf KJ, Schmidt LG. Dopaminergic responsivity in alcoholism: trait, state, or residual marker? Am J Psychiatry 1995; 152:1317–1321.

Diagnostic and Statistical Manual, 4th ed (DSM-IV). American Psychiatric Association Press, 1994.

Ebert D, Frestel H, Loew T, Pirner A. Dopamine and depression-striatal dopamine D2 receptor SPECT before and after antidepressant therapy. Psychopharmacology 1996; 126:91–94.

Elgerot A. Psychological and physiological changes during tobacco-abstinence in habitual smokers. J Clin Psychol 1978; 34:759–764.

Evans K, Sullivan JM. Dual Diagnosis: Counseling the Mentally Ill Substance Abuser. New York: The Guilford Press, 1990.

Farren CK, Clare AW, Hameedi FA, Ziedonis D, Dinan TG. Evidence for reduced dopamine D2 receptor sensitivity in postwithdrawal alcoholics. Alcoholism Clin Exp Res 1995a; 19:1520–1524.

Farren CK, Ziedonis D, Clare AW, Hameedi FA, Dinan TG. D-Fenfluramine induced prolactin responses in post withdrawal alcoholics and controls. Alcoholism Clin Exp Res 1995b; 19(6):1578–1582.

Farren CK, Clare AW, Dinan TG. Basal serum cortisol and dexamethasone induced growth hormone release in the alcohol dependence syndrome. Hum Psychopharmacol Clin Exp 1995c; 10:207–213.

Ford J, Hillard JR, Giesler LJ, et al. Substance abuse/mental illness diagnostic issues. Am J Drug Alcohol Abuse 1989; 15:297–307.

Fowler JS et al. Brain monoamine oxidase A: inhibition in cigarette smokers. Proc Natl Acad Sci USA, 1996; 93:14065–14069.

Fung KY, Schmid MJ, Anderson TM, Lau Y-S. Effects of nicotine withdrawal on central dopaminergic systems. Pharmacol Biochem Behav 1996; 53:635–640.

Gawin FH, Kleber HD. Abstinence symptomatology and psychiatric diagnosis in cocaine abusers. Arch Gen Psychiatry 1986; 43:107–113.

George FR, Sanchez F, Chavez R, Westerberg V, Ritz MC, Eggerth D, Tuason V. Impact of sertraline on alcohol consumption in an open clinical trial. Presentation at Research Society on Alcoholism Annual Meeting, Hawaii, June 1994.

George TP, Sernyak MJ, Ziedonis DM, Woods SW. Effects of clozapine on smoking in chronic schizophrenic outpatients. J Clin Psychiatry 1995; 56:344–346.

George TP, Verrico CD, Roth RH. (1998). Effects of repeated nicotine pre-treatment on mesoprefrontal dopaminergic and behavioral responses to acute footshock stress. Brain Res (in press).

Giannini AJ, Malone DA, Giannini MC, Price WA, Loiselle RH. Treatment of depression in chronic cocaine and phencyclidine abuse with desipramine. J Clin Pharmacol 1986; 26:211–214.

Gibson S, Becker J. Changes in alcoholics self-reported depression. Quarterly J Studies on Alcohol 1973; 34:829–836.

Glassman AH, et al. Smoking, smoking cessation and major depression. JAMA 1990; 264:1546–1549.

Glassman AH, et al. Smoking cessation, clonidine, and vulnerability to nicotine among dependent smokers. Clin Pharmacol Ther 1993; 670–679.

Glassman AH. Cigarette smoking: implications for psychiatric illness. Am J Psychiatry 1993b; 150:546–553.

Grant I, Reed R. Neuropsychology of alcohol and drug abuse. In: Alterman A (ed), Substance Abuse and Psychopathology. New York: Plenum Press, 1985.

Halbreich U, Castaneda R, Galanter M. Low basal levels of cortisol distinguish detoxified alcoholics with major depressive disorder from non-MDDs. Alcoholism Clin Exp Res 1989; 13:834–836.

Hall SM, Munoz R, Reus V. Depression and Smoking Treatment: A Clinical Trial of an Affect Regulation Treatment. Abstract presented at CPDD Meeting, Palm Beach, Florida, 1991.

Hall SM, Munoz RF, Reus VI et al: Nicotine, negative affect and depression. J Consult Clin Psychol 1993; 61:761–767.

Hasegawa K, Mukasa H, Nakazawa Y, Kodama H, Nakamura K. Primary and secondary depression in alcoholism-clinical features and family history. Drug and Alcohol Depend 1991; 27:275–281.

Helzer JE, Pryzbeck TR. The co-occurrence of alcoholism and other psychiatric disorders in the general population and its impact upon treatment. J Studies on Alcohol 1988; 49:219–224.

Hemenway D, Solnick SJ, Colditz GA. Smoking and suicide among nurses. Am J Public Health 1993; 83:249–251.

Heninger GR, Charney DS, Sternberg DE. Serotonergic function in depression: prolactin responses to IV tryptophan in depressed patients and healthy subjects. Arch Gen Psychiatry 1984; 41:398–402.

Hesselbrock V, Tennen H, Stabenau J, Hesselbrock M. Affective disorder in alcoholism. International J Addiction 1993; 18:435–444.

Hildebrand BE, Nomikos GG, Panagis G, Hertel P, Schilstrom B, Svensson TH. Mesolimbocortical dopamine neurotransmission in nicotine abstinence. Soc Neurosci Abstr 1997; 23:1358.

Ho A, Cambor R, Bodner G, Kreek MJ. Intensity of craving is independent of depression in newly abstinent chronic cocaine users. Abstract presented at the CPDD Meeting, Palm Beach, Florida, 1991.

Humfleet G, Hall S, Reus V, Sees K, Mufloz R, Triffleman E. The efficacy of nortriptyline as an adjunct to psychological treatment for smokers with and without depressive histories. In: Harris LS, ed. Problems of Drug Dependence 1995: Proceedings of the 57th Annual Scientific Meeting, NIDA Research Monograph (Vol 162). Rockville, MD: National Institute on Drug Abuse, 1996, p. 334.

Humfleet G, et al. The efficacy of nortriptyline as an adjunct to psychological treatment for smokers with and without depressive histories. In: Harris LS, ed. Problems of Drug Dependence 1995: Proceedings of the 57th Annual Scientific Meeting, NIDA research Monograph (Vol. 162). Rockville, MD: National Institute on Drug Abuse, 1996, p. 334.

Hurt RD, et al. A comparison of sustained-release bupropion and placebo for smoking cessation. N Engl J Med 1997; 337:1195–1202.

Kantor J. 1996: Clinical depression during addiction recovery process diagnosis and treatment.

Katamura Y, Saito T, Takahata N. Changes in platelet adenylyl cyclase system in alcoholics. Arukoru Kenkyuoto Yakubutsu Ison 1996; 32:164–176.

Kaufman E. The psychotherapy of dually diagnosed patients. J Substance Abuse Treatment 1989; 6:9–18.

Kendler KS, et al. Smoking and major depression. Arch Gen Psychiatry 1993; 50:36–43.

Kessler RC, McGonagle KA, Shanyang Z, Nelson CB, Hughes M, Eshleman S, Wittchen H, Kendler KS. Lifetime and 12-month prevalence of DSM-III-R psychiatric disorders in the United States: results from the National Comorbidity Survey, 1994; Arch Gen Psychiatry 51:8–18.

Khantzian EJ. The self-medication hypothesis of addictive disorders: focus on heroin and cocaine dependence. Am J Psychiatry, 1985; 142:1259–1264.

Klerman GL, Weissman MM, Rounsaville BJ, Chevron ES. Interpersonal Psychotherapy of Depression. New York: Basic Books, 1984; 73–142.

Koob GF. The role of dopamine in the rewarding effects of drugs of abuse. Trends Pharmacol Sci 1992; 13:177–184.

Kosten TR, Rounsaville BJ, Kleber HD. A 2.5-year follow-up of depression, life crises, and treatment effects on abstinence among opioid addicts. Arch Gen Psychiatry 1986; 43:733–738.

Kosten TR. Pharmacotherapeutic interventions for cocaine abuse: matching patients to treatments. J Nervous and Mental Disease 1989; 177:379–389.

Kranzler HR, Burleson JA, Korner P, del Boca FK, John MJ, Brown J, Liebowitz N. Placebo-controlled trial of fluoxetine as an adjunct to relapse prevention in alcoholics. Am J Psychiatry 1995; 152:391–397.

Kranzler HR. (1998). Substance and Comorbidity and Psychiatry disorders Schizophrenia and Substance Abuse Ch 5 "Prevalence, Diagnosis and Treatment of Comorbidity Mood Disorder and Alcoholism."

Larsen E. Stage II recovery: life beyond addiction. San Francisco: Harper Collins, 1985.

Laustiola KE, Kotamaki M, Lassila R, Kallioniemi O-P, Manninen V. Cigarette smoking

alters sympatoadrenal regulation by decreasing the density of β-2 adrenoreceptors. A study of monitored smoking cessation. J Cardiovasc Pharmacol 1991; 17:923–928.
LeMarquand D, Pihl RO, Benkelfat C. Serotonin and alcohol intake, abuse and dependence: clinical evidence. Biol Psychiatry 1994; 36:326–337.
Levin ED, et al. Sertraline attenuates hyperphagia in rats following nicotine. Pharmacol Biochem Behav 1993; 44:51–61.
Lucey JV, O'Keane V, Butcher G, Clare AW, Dinan TG. Cortisol and prolactin responses to D-fenfluramine in non-depressed patients with obsessive-compulsive disorder: a comparison with depressed and healthy controls. Br J Psychiatry 1992; 161:517–521.
Manki H, Kanba S, Muramatse T, Higuchi S, Suzuki E, Matsushita S, Ono Y, Chiba H, Shitani F, Nakamura M, Yagi G, Asai M. Dopamine D2, D3 and D4 receptor and transport gene polymorphisms and mood disorders. J Affect Dis 1996; 40:7–13.
Margolin A, Kosten TR, Avants SK, et al. A multicenter trial of bupropion for cocaine dependence in methandone-maintained patients. 1995; 40:125–131.
Marlattm GA, Gordon JK (eds). Relapse prevention: maintenance strategies in the treatment of addictive behaviors. New York: Guilford Press, 1985.
Marzuk PM, Mann J. Suicide and substance abuse. Psychiatric Annals 1988; 18:639–645.
McDougle CJ, Naylor ST, Cohen DJ, et al. Effects of trytophan depletion in drug-free adults with autistic disorder. Arch Gen Psychiatry 1996; 53:993–1000.
Mello NK, Mendelson JH. Cocaine's effects on neuroendocrine systems: clinical and preclinical studies. Pharmacol Biochem Behav 1997; 57:571–599.
Merikangas KR, Gelernter CS. Comoribidity for alcoholism and depression. Psychiatr Clin North Am 1990; 13:613–632.
Miller WR, Rollnick S. Motivational Interviewing: Preparing People to Change Addictive Behavior. New York, NY: Guilford Press, 1991.
Miller WR, Zweben A, DiClemente CC, Rychtarik RG. Motivational enhancement therapy manual. Rockville, MD: DS Department of Health and Human Services Publication NO. (ADM) 92-1894. 1992.
Myrsten A-L, Elgerot A, Edgren B. Effects of abstinence from tobacco smoking on physiological and psychological arousal levels in habitual smokers. Psychosom Med 1977; 39:25–38.
Nisell M, Nomikosm GG, Svennson TH. Nicotine dependence, midbrain dopamine systems and psychiatric disorders. Pharmacol Toxicol 1995; 76:157–162.
Nunes EV, McGrath PJ, Quitkin FM, Stewart JP, Harrison W, Tricamo E, Ocepek-Welikson K. Imipramine treatment of alcoholism with co-morbid depression. Am J Psychiatry 1993; 150:963–965.
Nunes EV, McGrath PJ, Quitkin FM, Ocepek-Welikson K, Stewart JW, Koening T, Wager S, Klein DF. Imipramine treatment of cocaine abuse: possible boundaries of efficacy. Drug Alcohol Depend 1995; 39:185–195.
Nunes EV, Quitkin FM. Treatment of depression in drug-dependent patients: effects on mood and drug use. NIDA Research Monograph 172. Treatment of Drug-Dependent Individuals with Co-morbid Mental Disorders. NIH Publication NO. 97-4172, 1997:61–85.

Obuchowsky M, Zweben JE. Bridging the gap: the methadone client in 12-step programs. J Psychoactive Drugs 1987; 19(3):301–302.
O'Keane V, Dinan TG. Prolactin and cortisol responses to *d*-fenfluramine in major depression: evidence for diminished responsivity of central serotonergic function. Am J Psychiatry 1992; 148:1009–1015.
O'Malley SS, Jaffe AJ, Chang G, Schottenfeld RS, Meyer RE, Rounsaville B. Naltrexone and coping skills therapy for alcohol dependence. A controlled study. Arch Gen Psychiatry 1992; 49:881–887.
O'Sullivan K, Whillans P, Daly M, Carroll B, Clare A, Cooney J. A comparison of alcoholics with and without coexisting affective disorder. Br J Psychiatry 1983; 143:133–138.
Petrakis I, Carroll K, Gordon L, Cushing G, Rounsaville B. Fluoxetine treatment for dually diagnosed methadone maintained opioid addicts: a pilot study. J Addict Disord 1994; 13:25–32.
Petty F, Kramer GL, Fulton M, Davis LL, Adinoff B. Plasma GABA as a predictor of relapse in alcohol dependent patients. Alcoholism Clin Exp Res 1996; 20(Suppl): 107A.
Pickworth WB, Baumann MH, Fant RB, Henningfield JE. Endocrine responses during acute nicotine withdrawal. Pharmacol Biochem Behav 1996; 55(3):433–437.
Post RM, Kotin J, Goodwin FR. The effects of cocaine on depressed patients. Am J Psychiatry 1974; 131:511–517.
Pottenger M, McKernon J, Patrie LE, Weismann MM, Ruben HL, Newberry P. The frequency of persistence of depressive symptoms in the alcohol abuser. J Nervous and Mental Disorders 1978; 166:562–570.
Rawson RA, Obert JL, McCann MJ, Smith DP, Ling W. Neurobehavioral treatment for cocaine dependency. J Psychoactive Drugs 1990; 22:159–171.
Regier DA, Farmer ME, Rae DS, Locke BZ, Keith SJ, Judd LL, Goodwin FK. Comorbidity of mental disorders with alcohol and drug abuse: results from the Epidemiologic Catchment Area (ECA) study. J Am Med Assoc, 1990; 264:2511–2518.
Rounsaville BJ, Anton SF, Carroll K, Budde D, Prusoff BA, Gawin F. Psychiatric diagnosis of treatment seeking cocaine abusers. Arch Gen Psychiatry 1991; 48:43–51.
Rounsaville BJ, Kosten TR, Weissman MM, Kleber HD. 1985.
Roy A, Pickar D, Linnoila M, Doran A, Ninan P, Paul S. Cerebrospinal fluid monoamines and monoamine metabolites in melancholia. Psychiatr Res 1985; 15:281–292.
Roy A, DeJong J, Lamparski D, George T, Linnoila M. Depression among alcoholics: relationship to clinical and cerebrospinal fluid variables. Arch Gen Psychiatry 1991; 48:428–432.
Schuckit MA, Monteiro MG. Alcoholism, anxiety, and depression. Br J Addictions 1988; 83:1373–1380.
Schuckit MA. Low level of response to alcohol as a predictor of future alcoholism. Am J Psychiatry 1994; 151:184–189.
Schuckit MA, Smith TL. An 8-year follow up of 450 sons of alcoholics and control subjects. Arch Gen Psychiatry 1996; 53:202–210.
Schuckit MA, Tipp JE, Bergman M, Reich W, Hesselbrock VM, Smith TL. Comparison

of induced and independent major depressive disorders in 2945 alcoholics. Am J Psychiatry 1996; 154:948–957.

Shaner A, Eckman TA, Roberts LJ, Wilkins JN, Tucker DE, Tsuang JW, Mintz J. Disability income, cocaine use, and repeated hospitalization among schizophrenic cocaine abusers—a government-sponsored revolving door? N Engl J Med, 1995; 333:777–783.

Staner L, Linkowski P, Mendlewicz J. Biological markers as classifiers for depression: a multivariate study. Progr Neuropsychopharmacol Biol Psychiatry 1994; 18:988–914.

Swartz CM, Dunner DJ. Dexamethasone suppression testing of alcoholics. Arch Gen Psychiatry 1982; 39:1309–1312.

Thakore JH, Dinan TG. Are blunted dexamethasone-induced growth hormone responses unique to depression? Psychol Med 1996; 26:1053–1059.

Volpicelli JR, Alterman AI, Hayashida M, O'Brien CP. Naltrexone in the treatment of alcohol dependence. Arch Gen Psychiatry 1992; 49:886–880.

Ward KD, Garvey AJ, Bliss RE, Young JB, Landsberg L. Changes in urinary catecholamine excretion after smoking cessation. Pharmacol Biochem Behav 1991; 40:937–940.

Weiss RD, Mirin SM, Griffin ML, Michael J. Psychopathology in cociane abusers: changing trends. J Nervous and Mental Disease 1988; 176:719–725.

West RJ, Russell MAH, Jarvis MJ, Pizzey T, Kadam B. Urinary adrenaline concentrations during 10 days of smoking abstinence. Psychopharmacology 1984; 84:141–142.

Whitworth AB, Fisher F, Lesch OM, Nimmerrichter A, Oberbauer H, Platz T, Potgieter A, Fleischhacker WW. Comparison of acamprosate and placebo in long-term treatment of alcohol dependence. Lancet 1996; 347:1438–1442.

Ziedonis DM, Kosten TR. Depression as a prognostic factor for pharmacological treatment of cocaine dependency. Psychopharmacol Bulletin 1991; 27(3):337–343.

Ziedonis DM, Kosten TR, Glazer WM, Frances RJ. Nicotine dependence and schizophrenia. Hosp Commun Psychiatry 1994; 45:204–206.

Ziedonis DM, Fisher W. Motivation-based assessment and treatment of substance abuse in patients with schizophrenia. Directions in Psychiatry, 1996; 16(11):1–8.

Ziedonis DM, George TP. Schizophrenia and nicotine use: report of a pilot smoking cessation program and review of neurobiological and clinical issues. Schizophrenia Bull 1997; 23(2):247–254.

Ziedonis DM, D'Avanzo K. Schizophrenia and substance abuse. In: Kranzler HR, Rounsaville BJ (eds). *Dual Diagnosis and Treatment: Substance Abuse and Comorbid Medical and Psychiatric Disorders*. New York: Marcel Dekker, 1998; 427–465.

Ziedonis DM, Wyatt SA, George TP. Current issues in nicotine dependence and treatment. In: McCance-Katz E, Kosten TR (eds). *New Treatments for Chemical Addictions*. Washington DC: American Psychiatric Press Inc, 1998; 1–34.

3

Depression in the Medically Ill

D. JEFFREY NEWPORT and CHARLES B. NEMEROFF
Emory University School of Medicine
Atlanta, Georgia

I. SIGNIFICANCE OF MEDICAL COMORBIDITY IN DEPRESSION

Comorbidity is defined as the co-occurrence of two or more disorders within a defined time frame. This is a relatively recent concept arising from the observation that the results of clinical research were often confounded by the presence of disorders other than those under study (1).

Interest in comorbidity in patients with psychiatric disorders has been driven in part by the difficulties presented by a diagnostic system based on descriptive grounds. Although recent revisions of the *Diagnostic and Statistical Manual of Mental Disorders* (DSM) have more clearly delineated psychiatric diagnoses, certain symptoms and disorders do not readily fit into a single diagnostic entity. Comorbidity is not limited to the coexistence of two psychiatric syndromes but includes the co-occurrence of a psychiatric disorder with a medical disorder.

Recognizing and accounting for the presence of comorbid medical illness is an especially critical factor in the evaluation and management of depression. Epidemiological studies typically are primary in the investigation of illness comorbidity. If high rates of comorbidity are demonstrated, the ramifications are quite extensive. Due to the often complex interactions between depression and medical disorders, the study of comorbidity ideally requires investigation into the pathophysiology of the comorbid illnesses, into the biological bases for the diagnostic systems, and into the longitudinal course of both the depression and the medical disorder. The findings of this inquiry are likely to have a marked impact upon disease prognosis, treatment selection, and, undoubtedly, the direction of future research.

II. DIAGNOSTIC ISSUES

A. Diagnostic Classification

Psychiatric diagnostic systems have historically been organized on one of two classification schemes: etiological and descriptive. Classification based upon etiology establishes diagnostic categories based upon the underlying pathophysiology of the disorder. Although etiology-based systems generally have fewer diagnostic categories and are therefore easy to use, the pathogenesis for most psychiatric disorders remains elusive. The usefulness of etiology-based systems is therefore limited in psychiatry. As a result, the science of psychiatric diagnosis, i.e., nosology, has evolved instead upon descriptive lines. The descriptive approach instead relies upon the clinical presentation of psychiatric disorders and attempts to identify clusters of symptoms that demonstrate cohesion and thereby define a syndrome. The descriptive system formed the primary basis of classification for DSM-III and subsequent revisions.

The presence of medical illness comorbid with a psychiatric syndrome does, however, raise etiological issues. Historically, the issue has been posed in the question "Is the psychiatric disorder functional or organic?" This etiological concern is reflected in DSM-III, which, for example, distinguishes major depression from organic mood syndrome. However, new findings regarding the neurobiological bases of psychiatric syndromes coupled with the advent of sophisticated neurodiagnostic tools such as positron emission tomographic (PET) scanning have led to the inescapable conclusion that the so-called functional psychiatric disorders have an "organic" basis. The question of functional versus organic is rendered obsolete as evidenced by the elimination of such terminology from DSM-IV. This does not, however, negate the fact that diagnostic issues based upon etiology arise when a psychiatric disorder is comorbid with a medical disorder. For this reason, diagnostic dilemmas with far-reaching implications arise on both descriptive and etiological grounds when the depressed patient with comorbid medical illness is assessed.

B. Diagnostic Validity

Evaluation of the medical patient who appears to be depressed raises important diagnostic difficulties. Even the legitimacy of the DSM-IV diagnostic criteria for depression can reasonably be called into question. In so doing, Cavenaugh (2) outlines four steps in the establishment of diagnostic validity. *Face validity*,

Table 1 Differential Diagnosis of Depression in the Medically Ill

Differential based upon descriptive criteria
Major depressive disorder
Adjustment disorder with depressed mood
Bipolar I/II disorder, depressed
No psychiatric diagnosis: grief
No psychiatric diagnosis: symptoms of medical illness resembling MDD
Psychological factors affecting general medical condition
Differential based upon etiological criteria
Major depressive disorder
Mood disorder due to general medical condition
Substance-induced mood disorder
Mental disorder affecting general medical condition

the first step, is the extent to which a cluster of symptoms demonstrate diagnostic cohesion and thereby accurately describe a syndrome. *Descriptive validity* is the second step and represents the degree to which the symptoms of a particular disorder are unique to that disorder and thereby differentiate it from other disorders. Third is *predictive validity* through which the arrival at a diagnosis accurately forecasts the course of the illness and recommends its treatment. Finally, *construct validity* is the degree to which a rational theory can be built to explain the etiology and pathophysiology of the disorder. The phenomenological basis for diagnosis in DSM-IV emphasizes face and descriptive validity with a view to predictive validity but eschews construct validity, which, from the perspective of the traditional medical model, is seen as critical to treatment optimization.

Most of the oft-debated issues encountered in diagnosing depression in the medically ill patient directly address the face and descriptive validity of depression (3–7). Namely, can depression be reliably diagnosed and reliably distinguished from other disorders in the medically ill patient using DSM-IV diagnostic criteria? However, the presence of the comorbid medical illness also raises etiological issues that address the construct validity of the diagnosis. The result is that a differential diagnosis of the medically ill patient who is apparently depressed can be constructed on both descriptive and etiological grounds (see Table 1).

C. Descriptive Differential

1. Major Depressive Disorder

The term "depression" is imprecisely used both in lay circles and in the psychiatric community. Depression may refer to a transient feeling of sadness that is commonly experienced and not pathological. Conversely, the term may refer to a mood disturbance characterized by profound despair persisting over time and thus representing the primary symptom of a psychiatric disorder. Additionally, depression in psychiatric nomenclature refers not only to the symptom of depressed mood but to a syndrome itself.

Paradigmatic of the psychiatric depressive syndromes is major depressive disorder (MDD). Depressed mood is the hallmark symptom of the disorder but is neither sufficient nor required to make a diagnosis of MDD. MDD is defined in DSM-IV by the presence of depressed mood *or* anhedonia for 2 weeks coinciding with a specified number of neurovegetative and cognitive symptoms.

MDD is a debilitating and potentially fatal illness, which typically responds well to therapeutic intervention. Timely and accurate diagnosis of MDD is therefore of utmost importance. As previously noted, however, difficulties arise on descriptive grounds when attempting to diagnose MDD in a medically ill patient. For example, is the patient's depressed mood an expected and nonpathological grieving response to the medical diagnosis and its consequences? Conversely, could it be that symptoms of the medical illness mimic the neurovegetative symptoms of depression creating the false impression of depression where none exists? Finally, can MDD be descriptively distinguished from other psychiatric syndromes such as adjustment disorder in a medically ill patient?

2. *Grief*

Grief is an expected reaction to any significant loss. The term is often used synonymously with bereavement although the latter is specifically associated with the response to the death of a loved one. The diagnosis and subsequent consequences of many medical illnesses frequently threaten a host of losses and thus naturally precipitate a grief reaction.

The experience of grief can encompass a variety of emotional responses based upon the circumstances of the loss and the cultural setting. Nevertheless, the process of grieving can be considered a nonpathological syndrome with predictable signs and symptoms, a demonstrable course, and an anticipated conclusion. Several efforts have been made to characterize the natural progression of grieving and to predict its duration (8–15). Common in these depictions of the grieving process are phases of depressed mood and other symptoms typically associated with depression.

MDD and grief are two generally recognized syndromes therein exhibiting face validity. However, because depressed mood is a prominent aspect of grieving, clinical differentiation of the two syndromes can be challenging thus calling into question the descriptive validity of the diagnostic criteria. In fact, DSM-IV acknowledges that "some grieving individuals present with symptoms characteristic of a major depressive episode" (16).

While grief is an expected consequence of medical illness, MDD is not.

Indeed, a minority of severely medically ill patients suffer from any psychiatric disorder including MDD (7,17–20). Nevertheless, grief can take a pathological course in some individuals and evolve into a psychiatric syndrome such as MDD. Studies revealing that psychosocial interventions are beneficial for nondepressed medically ill patients (21–23) may in fact be demonstrating that such assistance has prophylactic value in averting the pathological evolution of grief.

The adverse consequences and need for aggressive treatment for MDD make clinical distinction from nonpathological grief imperative. Symptoms more suggestive of MDD than grief include profound psychomotor retardation, feelings of worthlessness, prolonged functional impairment, suicidal thoughts, or hallucinatory experiences. Even so, there remains no definitive descriptive validity distinguishing MDD from grief.

3. Symptoms of Medical Illness Resembling Depression

Patients who are medically ill frequently experience symptoms such as anorexia, insomnia, and fatigue, which approximate the neurovegetative symptoms of depression. This can arguably create the clinical impression of depression where none exists (4,6,7). The descriptive validity of the diagnostic criteria for MDD is again at issue. How, then, can depression be reliably diagnosed in a patient with debilitating medical illness? Four conceptual approaches have been reviewed by Cohen-Cole and colleagues (4). In each of these diagnostic strategies, a descriptive classification requiring five symptoms present for a period of 2 or more weeks is retained. The distinction between the various approaches lies in the theoretical basis for including or eliminating certain symptoms from the diagnostic list.

1. The *inclusive approach* is the simplest strategy and recommends including all symptoms toward a diagnosis of MDD even if they are plausibly secondary to the medical illness (24).
2. The *exclusive approach* advocates elimination of neurovegetative symptoms such as fatigue and anorexia from the diagnostic criteria for MDD in a medically ill patient (17,25). The result is that the patient must have more of the cognitive symptoms of MDD to fulfill the diagnostic criteria for the disorder.
3. The *substitutive approach* attempts to account for the possibility of underdiagnosis using the exclusive approach by suggesting the substitution of additional cognitive symptoms such as self-pity, brooding, crying spells, or pessimism to replace neurovegetative symptoms such as anorexia, insomnia, and anergia (2,26).
4. The *etiological approach* advocates that a symptom be counted toward the diagnosis of MDD only if it is clearly not due to the comorbid medical illness (27).

Numerous observations can be made regarding these four approaches. First, the inclusive and exclusive are the most straightforward and likely the easiest to implement. The inclusive approach is more sensitive for the diagnosis of MDD but potentially less specific, while the exclusive approach should be more specific but less sensitive. Second, the substitutive approach, which seems conceptually rational, has never been validated as diagnostically reliable. In addition, if diagnostic criteria such as those proposed by Endicott (26) are valid for substitutive purposes, should not those criteria be diagnostically valid in the absence of comorbid medical illness? Third, while the etiological approach may be theoretically defensible, it requires that the etiology of the patient's symptoms be determined thereby establishing construct validity of the diagnosis. As previously discussed, the etiology of psychiatric illness even in the absence of medical comorbidity remains largely obscure.

In summary, none of these four diagnostic approaches is ideal and without difficulty. The problems encountered in implementing the substitutive and etiological approaches render them unwieldy and thus unsatisfactory for conventional clinical practice. The descriptive validity of MDD in the medically ill patient is not ideal. Neither the inclusive nor the exclusive approach to diagnosis overcomes these problems. The result is a choice between two admittedly suboptimal diagnostic approaches and hinges upon whether diagnostic specificity or diagnostic sensitivity should be maximized.

Studies have consistently documented that nonpsychiatric physicians fail to diagnose depression in over half of their depressed patients (20,28–35). The consequences of untreated depression comorbid with medical illness include poor compliance with medical care (36), longer hospital stays (37), poorer quality of life (37), and increased mortality (18,37–40). These adverse outcomes in depressed, medically ill patients coupled with the benefits of appropriate treatment argue that the more sensitive inclusive approach is preferable in the clinical setting. Conversely, the more stringent exclusive approach is preferable in the research setting where the elimination of confounding variables is of paramount importance.

Although the neurovegetative symptoms of depression are most commonly mimicked by medical disorders, in certain neurological conditions dysregulation of emotional expression can cause a person to exhibit a depressed affect when he is indeed not depressed. It is not unusual for neurological disorders such as multiple sclerosis (MS) to elicit these so-called pseudobulbar phenomena, which are manifested by pathological weeping and laughing (41,42). While MS patients are admittedly at increased risk for developing depression, these pseudobulbar symptoms do not represent a disorder of mood. Such patients do not feel depressed but behave as if depressed because they are at times unable to control their affective presentation. As a result, these patients may weep uncontrollably when they are not depressed. Cross-sectionally, it may be difficult to distinguish pathological weeping from depression; however, serial evaluations usually clarify the diagnosis.

4. Adjustment Disorder with Depressed Mood

An adjustment disorder is by definition a stress-related phenomenon that occurs when a demonstrable psychosocial stressor precipitates the development of maladaptive psychiatric symptoms. The stress associated with medical illness has long been known to evoke adjustment disorders. The depressive symptoms of an adjustment disorder should theoretically exhibit clear descriptive validity with respect to MDD and grieving. An adjustment disorder is distinguished from MDD when in the face of a clear stressor, depressive symptoms are present and cause impairment but they do not meet diagnostic criteria for MDD. An adjustment disorder can be distinguished from grieving in that "the distress [of an adjustment disorder] is in excess of what would be expected" (16) whereas the distress of grieving is reasonable given the circumstances.

In practice, this theoretical descriptive validity has not always withstood scrutiny. For example, in a study of psychiatric consultation patients in an inpatient medical hospital, many patients initially diagnosed with MDD were rediagnosed with adjustment disorder at the time of discharge, and patients initially diagnosed with an adjustment disorder had no psychiatric diagnosis at the time of discharge (43).

5. Bipolar I/II Disorder, Most Recent Episode Depressed

The bipolar spectrum disorders can be readily distinguished from MDD even in the setting of a current depressive episode by the presence of a prior history of mania or hypomania. The bipolar disorders are mentioned here, however, because all too often in the case of a depressed medically ill patient the collection of the longitudinal and family psychiatric histories is neglected and misdiagnosis results. Because initiation of antidepressant pharmacotherapy can precipitate a manic episode in a bipolar patient, it is imperative that past history regarding mania and/or hypomania be collected.

In addition, some medical illnesses and treatments have been implicated in the precipitation of manic episodes. While beyond the scope of the present discussion, several helpful reviews of these so-called secondary manic syndromes are available (44–48).

6. Psychological Factors Affecting Medical Condition (PFAMC)

PFAMC is not a discrete diagnostic entity but instead gives a name to the long-recognized interactions of *soma* and *psyche* in the medically ill patient. This diagnosis is descriptively distinguished from MDD and adjustment disorders in that diagnostic criteria are not met for any Axis I psychiatric syndrome. Instead, the psychiatric symptoms experienced by the patient with PFAMC are contextually reasonable and expectable. Accordingly, PFAMC is not mutually exclusive with grief and may be a reasonable diagnosis in a medically ill patient who is experiencing a grief reaction.

Although the depressive symptoms are not themselves pathological, they may nonetheless impact the patient's medical illness either by directly exacerbating the medical disorder or by interfering with its treatment. As a result, psychiatric intervention may be warranted even in the absence of Axis I psychopathology. Conversely, it may be argued that the medical disorder and its treatment may cause or exacerbate the psychiatric syndrome. It is at this point that the causal relationship between the medical disorder and the psychiatric syndrome give rise to a differential diagnosis based upon etiology.

D. Etiological Differential

1. *Mood Disorder due to General Medical Condition (MDDGMC)*

In addition to distinguishing MDD from other diagnoses on a descriptive basis, MDD in the medically ill patient must be differentiated on etiological grounds as well. The depressive symptoms required to diagnose MDDGMC range from the single symptom of depressed mood or anhedonia to the full diagnostic criteria for a major depressive episode. On purely descriptive grounds, MDDGMC is often indistinguishable from MDD and differs only in that "the disturbance is the direct physiological consequence of a general medical condition" (16). Thus, the diagnostic issue is not face validity or descriptive validity because MDDGMC is not distinguished from MDD on the basis of an inventory of psychiatric symptoms. The emphasis is instead upon the construct validity of the two diagnoses; in other words, the contrast lies not in the clinically observed syndrome but in the etiology and underlying pathophysiology that is producing the syndrome.

A vast array of medical disorders may cause depression, including neurological disorders, metabolic and nutritional disturbances, endocrine disorders, autoimmune disorders, infectious diseases, and neoplastic diseases. In some cases, accurate diagnosis bears implications for predictive validity in that appropriate treatment is contingent upon accurate diagnosis. For example, when primary hypothyroidism is the medical illness causing the depression, appropriate management is not primarily antidepressant therapy but thyroxine replacement, though the former may be necessary as well. While the depression associated with many medical disorders seems to respond adequately to treatment with conventional antidepressants, further clarification of the underlying pathophysiology could lead to additional disease-specific therapies.

Although epidemiological studies may suggest that a particular medical disorder is associated with an increased prevalence rate of depression, this does not mean that the medical disorder directly causes the mood disturbance. Clarification of this causal relationship requires that the pathophysiology of the medical disorder and of depression be understood. Depression is a brain disease associated with aberrations in neurochemical, neuroendocrine, autonomic, and immunological function. Pathophysiological models portray a multifactorial disorder in which stressors actuate the neurobiological abnormalities and associated clinical symptoms of depression in vulnerable individuals. This vulnerability is defined by risk factors including a personal or family history of depression, female gender, history of suicide attempts, social isolation, substance abuse, socioeconomic pressure, an accommodating or pessimistic personality style, and concurrent medical illness (18,49–56).

Depression may be indirectly caused by a medical illness through the mediation of illness-associated psychosocial stressors such as chronic unremitting pain, loss of self-sufficiency, threatened loss of life, or declining physical status (56–59). In addition, surgical and radiological procedures that dramatically alter body image and body function, such as radical curative surgery for gastric carcinoma (60), colostomy (61), orchiectomy (62), and mastectomy (63–65), may induce stress leading to depression. Depression arising in this manner is not directly induced by the medical illness but occurs in reaction to illness-associated stressors. This type of depression is frequently termed a "reactive depression" in the medical and psychiatric literature and requires a diagnosis of MDD on etiological grounds.

Conversely, MDDGMC is the appropriate diagnosis when there is evidence that the depression has been caused by the medical disorder through direct biological means. A variety of medical disorders have been implicated in the production of MDDGMC (see Table 2). For some medical illnesses, such as hypothyroidism, there is incontrovertible evidence that the medical disorder causes

Table 2 Medical Disorders Associated with Depression

Endocrine disease	Infectious disease
Hyper-/hypothyroidism	HIV/AIDS
Hyper-/hypoparathyroidism	Hepatitis
Cushing's syndrome	Mononucleosis
Hyperprolactinemia	
Neurological disease	Neoplastic disease
Cerebrovascular disease	Pancreatic cancer
Dementia	Oropharyngeal cancer
Huntington's disease	Breast cancer
Multiple sclerosis	
Parkinson's disease	
Traumatic brain injury	
Metabolic/nutritional	Rheumatological disease
Vitamin B_{12} deficiency	Systemic lupus erythematosus
Uremia	Rheumatoid arthritis

the depression and that the depression resolves when the medical illness is treated. For other medical illnesses, there is considerable laboratory evidence to suggest this direct pathophysiological causation but no definitive proof. For example, direct causation of depression has been postulated in the case of pancreatic cancer, which has an extremely high association with depression and often presents with depressed mood. It has been suggested that pancreatic cancer may cause depression via tumor-secreted proteins that produce derangements in serotonergic neuronal activity by interacting with central nervous system (CNS) serotonin receptors (66–69) or via tumor-produced cytokines that produce hormonal derangements by potentiating release of corticotropin-releasing factor (CRF), which has long been postulated to be involved in the pathophysiology of depression (70). The former hypothesis is supported by the evidence that excretion of 5-hydroxyindoleacetic acid (5-HIAA) is increased in pancreatic cancer (71), though this may be peripheral in origin, and by a case report in which intractable depression in a pancreatic cancer patient resolved after partial pancreatectomy (72).

2. *Substance-Induced Mood Disorder*

Substance-induced mood disorder (SIMD) differs from MDD not on descriptive grounds but in that "medication use is etiologically related to the disturbance" (16). The notion that medications can induce mood disturbance is not new. In fact, it was the recognition that medications such as reserpine induced depression that served as one impetus for research leading to current neurochemical theories of depression (73).

Some researchers have attributed the association of medications with depression to the ineffectiveness of the medication in ameliorating the physical symptoms of the medical disorder (74) or to the production of treatment side effects that decrease the patient's sense of well-being (75). In such cases, the diagnosis of SIMD is probably unwarranted. However, more direct causation of depression has been postulated in the case of many medications and illicit substances (Table 3).

Intense clinical scrutiny is required to ascertain whether the medication caused the mood disturbance or whether a primary MDD coincidentally arose during the course of medical treatment. In the depressed medically ill patient, difficult clinical decisions arise when a medication is suspected of inducing depression. While the suspected medication may be necessary to achieve cure or palliate the symptoms of the medical disorder, the depression it may be inducing can counter these gains by increasing both suffering and mortality.

E. Depression Screening

Diagnostic screening for depression in the medically ill is often the purview of nonpsychiatric physicians who decide upon the need for psychiatric referral. A

Table 3 Medications Associated with Depression

Antineoplastic agents	Cardiovascular agents	Gastrointestinal agents
Cycloserine	α-Methyldopa	Cimetidine
Glucocorticoids	Reserpine	
Interferon-α	Propranolol	
L-Asparaginase		
Leuprolide		
Procarbazine		
Tamoxifen		
Vinblastine		
Vincristine		
Analgesics	Neurological agents	Antibiotics
Codeine	Levodopa	Amphotericin B
Indomethacin	Phenobarbital	
Oxycodone		

variety of screening instruments are available to physicians for the assessment of depression, which require varying amounts of time for completion and scoring. The ideal screening tool is reasonably sensitive and specific for the detection of depression, does not require an inordinate time investment by the physician or medical staff, and is minimally taxing to a medically ill patient.

Use of screening devices is not, however, without problems. First, the abbreviated questionnaires potentially most useful to nonpsychiatric physicians have not been validated in all comorbid medical disorders and therefore may not be reliable in these populations. Second, questions regarding somatic symptoms may skew the results of these devices in the medically ill population. For this reason, some researchers recommend screening tools that do not rely heavily upon assessment of somatic symptoms, such as the Montgomery-Asberg Depression Rating Scale (MADRS) (76). However, if an inclusive approach to diagnosing depression is adopted, then this argument may be less important. Finally, recent evidence suggests that the treatment decisions of primary-care physicians were only marginally influenced by depression-screening devices (77).

One recent study found that the single question "Are you depressed?" was both more sensitive and specific for detecting depression in a sample of terminally ill cancer patients than a screening questionnaire or visual analog scale (78). This reemphasizes the fact that although screening instruments may be useful adjuncts, the importance of perceptive physician/patient interaction is inestimable. Medically ill patients at increased risk for depression should be periodically asked, "Are you depressed?"

III. NEUROBIOLOGICAL ISSUES

A. Overview of Neurobiological Issues

The pathophysiology of depression has been extensively researched and debated with the bulk of the literature addressing the role of monoamines, including norepinephrine (NE), serotonin (5-HT), and to a lesser extent dopamine (DA). Accordingly, modulation of these neurotransmitters at the synaptic level has been the focus to date of pharmacotherapy for depression.

Recent attention has shifted to the burgeoning new fields of psychoneuroendocrinology and psychoneuroimmunology, which study the interaction of psychiatric syndromes with neurological, endocrine, and immune system function. The neuroendocrine and neuroimmunological "window strategy" is one impetus for these new lines of investigation. In this strategy it is believed that insight regarding CNS activity and dysfunction can be gleaned through study of the neuroendocrine axes and their interaction with the immune system in patients with psychiatric syndromes. Furthermore, in the context of the depressed, medically ill patient, additional insight can potentially be gained regarding disease causality, diagnostic assessment, and treatment.

B. Neurochemistry of Depression

It was long ago recognized that reserpine, a monoamine-depleting antihypertensive, caused depression in certain individuals. This was soon followed by the serendipitous discoveries that iproniazid, developed as an antitubercular agent, and imipramine, originally developed as an antipsychotic, were efficacious antidepressants and through different mechanisms increased the synaptic transmission of monoamine neurotransmitters. These insights led to early hypotheses that decreased noradrenergic and serotonergic neurotransmission play a primary role in the pathophysiology of depression (73,79–81).

However, synaptic depletion of monoamine neurotransmitters cannot alone explain the pathophysiology of depression or the mechanism of antidepressant response. First, most antidepressants rapidly increase synaptic levels of NE and/or 5-HT, but the therapeutic benefit of these agents comes only with continued administration over several weeks. Second, studies examining the clinical effect of NE- and 5-HT-depleting agents demonstrate that they were not associated with depression in normal individuals but that patients currently treated with 5-HT or NE reuptake inhibitors relapsed into depression after monoamine depletion (82–84).

Clearly, other biological factors play a role in the pathophysiology of depression. One hypothesis is that hypersensitivity of postsynaptic β-adrenergic and 5-HT_2 receptors may lead to depression (85,86). In support of this hypothesis is the recognition that many antidepressant treatments are associated with down-regulation of β-adrenergic and 5-HT_2 receptors (87–89). This hypothesis is also not entirely satisfying. First, the timing of receptor down-regulation precedes the onset of therapeutic benefit (90–92). Second, some efficacious antidepressants do not modulate receptor density or sensitivity (90). Third, electroconvulsive therapy (ECT) actually up-regulates 5-HT_2 receptor density (92).

Recent advances have enabled researchers to study the effect of stress and subsequent antidepressant administration upon intracellular second-messenger systems and target genes. These studies suggest that both stressful life experiences and antidepressant therapy impact the activity of the cAMP signal transduction pathway and the expression of neurotrophins (93). The significance of these new data is that depression and its treatment cannot be understood simply as a function of synaptic monoamine levels or monoamine receptor density. While these molecular studies open new horizons for study into the pathophysiology of depression, they continue to recognize the role of monoamine systems in the pathophysiology of mood disorders.

As it stands, the induction of aberrations in monoamine neurotransmission has been implicated as a vehicle for medical disorders and their treatments to induce depression. As previously mentioned, neoplasm-mediated derangements in serotonergic activity have been postulated to cause depression in patients with pancreatic cancer (66–69). Drug-induced mood disorders have also been attributed to derangements in monoamine neurotransmission iatrogenically induced by an ever-increasing number of pharmacological agents. Examples include the antineoplastic agents vincristine, vinblastine, and procarbazine. The vinca alkaloids inhibit dopamine β-hydroxylase, the neuronal enzyme responsible for converting dopamine to norepinephrine, and may therefore precipitate depression by decreasing norepinephrine stores available at the synapse (94–96). Procarbazine, typically characterized as a monoamine oxidase inhibitor, which should theoretically protect against depression, may instead potentiate the activity of monoamine oxidases through the activity of an active metabolite, monomethylhydrazine (97,98).

As understanding of the neurochemical basis for depression extends beyond the synapse to intraneuronal and molecular levels, this will hopefully lead to further evolution of the understanding of the etiological relationship between medical illness and depression.

C. Neuroendocrinology of Depression

Depression is also associated with certain well-documented aberrations in neuroendocrine function. Investigators have evaluated the function of most endocrine axes in depressed patients, with the hypothalamic-pituitary-adrenal (HPA) and the hypothalamic-pituitary-thyroid (HPT) axes being the most intensely scrutinized.

1. HPA Axis

Inquiry into the role of the HPA axis in depression began over 40 years ago when it was first reported that depressed patients have higher levels of adrenocortical hormones (99–101). Other early studies suggested that cortisol nonsuppression in the dexamethasone suppression test (DST), developed by Liddle as a diagnostic tool for the evaluation of Cushing's syndrome, was useful in the diagnostic assessment of depression as well (102).

Subsequently, hundreds of studies have confirmed these early reports of HPA axis hyperactivity in depressed patients. Included are anatomical studies demonstrating enlargement of the adrenal glands (103–107) and pituitary gland of depressed patients (108). The DST, initially envisioned as a breakthrough psychiatric diagnostic tool, would later become a point of controversy owing to its purported lack of specificity and sensitivity with respect to depression (109). While DST nonsuppression has admittedly not proven a definitive biological marker for depression, this misses the more important issue. The DST, like other functional HPA measures, reliably demonstrates an association between severity of depression and HPA axis hyperactivity (110–113).

While pituitary and adrenal hypertrophy may in part explain the adrenocortical hyperactivity associated with depression, recent evidence suggests that hypersecretion of corticotropin-releasing factor (CRF) may be the primary pathophysiological derangement of the HPA axis in depressed patients. The evidence for hypersecretion of CRF in these patients includes the elevation of CRF concentrations in cerebrospinal fluid (CSF) (114–118), blunting of the ACTH response after a standard CRF stimulation test (119–123), and increases in the number of CRF-staining cells and CRF mRNA expression in the hypothalamus (124). In addition, the elevation of CSF CRF levels (125–127) and the blunting of the ACTH response to exogenous CRF (119) are state-dependent variables that normalize when the depression resolves.

Perhaps more illuminating is the finding that CRF neurons are present not only in the hypothalamus but in extrahypothalamic regions of the CNS as well. Limbic projections of CRF neurons may mediate some of the neurovegetative symptoms of depression including decreased libido, insomnia, anorexia, and psychomotor retardation (128). Additionally, maternal deprivation studies using laboratory animals suggest that early untoward life experiences may produce a kindling-like phenomenon by sensitizing CRF neurons thereby leaving the individual susceptible to persistent derangements in CRF signaling and theoretically at increased risk for depression (128).

The HPA axis in general and CRF in particular clearly play a prominent role in the pathophysiology of depression; however, HPA axis activity has not been well characterized in depressed patients with comorbid medical illness or in nondepressed patients with nonendocrine medical illness. The DST has been utilized in three controlled studies of depressed patients with cancer confirming an association between depression and nonsuppression of cortisol in the DST. However, in these studies cortisol nonsuppression was also found in cancer patients who were not depressed (129–131). In another controlled study, nondepressed patients with metastatic breast cancer at various stages were given a "behavioral challenge" after which they exhibited higher cortisol levels and a blunted ACTH response to the challenge as compared with control subjects (132).

2. *HPT Axis*

Early evidence that thyroid disease is often associated with a host of neuropsychiatric symptoms coupled with the utility of triiodothyronine (T_3) as an antidepressant adjuvant (133–135) led to further scrutiny of the HPT axis in depressed patients.

Like CRF, TRH functions not only to release a pituitary hypophysiotropic hormone but also as a CNS neurotransmitter with extrahypothalamic projections (131). Two studies have demonstrated elevated CSF TRH concentrations (136,137), which is postulated to reflect central TRH hypersecretion (138). Additionally, several investigators have found that approximately 25% of euthyroid depressed patients exhibit a blunted TSH response after exogenous TRH administration (139–141). Chronic TRH hypersecretion resulting in down-regulation of pituitary TRH receptors could arguably explain this blunted response to TRH stimulation as well.

In some depressed patients, the TSH response to TRH stimulation is not blunted but exaggerated (142), often in association with the abnormal presence of antithyroglobulin antibodies or antimicrosomal antibodies (143). Additionally, these antibodies are sometimes detectable in patients with no measured abnormality of HPT axis function, a condition known as symptomless autoimmune thyroiditis (SAT) or grade IV hypothyroidism.

These insights, and others, have led to reexamination of the definition of hypothyroidism. Traditional definitions have been established by endocrinologists, who are most likely to recognize the degree of thyroid abnormality necessary to produce somatic symptoms. These definitions may not sufficiently detect lesser degrees of thyroid dysfunction that could contribute to the pathophysiology of depression. It is these less severe or higher grades of hypothyroidism that complicate study of the interrelationship of depression and thyroid disease. As seen in Table 4, three grades of hypothyroidism have long been recognized based upon laboratory measures of thyroid function with a fourth grade now recommended (144).

These "subclinical" measures of thyroid dysfunction in the depressed patient raise several questions. First, what is the etiological relationship of the interaction that has been reported between thyroid hormone and catecholamines (145)? Second, is thyroid hormone a necessary and/or sufficient treatment when depres-

Table 4 Grades of Hypothyroidism

Grade	TSH	T_3,T_4	TSH response[a]	Antibodies[b]
1	Increased	Decreased	Increased	Positive/negative
2	Increased	Normal	Increased	Positive/negative
3	Normal	Normal	Increased	Positive/negative
4	Normal	Normal	Normal	Positive

[a]TSH response in a standard TRH stimulation test.
[b]Presence of antithyroglobulin antibodies or antimicrosomal thyroid antibodies.

sion occurs in the context of these so-called subclinical abnormalities of thyroid function? Finally, when hormone supplementation is used as monotherapy or adjuvant therapy in these patients, should the hormone supplement be discontinued when the depression resolves? These questions should be considered in the context of the long-held clinical observations that antidepressants are not effective in hypothyroid patients, and moreover that T_3 supplementation is effective in converting antidepressant nonresponders to responders.

D. Neuroimmunology of Depression

The impact of depression and stress upon immune system function is also a focus of investigation. Animal studies have clearly demonstrated the prominent impact of stress on immune system physiology (146–148), but human studies have been less consistent. Investigations of the association between depression and immunological disturbance include cellular enumeration and immune function studies. The enumerative measures include total leukocyte, total neutrophil, total lymphocyte, and lymphocyte subset cell counts; the functional studies include natural killer cell activity (NKA) assays and mitogen assays, which measure the lymphocyte proliferative response to a variety of mitogens. Although a recent review of these data found evidence of an association between depression and changes in functional immune measures (149), an earlier review regarded these findings as inconclusive and argued that confounding methodological variables such as assay technique, diagnostic heterogeneity, and limited sample sizes complicated any attempt at meta-analysis (150).

A decrease in NKA, however, has been one largely consistent finding from these human studies. Two breast cancer studies found that those patients with symptoms of depression, fatigue, and poor social support exhibited a 30% decrease in NKA and had more metastatic nodes on follow-up (151), while patients who received high-quality emotional support had higher measures of NKA (152).

New evidence suggests that attempts to demonstrate immunosuppression in depressed patients may oversimplify the underlying pathophysiology. On the contrary, increasing evidence shows that the immune system may in fact be activated in an acute-phase response during depression. These studies reveal increases in concentrations of a variety of acute-phase proteins and in cytokine production (153–157). How can results such as decreased NKA which suggest immunosuppression in depressed patients be reconciled with this apparently contradictory evidence of immunoactivation? One hypothesis is that bidirectional, homeostatic interactions between the neuroendocrine and neuroimmunological systems may explain this seeming discrepancy (158–164).

HPA axis activation and increased CRF secretion have been associated with measures of immunoactivation including increased IL-1 (165–166), IL-2 (154, 167), and IL-6 (154). Conversely, HPA hyperactivity may also elicit immunosuppressive changes as evidenced by animal studies in which intracerbroventricular administration of CRF produces decreased NKA and a reduced response to mitogen exposure (168–169).

In summary, depressed patients demonstrate evidence of immunological activation, immunological suppression, and HPA axis hyperactivity. The measures suggestive of immunoactivation may represent an acute-phase response to depression initiating cytokine release, which in turn stimulates CRF secretion and thereby activates the HPA axis. Furthermore, CRF hypersecretion may produce immunosuppressive changes such as decreased NKA. But even this explanation, though plausible, is likely an oversimplification in that it does not account for noradrenergic modulation (170) or circadian and ultradian rhythms (171) of the neuroendocrine and neuroimmunological systems.

Nonetheless, the immunosuppression associated with depression can have untoward consequences for the medically ill patient. Both human and animal studies reveal an association between stress, decreased NKA, and increases in tumor metastasis (152,172–174). Perhaps equally important for patient outcome is the observation that NKA responds to psychosocial support (175).

E. Summary of Neurobiological Issues

The neurobiological changes associated with depression are indeed interdependent and complex. It remains unclear which is the primary abnormality, the neurochemical disturbance, the neuroendocrine disturbance, or the neuroimmunological disturbance. Some researchers contend that a neuroendocrine abnormality, such as CRF hypersecretion, may be the prime pathogenetic event leading to major depression. Others argue that the neurochemical changes accompanying the mood disturbance in some way induce the associated neuroendocrine and neuroimmunological changes. Clearly, depression is associated with aberrations in each of these functional systems; however, the causal relationships have not yet been well defined.

When consideration of the impact of a comorbid medical illness is added, these interactions become even more complex. Many medical illnesses frequently associated with depression, such as AIDS, cancer, systemic lupus erythematosus (SLE), and MS, are associated with abnormalities in immune system function. Conversely, some of the therapies for these disorders can lead to both immunological compromise and iatrogenic depression. As a result, investigating the pathophysiology underlying the relationship of medical illnesses and their treatments with depression, and the accompanying neurobiological changes, can be a daunting task. As previously noted, it can be difficult to reach a definitive diagnosis of depression in a medically ill patient on both descriptive and etiological grounds. However, the causal uncertainty between depression and medical illness extends even further. While medical disorders can elicit depression through mediation of both direct pathophysiological means and illness-associated psychosocial stressors, depression can increase the risk for developing medical illness or can exacerbate preexisting medical illness via induction of neuroendocrine and neuroimmunological dysfunction (176).

The clinical significance of the neurobiology of depression in the context of comorbid medical disease is twofold. First, these studies may ultimately produce more sensitive and specific biological markers for depression, which will be of value when diagnosis on descriptive grounds is problematic. Second, further elucidation of the underlying pathophysiology may lead to more disease-specific treatment modalities both to increase efficacy and to minimize medical complications of antidepressant pharmacotherapy.

IV. TREATMENT ISSUES

A. Somatic Therapies

1. Antidepressant Selection

Antidepressant pharmacotherapy among medically ill patients is both widespread (177) and effective (178). Psychiatric consensus holds that all antidepressants are equally efficacious in the treatment of depression. However, this should not be understood to imply that an antidepressant can be chosen haphazardly. There are, in fact, numerous factors that should guide antidepressant selection:

1. An agent that has previously been efficacious in the patient or a family member has an increased likelihood of being efficacious in a repeat trial and is thus preferred.
2. An antidepressant that has in the past produced intolerable side effects will likely do so again and therefore should be avoided.
3. An antidepressant with a known mechanism of action or side effect that

could theoretically exacerbate the comorbid medical illness should be avoided. Examples include tricyclic antidepressants (TCAs), which should not be used in post–myocardial infarction (MI) depressed patients because their quinidine-like properties can potentiate cardiac arrhythmias, and bupropion, which should not be used in patients with structural brain lesions or recent strokes because it may further increase the risk of seizure.

4. An agent that could theoretically both treat the depression and alleviate symptoms of the comorbid medical disorder is preferred. For example, the dopaminergic properties of bupropion theoretically make it an excellent antidepressant for the depressed patient with Parkinson's disease (PD).
5. An antidepressant with a pharmacokinetic profile that could theoretically interact adversely with a medication needed to treat the medical condition should be avoided.

Selection of an antidepressant should be guided by an effort to maximize efficacy and minimize the potential for adverse effects. The axiom "start low and go slow" is the appropriate strategy for dose titration in medically ill patients. This is because these patients are at increased risk for developing adverse side effects from medications, are at increased risk for untoward medication interactions due to polypharmacy, and often respond to lower doses because they may not clear the medications as well as otherwise healthy patients.

Antidepressant medications are grouped into four classifications based upon proposed mechanism of action. These include the older tricyclic (TCA) and related tetracyclic antidepressants and monoamine oxidase inhibitors (MAOIs) in addition to the recently developed selective serotonin reuptake inhibitors (SSRIs) and a heterogeneous group of atypical antidepressants.

2. Heterocyclic Antidepressants

The first TCA, imipramine, was originally developed for use as an antipsychotic medication. Although ineffective as an antipsychotic, imipramine was soon discovered to have antidepressant properties leading to the development of a host of other structurally similar compounds such as nortriptyline and clomipramine. Imipramine and the other TCAs soon became first-line antidepressant agents and even today remain the gold standard of efficacy for comparative clinical research purposes.

Today, the utility of TCAs is limited by their lethality in overdose and their prominent side effect profile. Side effects of TCAs include sedation, orthostatic hypotension, potentiation of cardiac arrhythmias, lowering of the seizure threshold, and potent anticholinergic properties. For these reasons, TCAs should in particular be avoided in patients with known coronary artery disease (CAD), cardiac conduction defects, or a history of arrhythmias, in patients with a history of seizures, cerebrovascular accident (CVA), or intracranial lesion, which increase the risk of seizure, or in patients with conditions such as narrow-angle glaucoma and benign prostatic hypertrophy (BPH), which are exacerbated by anticholinergic medications. In addition, the antihistaminic and anticholinergic properties of these medications can precipitate delirium in medically ill individuals. For these reasons, TCAs are no longer considered first-line agents in depressed patients with comorbid medical disorders.

3. Monoamine Oxidase Inhibitors

The first antidepressant, iproniazid, was developed as an antitubercular agent but was also found to be an efficacious antidepressant. Its mechanism of action was nonselective, irreversible inhibition of the monoamine oxidase enzymes. Unfortunately, iproniazid was associated with development of hepatic necrosis and was removed from the market.

Other MAOIs have since been developed and remain useful agents. Currently MAOIs approved in the United States are nonselective and nonreversible inhibitors of the MAO-A and MAO-B isoenzymes. Although these agents are effective antidepressants, their utility in medically ill patients is limited owing to their prominent side effects, dietary restrictions, and potentially dangerous interactions with a variety of commonly used medications including meperidine and indirectly acting sympathomimetics such as pseudoephedrine. In addition, these agents may directly exacerbate some medical illnesses. For example, MAOIs can produce episodes of profound hypoglycemia in diabetic patients and lower seizure threshold in epilepsy patients. MAOIs, like TCAs, are not considered first-line agents in depressed patients with comorbid medical illness.

Moclobemide, a reversible inhibitor of the MAO-A isoenzyme available in Europe and Canada, may prove to be more useful in medically ill patients than its counterparts. The only prominent side effect with this agent is nausea. In addition, dietary restrictions may not apply and drug interactions are not as problematic as with other MAOIs.

4. Selective Serotonin Reuptake Inhibitors and Atypical Antidepressants

Research efforts to design effective antidepressants with side effect and toxicity profiles more favorable than those of the TCAs and MAOIs have resulted in development of the SSRIs (fluoxetine, fluvoxamine, paroxetine, sertraline, citalopram) and atypical antidepressants (bupropion, mirtazapine, nefazodone, trazodone, venlafaxine, mianserin). The side effects associated with these medications with a few exceptions should seldom exacerbate comorbid medical illness. Two noteworthy exceptions are bupropion, which may induce seizures in vulnerable patients, and mirtazapine, which in premarketing trials induced agranulocytosis, albeit rarely, and should thus be avoided in patients with immunodeficiency syndromes or hematological malignancies.

Potential drug interactions may be more problematic for medical patients taking the newer antidepressants (179,180). This is particularly true if the antidepressants interact with medications having low therapeutic indices thereby risking dangerous toxicities from unanticipated drug interactions.

Drug interaction may occur via competition for plasma protein–binding sites. With the exception of venlafaxine, antidepressants are all relatively highly protein bound and may displace other medications from their protein-binding sites thereby increasing the free and active concentration of the compound and risking toxicity. Another potential route for drug interaction is through inhibition of hepatic metabolism via the cytochrome P450 system. As shown in Table 5, many of these new antidepressants inhibit various P450 isoenzymes, and the list of medications known to be metabolized by these enzymes is ever growing.

5. *Psychostimulants*

Psychostimulants provide a reasonable alternative in medically compromised patients who require a brisk clinical response. These agents, including methylphenidate, dextroamphetamine, and pemoline, can be used as monotherapy or as adjuvants to conventional antidepressants. Response rates in noncontrolled studies of medically ill patients have rivaled that of TCAs (181–186). In addition, rapid clinical response within 1 or 2 days has been reported (185). While anorexia is a commonly reported side effect of stimulants, studies of these medications in medically ill patients have paradoxically found increases in appetite.

Table 5 Pharmacokinetics of Newer Antidepressants Available in the United States

Generic name	Trade name	Protein binding	1A2 inhibition	2C9[a] inhibition	2D6 inhibition	3A4 inhibition
Bupropion	Wellbutrin	80%				
Fluoxetine	Prozac	94%		I	I	
Fluvoxamine	Luvox	80%	I	I		I
Mirtazapine	Remeron	85%				
Nefazodone	Serzone	99%				I
Paroxetine	Paxil	95%			I	
Sertraline	Zoloft	98%		i	I	
Venlafaxine	Effexor	27%				

[a]The 2C9 isoenzyme is the least studied of the P450 isoenzymes listed above. Although preliminary evidence suggests that fluoxetine, fluvoxamine, and sertraline may inhibit this isoenzyme, more definitive studies remain to be completed.

I = potent inhibition; i = low to moderate inhibition.

6. *Electroconvulsive Therapy (ECT)*

ECT was introduced by Meduna in 1934 to treat schizophrenia with the mistaken notion that schizophrenia and epilepsy were mutually exclusive disorders (187). Despite this faulty rationale, ECT was soon discovered to be a highly efficacious treatment for a variety of psychiatric syndromes including depression (188) and became a mainstay of psychiatric treatment until the proliferation of psychopharmacological therapies in the 1950s.

Thereafter, ECT utilization subsided until interest resurfaced in the early 1980s with the growing recognition of the limitations of pharmacological treatments. In recent years, approximately 80% of patients receiving ECT suffer from MDD (189) and response rates to ECT exceed those to antidepressant medications (190–192).

In addition to being an effective treatment for depression and other psychiatric syndromes, ECT can also provide symptomatic improvement for certain medical disorders. In particular, ECT has proven beneficial in the treatment of neuroleptic malignant syndrome (193–196), PD (197), and possibly medication-resistant epilepsy (198–199).

While there are no absolute contraindications to ECT, there are clinical situations where increased risk of complications warrants careful justification of the use of ECT. Relative contraindications to ECT include recent MI, intracranial space-occupying lesions, recent intracerebral hemorrhage, retinal detachment, pheochromocytoma, and unstable vascular aneurysm (200).

ECT treatment produces transient but marked hemodynamic changes that can be problematic for patients with cardiovascular or cerebrovascular disease. The electrical stimulus triggers an increase in parasympathetic tone with resultant bradycardia. Conversely, the subsequent seizure induces an increase in sympathetic output resulting in tachycardia and hypertension (201). Prophylactic utilization of β-blockers such as labetolol or esmolol is now routine to moderate the cardiovascular effects of seizure induction (202), but the clinical utility in reducing morbidity has not been documented.

B. Psychosocial Therapies

A variety of psychosocial interventions have proven effective in alleviating the symptoms of depression in medically ill patients. The diverse psychosocial treatment offerings studied in medically ill patients include group psychotherapy, several modalities of individual psychotherapy, hypnotherapy, multimedia psychoeducation, biofeedback, and relaxation training (203–213).

The impact of psychosocial interventions extends beyond relief of the depression. Psychosocial therapies for depressed medical patients lengthen survival time (214–217), improve compliance with medical care (216), enhance subjective measures of quality of life (218), and even produce improvement in measures of immune function (23,219).

V. DEPRESSION IN SELECTED MEDICAL DISORDERS

A. Neurological Disorders

1. Cerebrovascular Disease

Depression frequently complicates poststroke recovery. The clinical presentation of depression in the aftermath of a cerebrovascular accident (CVA) has generally been found to be indistinguishable from depression in other patients except that psychomotor retardation is more common while anhedonia and poor concentration are less common in poststroke depression (220).

Depression occurring in the immediate poststroke period is most frequently associated with lesions located in the left anterior cortex and left basal ganglia (221–223). Depression remains a significant problem up to at least 2 years after a stroke (223–226). These delayed depressions do not demonstrate an association with lesion location (224,226) but are associated with a poor social support network (227,228).

A wide variety of antidepressant agents have been used in poststroke depression including TCAs, SSRIs, and atypical antidepressants. Psychostimulants have also been used with promising results. A retrospective study of methylphenidate in poststroke depression suggested a brisk clinical response (229), and a controlled study of dextroamphetamine demonstrated improvement in both mood and motor function in stroke patients (230). Finally, ECT is a safe and efficacious treatment for depressed stroke patients, though it is preferable to wait for the resolution of cerebral edema before initiating a course of treatment.

2. Epilepsy

While depression has been reported in association with many variants of status epilepticus (231), depression is typically not a peri-ictal but an interictal phenomenon. Risk factors for depression in seizure patients include a complex partial seizure disorder and a left-sided seizure focus (232–235). Conflicting results have been found in studies of other risk factors such as gender (233,235,236) and seizure frequency (232,233,237,238).

Antidepressant selection is particularly important in epilepsy patients. Bupropion, MAOIs, and most of the TCAs, in particular amitriptyline, imipramine, clomipramine, maprotiline, and amoxapine, lower the seizure threshold and should be avoided in seizure patients. Of the TCAs, doxepin may be the least likely to increase seizure frequency (239).

Drug interactions, through both competitive protein binding and inhibition of particular cytochrome P450 isoenzymes, are another significant concern in depressed seizure patients. Of the anticonvulsants, phenytoin is known to be a substrate of the P450 2C9 isoenzyme while carbamazepine is a 3A4 substrate. Preliminary studies suggest that fluoxetine, fluvoxamine, and sertraline may inhibit the 2C9 isoenzyme and could theoretically elevate phenytoin levels, though alternate metabolic pathways for phenytoin exist. Carbamazepine levels may be elevated by 3A4 inhibitors such as nefazodone and fluvoxamine.

Finally, ECT is a safe treatment for epilepsy patients and may help to reduce seizure frequency by raising the seizure threshold temporarily (198,199). It is generally recommended that anticonvulsants be continued during a course of ECT in an epileptic patient.

3. *Multiple Sclerosis*

MS, the most common of the demyelinating disorders, is associated with a high rate of depression. As previously noted, depression in MS patients must be carefully distinguished from pseudobulbar phenomena such as pathological crying. Growing evidence suggests that depression in MS patients is not always "reactive" but may be a direct pathophysiological result of demyelination. This evidence includes the fact that the onset of depression in MS patients sometimes antedates the onset of neurological impairment (240–243), is often coincidental with disease exacerbation (244,245), and occurs at a higher rate with involvement of the temporal lobe or anterior white matter (246,247). No antidepressants are specifically contraindicated in MS patients, but the side effects of TCAs and MAOIs may render them poorly tolerated.

4. *Dementia*

Patients commonly present with cognitive impairment coincidental with depressive symptoms. Differentiating a depression with pseudodementia from an apathetic dementia can be a difficult task. Moreover, dementia can produce pseudobulbar symptoms such as pathological crying in the same manner as MS (248), or a genuine depression can be comorbid with dementia. Depression has in fact been reported in patients with a variety of dementing illnesses including Alzheimer's dementia (AD), multi-infarct dementia (MID), dementia associated with PD, and HIV-related dementia. While there is no definitive diagnostic test to discriminate dementia from depression, the DST may be a helpful diagnostic aid in that a depressed patient would be more likely to exhibit cortisol nonsuppression than a demented patient without depression. However, later in the course of AD, probably secondary to the loss of glucocorticoid feedback sites in the hippocampus, hypercortisolemia and DST nonsuppression are common even in the absence of depression.

In patients presenting with this clinical picture, a trial of antidepressant therapy is warranted. Medications with anticholinergic properties such as the TCAs and perhaps paroxetine may worsen cognition or precipitate delirium in demented patients. This is particularly true in patients with dementia of the Alzheimer's type in which diminution of acetylcholine neurotransmission is a key to the underlying pathophysiology. ECT is another therapeutic alternative in these patients with the caveat that posttreatment confusion can be more severe and prolonged in demented patients.

5. *Parkinson's Disease*

Depression is the most common psychiatric disturbance associated with PD and was first noted by Parkinson himself (249). Depressed PD patients are reported to have prominent symptoms of hopelessness, sadness, and suicidal ideation, but less frequently exhibit guilt or self-reproach (250–252).

The etiology of depression is unclear but may directly result from depletion of central monoamines, especially DA and 5-HT, or be indirectly attributable to stress arising from the physical impairment of PD (249). In addition, several antiparkinsonian medications, notably amantidine, bromocriptine, carbidopa, and levodopa, have been implicated in the development of depression (253).

The diagnosis and monitoring of depression in the patient with PD can be aided by the Beck Depression Inventory (BDI), which has been found not to be unduly influenced by any crossover somatic symptoms of PD (251,254). Unfortunately, studies of biological markers, including the DST, TRH stimulation test, and CSF 5-HIAA, have been inconclusive (255).

Careful antidepressant selection is of paramount importance in the patient with PD. The dopaminergic properties of bupropion and sertraline and the anticholinergic properties of the TCAs and to a lesser extent paroxetine may improve the motor symptoms of PD in addition to treating the depression. ECT has also been shown to improve both the depression associated with PD and its motor symptoms (256). Conversely, serotonergic antidepressants, including clomipramine, the SSRIs, nefazodone, and trazodone, may theoretically worsen symptoms of PD through serotonin-mediated inhibition of dopamine neurotransmission, though there is little clinical evidence for this.

The potential for adverse drug-drug interactions should also guide antidepressant selection in PD patients. MAOIs should be avoided in patients taking levodopa or other dopaminergic medications owing to the risk of hypertensive crisis. Coadministration of selegiline, a selective MAO-B inhibitor used to treat PD, with serotonergic antidepressants should theoretically be avoided owing to the risk of precipitating serotonin syndrome. In practice, however, this combination is apparently frequently used with few untoward effects noted.

B. Endocrine Disorders

1. *Diabetes Mellitus (DM)*

The prevalence of depression in diabetic patients may not be significantly higher than that of the general population (257–259), but when present, depression can have a profound impact on the course of DM with impairment of glycemic control (260,261) and noncompliance with diet and medication (262).

Depression can present diagnostic difficulties in diabetic patients as in patients with other medical disorders owing to the presence of neurovegetative symptoms such as fatigue and lethargy commonly associated with DM. However, the BDI has been posited as a reliable diagnostic instrument in DM patients (263).

Antidepressant selection is of key importance in DM patients. Noradrenergic medications such as the TCAs tend to elevate serum glucose levels by inducing carbohydrate craving and by inhibiting glucose-mediated insulin release (264–268); they should therefore be eschewed in DM patients. MAOIs should also be avoided in these patients because they can produce episodes of profound hypoglycemia by inhibiting the gluconeogenesis enzyme carnitine acetyltransferase (269,270).

Serotonergic medications including reuptake inhibitors, 5-HT precursors, and 5-HT-releasing agents have all demonstrated moderate and sustained reductions in plasma glucose levels (271–276). As a result, serotonergic medications, of which fluoxetine is the best studied, are recommended first-line agents in DM patients. In addition, a recent open study suggests that paroxetine provides the same analgesic benefits of TCAs for patients with painful diabetic neuropathy (277).

2. *Thyroid Disorders*

Depression frequently complicates the clinical course of both hypothyroidism and hyperthyroidism. As previously discussed, the HPT axis has been extensively investigated in depressed patients and may play a key role in the pathophysiology of depression even in the absence of overt thyroid dysfunction.

First-line treatment for depression in hypothyroid patients is thyroxine supplementation. Typically, when euthyroidism is achieved, psychiatric symptoms such as depression also resolve. Unclear, however, is the role of thyroid hormone supplementation in the treatment of depression in patients with "subclinical" measures of hypothyroidism.

If depression does not resolve with the attainment of euthyroid measures, then conventional antidepressants should be considered. Because hypothyroid patients are particularly sensitive to sedating and anticholinergic effects of medication, newer agents with less prominent side effects are recommended. In addition, reports that TCAs induce rapid cycling in hypothyroid patients (278) further preclude their usage.

In hyperthyroid patients, conventional antidepressants may be used to treat depression while thyroid-suppressing therapy is initiated. TCAs should be avoided in these patients, however, as they may induce tachyarrhythmias (279).

3. *Cushing's Syndrome*

Depressive disorders are common in cushingoid states with the most frequent presentation being a mixed depression/anxiety syndrome (280,281). The mood disturbance may occur early in the course of Cushing's syndrome and may even be the presenting symptom (282). Treatment of the underlying medical condition tends to resolve the depression as cortisol levels normalize.

Depression is also associated with iatrogenic Cushing's syndrome induced by exogenous administration of corticosteroids. In such cases, reduction of the corticosteroid dose, if possible, may reduce the depressive symptoms (283). Treatment with lithium or valproic acid has been reported to be helpful in treating steroid-induced mood disorders (284,285). Conversely, TCAs are reported to have worsened the clinical course of patients taking exogenous corticosteroids (286).

4. *Hyperprolactinemia*

The most common cause of elevated prolactin is a pituitary adenoma. Other causes include medication-induced hyperprolactinemia and secretion of prolactin in association with other endocrinopathies. The predominant clinical feature of prolonged elevation of prolactin is gonadal dysfunction. Depression is not an uncommon complication of hyperprolactin states (287) and presents as an irritable, hostile and at times agitated depression.

Bromocriptine, a dopamine agonist used to treat both hyperprolactinemia and PD, has been reported to improve both the physical and psychiatric symptoms associated with the disorder (288,289). While no studies have evaluated the use of bupropion or sertraline in this setting, their dopaminergic activity theoretically makes either a wise choice.

C. Cardiovascular Disease

Depression occurs frequently in patients with coronary artery disease (CAD) and can seriously complicate the clinical course after MI by delaying physical and functional recovery, and increasing the risk of subsequent mortality (290–292). While the high frequency of smoking among depressed patients may in part explain this association, a large prospective study demonstrated increased rates of fatality in both depressed smokers and depressed nonsmokers (293). In the largest study of post-MI patients with depression, the combination of elevated BDI score and frequent premature ventricular contractions (PVCs) was most predictive of mortality within the 18-month period following the index MI (294). While the adverse impact of depression upon medical compliance may contribute to this outcome, new evidence suggests that depression may increase the risk for mortality after MI more directly. Studies suggest that depression impairs parasympathetic modulation of heart rate and contractility (290,295,296) and increases the likelihood of thrombus formation (297,298).

Treatment of post-MI depression is essential to appropriate management. TCAs have been extensively studied in this population and are efficacious for treatment of depression after MI. However, they should be avoided post-MI because medications with quinidine-like type IA antiarrhythmic effects have been shown to increase mortality after MI by sudden cardiac death (299). MAOIs should also be eschewed in these patients because their potential for hypertensive crises renders their use ill advised in patients with CAD.

The cardiovascular side effects of the newer agents are generally negligible and make them preferable for use post-MI. An exception is trazodone, which often produces significant orthostasis and exacerbates preexisting PVCs (300). Unfortunately, the newer agents have not been well studied in depressed post-MI patients to date.

Potential drug interactions are an important factor in antidepressant selection for patients with cardiovascular disease. Digoxin and warfarin, commonly used in patients with certain cardiac arrhythmias or cardiomyopathy, are highly protein-bound compounds that can theoretically be displaced from serum-binding proteins by antidepressants. Venlafaxine is unique among the antidepressants for its low binding affinity for plasma proteins (27%) and thus may be less likely to produce an adverse event via this mechanism.

Furthermore, many cardiovascular medications are metabolized by hepatic cytochrome P450 isoenzymes, which are inhibited by a variety of antidepressants. Warfarin is metabolized by isoenzyme 2C9, which may be inhibited by fluoxetine, fluvoxamine, and sertraline. The 2D6 isoenzyme is inhibited by fluoxetine, paroxetine, and sertraline and is responsible for the metabolism of various β-blockers and the antiarrhythmics encainide, flecainide, and mexilitine. Finally, the 3A4 isoenzyme, which metabolizes lidocaine, quinidine, and numerous calcium channel antagonists, is inhibited by fluvoxamine and nefazodone.

D. HIV

Mood disturbance commonly affects seropositive HIV patients. The etiology for HIV-associated depression can be attributable to psychological stressors such as receiving the initial report of seropositivity, recognizing the first somatic symptoms of AIDS (301), or enduring the societal and familial rejection that often accompanies the diagnosis (302). It is perhaps equally important that the groups at greatest risk for contracting HIV infection in the United States, homosexual men and IV drug users, are at high risk for depression even in the absence of HIV infection (303). In fact, one recent study found the rate of depression in the asymptomatic stage of HIV infection to be no higher than the rate of depression in noninfected homosexual men (304). Evidence suggests that depression may also be the direct result of virus-induced neuropathological changes in the CNS (304).

Controlled studies have repeatedly demonstrated the efficacy of TCAs in treating depressed HIV patients (305–306). Open trials of fluoxetine and sertraline have also produced promising results (307–308). Psychostimulants have also been suggested as efficacious agents in numerous case studies and one blind trial comparing methylphenidate with desipramine (309).

Antidepressant side effects can be particularly problematic for the depressed HIV patient. The anticholinergic properties of TCAs may worsen cognition and dry mucous membranes predisposing the patient to development of oral candidiasis. Due to nutritional restrictions and potential adverse interactions with zidovudine, MAOIs should not be used in depressed HIV patients (310). SSRIs are generally well tolerated by AIDS patients except those with chronic diarrhea.

Potential drug interactions are a concern for the depressed HIV patient taking protease inhibitors such as ritonavir, saquinavir, delavirdine, and indinavir. These protease inhibitors are all substrates of the cytochrome P450 3A4 isoenzyme and to varying degrees all inhibit the 3A4 isoenzyme (311–315) making them susceptible to adverse interactions with nefazodone and fluvoxamine, which also inhibit the 3A4 isoenzyme. In addition, the antitubercular agents rifampicin and rifabutin, which are frequently used in the HIV patient population, are also substrates of the 3A4 isoenzyme (316–317) and therefore may interact adversely with fluvoxamine and nefazodone.

E. Cancer

Rates of depression in cancer are highly variable. Some cancers have rates of depression only slightly higher than that of the general population, whereas other cancers have extremely high rates of comorbid depression. In particular, cancer of the pancreas, oropharynx, and breast have remarkably high rates of depression. In addition to these primary tumor sites, other risk factors for the development of depression in cancer patients include an advanced disease state with declining physical status (17,18,50,52,59), certain chemotherapeutic regimens (318–319), surgical procedures, and radiotherapy.

Depression in cancer may be precipitated by cancer-associated psychosocial stressors such as unremitting pain, loss of autonomy, or threatened loss of life. Additionally, depression may be a direct pathophysiological consequence of the cancer representing a paraneoplastic syndrome. In fact, the high rate of depression in certain cancers may be a consequence of previously unrecognized paraneoplastic syndromes.

The two major controlled studies evaluating the use of antidepressants in cancer have studied TCAs. These two studies found the TCAs efficacious in alleviating depression and improving quality of life (24,320). Unfortunately,

TCAs are often not well tolerated in cancer patients owing to their prominent side effect profiles. Likewise, MAOIs are of limited usefulness in cancer patients because of their side effects and dietary restrictions. The only non-TCA-controlled study in depressed cancer patients found mianserin, a structural analog to mirtazapine, to be more efficacious than and as safe as placebo (321).

SSRIs and atypical antidepressants have become first-line agents in treating depressed cancer patients despite a lack of controlled studies to confirm their efficacy. At present, a multicenter, double-blind, placebo-controlled trial evaluating the efficacy of paroxetine in comparison with desipramine is underway. While there are no specific contraindications to using any of the newer antidepressants in cancer patients, mirtazapine, which was associated with the rare development of agranulocytosis in premarketing trials, should probably be avoided in patients with hematological malignancies or patients taking marrow-suppressing chemotherapy. Psychostimulants such as methylphenidate, dextroamphetamine, and pemoline are also useful in depressed cancer patients. Non-controlled studies of these medications in cancer suggest that they are not only effective but may provide a brisker clinical response than conventional antidepressants. In general, the newer antidepressants should now be considered first-line treatment for depressed cancer patients because of their favorable side effect and toxicity profiles. Stimulants are useful for adjuvant therapy or as first-line agents in medically compromised patients who require a fast clinical response.

While the relatively benign side effect profiles of these newer agents have expanded the treatment options for depressed cancer patients, the risk of significant drug interactions remains a cause for concern (322,323). Cytotoxic antineoplastic agents have low therapeutic indices and serious toxicities can occur from unanticipated drug interactions.

One potential mechanism for drug interaction lies in competition for protein-binding sites (324). Many chemotherapeutic medications are highly protein bound, and the addition of other highly bound medications, such as antidepressants, can lead to higher free concentrations of the cytotoxic medications thereby risking unanticipated toxicity.

Drug interaction with chemotherapeutic agents may also be mediated by the hepatic cytochrome P450 system (325). The 3A4 isoenzyme appears to be most involved in metabolism of chemotherapeutic agents including doxorubicin, cyclophosphamide, ifosfamide, etoposide, teniposide, tamoxifen, taxol, and the vinca alkaloids. Antidepressants that inhibit the 3A4 isoenzyme include fluvoxamine and nefazodone (322,323). In addition, some cytochrome P450 3A4 substrates have been implicated as inhibitors of P-glycoprotein, which normally serves to mediate drug elimination from the cell (325). If antidepressants that are metabolized by the 3A4 isoenzyme also prove to act as P-glycoprotein inhibitors, this may further increase the risk of unexpected drug toxicity by impeding antineoplastic drug elimination.

VI. CONCLUSION

The comorbidity of medical illness with depression has far-reaching implications. It raises challenges for the psychiatric diagnostician faced with symptoms of uncertain genesis, for the treating physician faced with myriad therapeutic options, and for the scientist striving to understand the neurobiology of depression in the context of dynamically changing organ systems.

While there remain difficulties in achieving accurate diagnoses in medically ill patients who appear to be depressed, the importance of appropriate diagnosis and treatment of these patients cannot be overestimated. Treatment of depression in the medically ill patient not only alleviates emotional suffering; it can help relieve physical pain, improve compliance with medical care, and extend life.

Treatment options include both psychosocial and pharmacological modalities, which should not be chosen capriciously but should be selected with a view to maximizing treatment efficacy and minimizing adverse interactions with the medical illness or its treatment.

REFERENCES

1. Feinstein AR. The pre-therapeutic classification of comorbidity and chronic disease. J Chronic Dis 1970; 23:455–468.
2. Cavanaugh S. Depression in the medically ill: critical issues in diagnostic assessment. Psychosomatics 1995; 36:48–59.
3. Cassem EH. Depressive disorders in the medically ill: an overview. Psychosomatics 1995; 36(Suppl):2–10.
4. Cohen-Cole SA, Brown FW, McDaniel S. Diagnostic assessment of depression in the medically ill. In: Stoudemire A, Fogel B, eds. Principles of Medical Psychiatry. New York: Oxford University Press, 1993:53–68.
5. Federoff JP, Starkstein SE, Parikh RM, et al. Are depressive symptoms nonspecific in patients with acute stroke? Am J Psychiatry 1991; 148:1172–1176.
6. Kathol RG, Mutgi A, Williams J, Clamon G, Noyes R. Diagnosis of major depression in cancer patients according to four sets of criteria. Am J Psychiatry 1990; 147:1021–1024.
7. Kathol RG, Noyes R, Williams J, Mutgi A, Carroll B, Perry A. Diagnosing depression in patients with medical illness. Psychosomatics 1990; 31:434–440.
8. Brown JT, Stoudemire GA. Normal and pathological grief. JAMA 1983; 250: 378–382.
9. Clayton PJ. Course of depressive symptoms following the course of bereavement. J Clin Psychiatry 1990; 51(Suppl):34–40.
10. Clayton PJ, Desmaris L, Winokur G. A study of normal bereavement. Am J Psychiatry 1968; 125:168–178.
11. Dworetzky JP. Human Development. St Paul, MN: West Publishing, 1995.
12. Kubler-Ross E. On Death and Dying. New York: Macmillan, 1969.

13. National Institute of Mental Health: Health Professionals and the Bereaved. Washington, DC: National Academy Press, 1988.
14. Parkes CM. The first year of bereavement: a longitudinal study of the reaction of London widows to the deaths of their husbands. Psychiatry 1970; 33:444–467.
15. Schulz R. The Psychology of Death, Dying and Bereavement. Reading, MA: Addison-Wesley, 1978.
16. Diagnostic and Statistical Manual of Mental Disorders, 4th ed. Washington, DC: American Psychiatric Press, 1994.
17. Bukberg J, Penman D, Holland JC. Depression in hospitalized cancer patients. Psychosom Med 1984; 46:199–212.
18. Rodin GM, Voshart K. Depression in the medically ill: an overview. Am J Psychiatry 1986; 143:696–705.
19. Stoudemire A. Depression in the medically ill. In: Cavenar J, ed. Psychiatry, Vol 2. Philadelphia: JB Lippincott, 1985:section 99, pp 1–8.
20. Wells KB, Hays RD, Burnam A, Rogers W, Greenfield S, Ware JE. Detection of depressive disorders for patients receiving prepaid or fee-for-service care. JAMA 1989; 262:3298–3302.
21. Spiegel D, Bloom JR, Yalom I. Group support for patients with metastatic cancer. Arch Gen Psychiatry 1981; 38:527–533.
22. Spiegel D, Bloom JR, Kraemer HC, Gottheil E. Effect of psychosocial treatment on survival of patients with metastatic breast cancer. Lancet 1989; 2:888–891.
23. Fawzy FI, Cousins N, Fawzy NW, Kemeny ME, Elashoff R, Morton D. A structured psychiatric intervention for cancer patients. I. Changes over time in methods of coping and affective disturbance. Arch Gen Psychiatry 1990; 47: 720–725.
24. Rifkin A, Readon G, Siris S, et al. Trimipramine in physical illness with depression. J Clin Psychiatry 1985; 46:4–8.
25. Plumb MM, Holland J. Comparative studies of psychological function in patients with advanced cancer. I. Self-reported depressive symptoms. Psychosom Med 1981; 39:264–276.
26. Endicott J. Measurement of depression in patients with cancer. Cancer 1984; 53: 2243–2248.
27. Spitzer RL, Williams J, Gibbons M, et al. Structured Clinical Interview for DSM-III-R (SCID). Users Guide for the Structured Clinical Interview for DSM-III-R. Washington, DC: American Psychiatric Press, 1990.
28. Cavenaugh S, Clark D, Gibbons R. Diagnosing depression in the hospitalized medically ill. Psychosomatics 1983; 24:809–815.
29. Cavenaugh S, Kennedy S. A successful training program for medical residents. Gen Hosp Psychiatry 1986; 8:73–80.
30. Cohen-Cole SA, Bird J, Freeman A. Psychiatry for internists: a study of needs. J Operat Psychiatry 1982; 13:100–115.
31. Knights E, Folstein M. Unsuspected emotional and cognitive disturbance in medical patients. Ann Intern Med 1977; 87:723–724.
32. Neilsen AC, Williams TA. Depression in ambulatory medical patients: prevalence by self-report questionnaire and recognition by non-psychiatric physicians. Arch Gen Psychiatry 1980; 37:999–1004.

33. Schulberg HC, Saul M, McClelland M, Ganguli M, Christy W, Frank R. Assessing depression in primary medical and psychiatric practices. Arch Gen Psychiatry 1985; 42:1164–1170.
34. Thompson TL, Stoudemire A, Mitchell WE. Underrecognition of patients' psychosocial distress in a university hospital medical clinic. Am J Psychiatry 1983; 140:158–161.
35. Hardman A, Maguire P, Crowther D. The recognition of psychiatric morbidity on a medical oncology ward. J Psychosom Res 1981; 25:237–243.
36. Stoudemire A, Thompson TL. Medication non-compliance: systematic approaches to evaluation and intervention. Gen Hosp Psychiatry 1983; 5:233–239.
37. Koenig HG, Shelp F, Goli V, Cohen HJ, Blazer DG. Survival and health care utilization in elderly medical inpatients with major depression. J Am Geriatr Soc 1989; 37:599–606.
38. Abram HS, Moore GL, Westervelt FB. Suicidal behavior in chronic dialysis patients. Am J Psychiatry 1971; 127:1199–1204.
39. Hawton K. The long term outcome of psychiatric morbidity detected in general medical patients. J Psychosom Res 1981; 25:237–243.
40. Murphy E, Smith R, Slatter J. Increased mortality rates in late-life depression. Br J Psychiatry 1988; 152:347–353.
41. Surridge D. An investigation into some psychiatric aspects of multiple sclerosis. Br J Psychiatry 1969; 115:749–764.
42. Ron MA. Multiple sclerosis: psychiatric and psychometric abnormalities. J Psychosom Res 1986; 30:3–11.
43. Snyder S, Strain JJ. Differentiation of major depression and adjustment disorder with depressed mood in the medical setting. Gen Hosp Psychiatry 1989; 12: 159–165.
44. Khouzam HR, Emery PE, Reaves B. Secondary mania in late life. J Am Geriatr Soc 1994; 42:85–87.
45. Krauthammer C, Clerman GL. Secondary mania. Arch Gen Psychiatry 1978; 35: 1333–1339.
46. Larson EW. Organic causes of mania. Mayo Clin Proc 1988; 63:906–912.
47. McDonald WM, Nemeroff CB. The diagnosis and treatment of mania in the elderly. Bull Menninger Clin 1996; 60:174–196.
48. West SA. Medical disorders associated with mania: a review of the literature. Med Update Psychiatrists 1996; 1:28–31.
49. Depression Guideline Panel: Depression in Primary Care, Vol 1, Detection and Diagnosis. Clinical Practice Guideline, No. 5. Rockville, MD: U.S. Department of Health and Human Services, Agency for Health Care Policy and Research, 1993. AHCPR publication 93-0550.
50. Cassileth BR, Lusk EJ, Strouse TB, et al. Psychosocialstratus in chronic illness: a comparative analysis of six diagnostic groups. N Engl J Med 1984; 311:506–511.
51. Grassi L, Rosti G. Psychosocial morbidity and adjustment to illness among long-term cancer survivors. Psychosomatics 1996; 37:523–532.
52. Noyes R, Kathol RG. Depression and cancer. Psychiatry Dev 1986; 2:77–100.
53. Parle M, Jones B, Maguire P. Maladaptive coping and affective disorders among cancer patients. Psychol Med 1996; 26:735–744.

54. Spiegel D, Kato PM. Psychosocial influences on cancer incidence and progression. Harvard Rev Psychiatry 1996; 4:10–26.
55. Mayou RA. Depression and types of physical disorder and treatment. In: Robertson MM and Katona CLE, eds. Depression and Physical Illness. New York: John Wiley and Sons, 1997:21–38.
56. Weissman A, Worden J. The existential plight in cancer: significance of the first 100 days. Psychiatry Med 1976; 7:1–15.
57. Breitbart W. Identifying patients at risk for, and treatment of major psychiatric complications of cancer. Support Care Cancer 1995; 3:45–60.
58. Cassileth BR, Lusk EJ, Brown LL, et al. Factors associated with psychological distress in cancer patients. Med Pediatr Oncol 1986; 14:251–254.
59. Noyes R, Kathol RG, Debelius-Enemark P, et al. Distress associated with cancer as measured by the Illness Distress Scale. Psychosomatics 1990; 31:321–330.
60. Everitt NJ, Noble TW, Hosie KB, Rogers K. Psychiatric consequences of radical curative surgery for gastric cancer. J Roy Soc Med 1995; 88:516–517.
61. Sutherland AM, Orbach CD, Dyk RB, Bard M. The psychological impact of cancer and cancer surgery. I. Adaptation to the dry colostomy. Cancer 1952; 5: 857–872.
62. Aase N, Grunfeld B, Kaalhus O, Fossa SD. Pre- and post-treatment sexual life in testicular cancer patients: a descriptive investigation. Br J Cancer 1993; 67: 1113–1117.
63. Morris T, Greer HS, White P. Psychological and social adjustment to mastectomy. Cancer 1977; 40:2381–2387.
64. Omne-Ponten M, Holmberg L, Bergstrom R, Sjoden PO, Burns T. Psychosocial adjustment among husbands of women treated for breast cancer: mastectomy vs. breast-conserving surgery. Eur J Cancer 1993; 29:1393–1397.
65. Omne-Ponten M, Holmberg L, Burns T, Adami HO, Bergstrom R. Determinants of the psychosocial outcome after operation for breast cancer: results of a prospective comparative interview study following mastectomy and breast conservation. Eur J Cancer 1992; 28:1062–1067.
66. Brown JH, Paraskevas F. Cancer and depression: cancer presenting with depressive illness: an autoimmune disease. Br J Psychiatry 1982; 141:227–232.
67. Joynt RJ. The brain's uneasy peace with tumors. Ann NY Acad Sci 1974; 230: 342–347.
68. Petty F, Noyes R. Depression secondary to cancer. Bio Psychiatry 1981; 16: 1203–1220.
69. Schnider B, Manolo A. Paraneoplastic syndromes' unusual manifestations of malignant disease. Dis Month 1979; 25:1–59.
70. Green AI, Austin CP. Psychopathology of pancreatic cancer: a psychobiologic probe. Psychosomatics 1993; 34:209–221.
71. McMullen FF, Hanson HH. Excessive urinary 5-hydroxy-3 indoleacetic acid in the absence of metastatic carcinoid. Circulation 1958; 18:883–886.
72. Pomara NP, Gershon S. Treatment-resistant depression in an elderly patient with pancreatic carcinoma: case report. J Clin Psychiatry 1984; 45:439–440.
73. Schildkraut JJ. The catecholamine hypothesis of affective disorders: a review of supporting evidence. Am J Psychiatry 1965; 122:509–522.

74. Medical Research Council Lung Cancer Working Party. Randomized trial of four-drug vs. less intensive two-drug chemotherapy in the palliative treatment of patients with small cell lung cancer and poor prognosis. Br J Cancer 1996; 73: 406–413.
75. Love RR, Leventhal H, Easterling DV, Nerenz DR. Side effects and emotional distress during cancer chemotherapy. Cancer 1989; 63:604–612.
76. Bech P, Malt UF, Dencker SJ, Allfors UG, Elgen K, Lewander T, Lundell A, Simpson GM, Lingjaerde O. Scales for depression. Acta Psychiatr Scand 1993; 87(Suppl 372):37–40.
77. Dowrick C. Does testing for depression influence diagnosis or management by general practitioners? Fam Pract 1995; 12:461–465.
78. Chochinov HM, Wilson KG, Enna M, et al. "Are you depressed?" Screening for depression in the terminally ill. Am J Psychiatry 1997; 154:674–676.
79. Bunney WE, Davis J. Norepinephrine in depressive reactions: a review. Arch Gen Psychiatry 1965; 13:483–494.
80. Coppen A. The biochemistry of affective disorders. Br J Psychiatry 1967; 113: 1237–1264.
81. Coppen A, Prange AJ, Whybrow PC, et al. Abnormalities of indoleamines in affective disorders. Arch Gen Psychiatry 1972; 26:474–478.
82. Shopsin B, Gershon S, Goldstein M, Friedman E, Wilk S. Use of synthesis inhibitors in defining a role for biogenic amines during imipramine treatment in depressed patients. Psychopharmacol Commun 1975; 1:239–249.
83. Delgado PL, Price LH, Miller HL, Salomon RM, Aghajanian G, Heninger GR, Charney D. Serotonin and the neurobiology of depression. Arch Gen Psychiatry 1994; 51:865–874.
84. Miller HL, Delgado PL, Salomon RM, Berman R, Krystal JH, Heninger GR, Charney D. Clinical and biochemical effects of catecholamine depletion of antidepressant-induced remission of depression. Arch Gen Psychiatry 1995; 53:117–128.
85. Susler F, Vetulani J, Mobley P. Mode of action of antidepressant drugs. Biochem Pharmacol 1978; 27:257–261.
86. Charney DS, Menkes DB, Heninger GR. Receptor sensitivity and the mechanism of action of antidepressant treatment: implications for the etiology and therapy of depression. Arch Gen Psychiatry 1981; 38:1160–1180.
87. Vetulani J, Sulser F. Action of various antidepressant treatments reduces reactivity of noradrenergic cAMP-generating system in limbic forebrain. Nature 1975; 257:495–496.
88. Banerjee SP, Kung LS, Riggi SJ, Chanda SK. Development of β-adrenergic receptor subsensitivity by antidepressants. Nature 1977; 268:455–456.
89. Peroutka SL, Snyder SH. Long-term antidepressant treatment decreases spiroperidol-labeled serotonin receptor binding. Science 1980; 210:88–90.
90. Heninger GR, Charney D. Mechanisms of action of antidepressant treatments: implications for the etiology and treatment of depressive disorders. In: Meltzer HY, ed. Psychopharmacology: The Third Generation of Progress. New York: Raven Press, 1987:535–544.
91. Riva MA, Creese I. Re-evaluation of the regulation of β-adrenergic receptor binding by desipramine treatment. Mol Pharmacol 1989; 36:211–218.

92. Butler MO, Morinobu S, Duman RS. Chronic electroconvulsive seizures increase the expression of serotonin-2 receptor mRNA in rat frontal cortex. J Neurochem 1993; 61:1270–1276.
93. Duman RS, Heninger GR, Nestler EJ. A molecular and cellular theory of depression. Arch Gen Psychiatry 1997; 54:597–606.
94. Poisner AM, Bernstein J. A possible role of microtubules in catecholamine release from the adrenal medulla: effect of colchicine, vinca alkyloids and deuterium oxide. J Pharmacol Exp Ther 1971; 177:102–108.
95. Silberfarb PM, Holland JC, Aubar D, Bahna G, Mauser LH, Chakinian AP, Comis R. Psychological response of patients receiving two drug regimens for lung carcinoma. Am J Psychiatry 1983; 140:110–111.
96. Thoa NM, Wooten GF, Axelrod J, et al. Inhibition of release of dopamine beta-hydroxylase and norepinephrine from sympathetic nerves by colchicine, vinblastine, and cytochalasin-B. Proc Natl Acad Sci USA 1972; 69:520–522.
97. Holt A, Callingham BA. Further studies on the ex-vivo effects of procarbazine and monomethylhydrazine on rat semicarbazide-sensitive amine oxidase and monoamine oxidase activities. J Pharm Pharmacol 1995; 47:837–845.
98. Holt A, Sharman DF, Callingham BA, Kettler R. Characteristics of procarbazine as an inhibitor in-vitro of rat semicarbazide-sensitive amine oxidase. J Pharm Pharmacol 1992; 44:478–493.
99. Board F, Persky H, Hamburg DA. Psychological stress and endocrine functions: blood levels of adrenocortical and thyroid hormones in acutely disturbed patients. Psychosom Med 1956; 18:324–333.
100. Carpenter W, Bunney W. Adrenal cortical activity in depressive illness. Am J Psychiatry 1971; 128:31–40.
101. Sachar E, Hellman L, Fukushima D, Gallagher T. Cortisol production in depressive illness. Arch Gen Psychiatry 1970; 23:289–298.
102. Carroll BJ. Pituitary-adrenal function in depression. Lancet 1968; 556:1373–1374.
103. Amsterdam JD, Marinelli DL, Arger P, Winokur A. Assessment of adrenal gland volume by computed tomography in depressed patients and healthy volunteers: a pilot study. Psychiatry Res 1987; 21:189–197.
104. Nemeroff CB, Krishnan KRR, Reed D, Leder R, Beam C, Dunnick NR. Adrenal gland enlargement in major depression: a computed tomographic study. Arch Gen Psychiatry 1992; 49:384–387.
105. Rubin RT, Phillips JJ, Sadow TF, McCracken JT. Adrenal gland volume in major depression: increase during the depressive episode and decrease with successful treatment. Arch Gen Psychiatry 1995; 52:213–218.
106. Szigethy E, Conwell Y, Forbes NT, Cox C, Caine ED. Adrenal weight and morphology in victims of completed suicide. Bio Psychiatry 1994; 36:374–380.
107. Zis KD, Zis A. Increased adrenal weight in victims of violent suicide. Am J Psychiatry 1987; 144:1214–1215.
108. Krishnan KRR, Doraiswamy PM, Lurie SN, Figiel GS, Husain MM, Boyko OH, Ellinwood EH, Nemeroff CB. Pituitary size in depression. J Clin Endocrinol Metab 1991; 72:256–259.
109. Arana GW, Mossman D. The DST and depression: approaches to the use of a laboratory test in psychiatry. Neurol Clin 1988; 6:21–39.

110. Arana GW, Baldesarrini RJ, Ornsteen M. The dexamethasone suppression test for diagnosis and prognosis in psychiatry. Arch Gen Psychiatry 1985; 42:1192–1204.
111. Evans DL, Nemeroff CB. Use of dexamethasone suppression test using DSM III criteria on an inpatient psychiatric unit. Biol Psychiatry 1983; 18:505–511.
112. Krishnan KRR, France PD, Pelton S, McCann UD, Manepalli AN, Davidson JRT. What does the dexamethasone suppression test identify? Biol Psychiatry 1985; 20:957–964.
113. Schatzberg AF, Rothschild AJ, Bond TC, Cole JO. The DST in psychotic depression: diagnostic and pathophysiologic implications. Psychopharmacol Bull 1984; 20:362–364.
114. Arato M, Banki CM, Nemeroff CB, Bissette B. Hypothalamic-pituitary-adrenal axis and suicide. Ann NY Acad Sci 1986; 487:263–270.
115. Banki CM, Bissette G, Arato M, O'Connor L, Nemeroff CB. Cerebrospinal fluid corticotropin-releasing factor-like immunoreactivity in depression and schizophrenia. Am J Psychiatry 1987; 144:873–877.
116. France RD, Urban B, Krishnan KRR, Bissette G, Banki CM, Nemeroff CB, Balleyer JC. CSF corticotropin-releasing factor-like immunoreactivity in chronic pain patients with and without major depression. Biol Psychiatry 1988; 23:86–88.
117. Nemeroff CB, Widerlov E, Bissette G, Walleus H, Karlsson I, Eklund K, Kilts CD, Loosen PT, Vale V. Elevated concentrations of CSF corticotropin-releasing factor-like immunoreactivity in depressed patients. Science 1984; 226:1342–1344.
118. Risch SC, Lewine RJ, Kalin NH, Jewart RD, Risby ED, Caudle JM, Stipetic M, Turner J, Eccard MB, Pollard WE. Limbic-hypothalamic-pituitary-adrenal axis activity and ventricular-to-brain ratio studies in affective illness and schizophrenia. Neuropsychopharmacology 1992; 6:95–100.
119. Amsterdam JD, Maislin G, Winokur A, Berwish N, Kling M, Gold P. The oCRH test before and after clinical recovery from depression. J Affect Dis 1988; 14:213–222.
120. Gold PW, Chrousos GP, Kellner C, Post RM, Roy A, Augerinas P, Schulte H, Oldfield EH, Loriaux DL. Psychiatric implications of basic and clinical studies with corticotropin-releasing factor. Am J Psychiatry 1984; 141:619–627.
121. Holsboer F, Von Bardeleben U, Gerken A, Muler D. Blunted corticotropin and normal cortisol response to human corticotropin-releasing factor in depression. N Engl J Med 1984; 311:1127.
122. Kathol RG, Jaeckle RS, Lopez JR, Mullter WH. Consistent reduction of ACTH responses to stimulation with CRH, vasopressin and hypoglycaemia in patients with depression. Br J Psychiatry 1989; 155:468–478.
123. Young EA, Watson SJ, Kotun J. Beta-lipotropin-beta-endorphin response to low-dose ovine corticotropin releasing factor in endogenous depression. Arch Gen Psychiatry 1990; 47:449–457.
124. Raadsheer F, Hoogendijk WJG, Stam FC, Tilders FJH, Swaab DF. Increased number of corticotropin-releasing hormone expressing neurons in the hypothalamic paraventricular nucleus of depressed patients. Neuroendocrinology 1994; 60:436–444.

125. DeBellis MD, Gold PW, Geracioti TD, Listwak S, Kling MA. Fluoxetine significantly reduces CSF CRH and AVP concentrations in patients with major depression. Am J Psychiatry 1993; 150:656–657.
126. Nemeroff CB, Bissette G, Akil H, Fin M. Neuropeptide concentrations in the cerebrospinal fluid of depressed patients treated with electroconvulsive therapy: corticotropin-releasing factor, beta-endorphin and somatostatin. Br J Psychiatry 1991; 158:59–63.
127. Veith RC, Lewis N, Langohr JI, Murburg MM, Ashleigle EA, Castillo S, Peskind ER, Pascialy M, Bissette G, Nemeroff CB, Raskin J. Effect of desipramine on cerebrospinal fluid concentrations of corticotropin-releasing factor in human subjects. Psychiatry Res 1992; 46:1–8.
128. Nemeroff CB. The corticotropin-releasing factor (CRF) hypothesis of depression: new findings and new directions. Mol Psychiatry 1996; 1:336–342.
129. Evans DL, McCartney LF, Nemeroff CB, Raft D, Quade D, Golden RN, Haggerty JJ, Holmes V, Simon JS, Droba M, Mason GA, Fowler WC. Depression in women treated for gynecological cancer: clinical and neuroendocrine assessment. Am J Psychiatry 1986; 143:447–452.
130. Joffe RT, Rubinow DR, Denicoff KD, Maher M, Sindelau WF. Depression and cancer of the pancreas. Gen Hosp Psychiatry 1986; 8:241–245.
131. Musselman DL, Nemeroff CB. Neuroendocrinology of depression. Clin Neurosci 1993; 1:115–121.
132. van der Pompe G, Antoni MH, Heihnen CJ. Elevated basal cortisol levels and attenuated ACTH and cortisol responses to a behavioral challenge in women with metastatic breast cancer. Psychoneuroendocrinology 1996; 21:361–374.
133. Prange AJ, Wilson IC, Rabon AM, Lipton MA. Enhancement of imipramine antidepressant activity by thyroid hormone. Am J Psychiatry 1969; 126:457–469.
134. Prange AJ, Loosen PT, Wilson I, Lipton MA. The therapeutic use of hormones of the thyroid axis in depression. In: Post CR, Ballenger J, eds. Neurobiology of Mood Disorders. Baltimore: Williams & Wilkins, 1980:311–322.
135. Joffe RT, Singer W, Levitt AJ, MacDonald C. A placebo-controlled comparison of lithium and triiodothyronine augmentation of tricyclic antidepressants in unipolar refractory depression. Arch Gen Psychiatry 1993; 50:387–394.
136. Kirkegaard CJ, Faber J, Hummer L, Rogowski P. Increased levels of TRH in cerebrospinal fluid from patients with endogenous depression. Psychoneuroendocrinology 1979; 4:227–235.
137. Banki CM, Bissette G, Arato M, Nemeroff CB. Elevation of immunoreactive CSF TRH in depressed patients. Am J Psychiatry 1988; 145:1526–1531.
138. Post RM, Gold P, Rubinow DR, Ballenger JC, Bunney WE, Goodwin FK. Peptides in cerebrospinal fluid of neuropsychiatric patients: an approach to central nervous system peptide function. Life Sci 1982; 31:1–15.
139. Prange AJ, Wilson IC, Lara PP, Alltop LB, Breese GR. Effects of thyrotropin-releasing hormone in depression. Lancet 1972; 2:999–1002.
140. Nemeroff CB, Evans DL. Thyrotropin-releasing hormone (TRH), the thyroid axis and affective disorder. Ann NY Acad Sci 1989; 553:304–310.
141. Kastin AJ, Schalch DS, Ehrensing RH, Anderson MS. Improvement in mental

depression with decreased thyrotropin response and administration of thyrotropin-releasing hormone. Lancet 1972; 2:740–742.
142. Extein I, Pottash AC, Gold MS. The thyrotropin-releasing hormone test in the diagnosis of unipolar depression. Psychiatry Res 1981; 5:311–316.
143. Gold MS, Pottash AC, Extein I. Symptomless autoimmune thyroiditis in depression. Psychiatry Res 1982; 6:261–269.
144. Haggerty JJ, Evans DL, Golden RN, Pedersen CA, Simon JS, Nemeroff CB. The presence of anti-thyroid antibodies in patients with affective and non-affective psychiatric disorders. Biol Psychiatry 1990; 27:51–60.
145. Whybrow PC, Prange AJ. A hypothesis of thyroid-catecholamine-receptor interaction: its relevance to affective illness. Arch Gen Psychiatry 1981; 33:106–113.
146. Coe CCL, Hall NR. Psychological disturbance alters thymic and adrenal hormone secretion in a parallel but independent manner. Psychoneuroendocrinology 1993; 21:237–247.
147. Weiss JM, Sundar S. Effects of stress on cellular immune responses in animals. In: Tasman A, Riba M, eds. American Psychiatry Press Review of Psychiatry. Washington, DC: American Psychiatric Press, 1992:145–168.
148. Moynihan JA, Ader R. Psychoneuroimmunology: animal models of disease. Psychosom Med 1996; 58:546–558.
149. Herbert TB, Cohen S. Depression and immunity: a meta-analytic review. Psychol Bull 1993; 13:472–486.
150. Stein M, Miller A, Trestman RL. Depression, the immune system, and health and illness. Arch Gen Psychiatry 1991; 48:171–177.
151. Levy SM, Herberman RB, Lippman M, D'Angelo T. Correlation of stress factors with sustained depression of natural killer cell activity and predicted prognosis in patients with breast cancer. J Clin Oncol 1987; 5:348–353.
152. Levy SM, Herberman RB, Whiteside T, Sanzo K, Lee J, Kirkwood J. Perceived social support and tumor estrogen/progesterone receptor status as predictors of natural killer cell activity in breast cancer patients. Psychosom Med 1990; 42:73–85.
153. Maes M. Evidence for an immune response in major depression: a review and hypothesis. Prog Neuropsychopharmacol Biol Psychiatry 1994; 19:11–38.
154. Maes M, Bosman E, Meltzer HY. Immunoendocrine aspects of major depression. Relationships between plasma IL-6 and soluble IL-2 receptor, prolactin and cortisol. Eur Arch Psychiatry Clin Neurosci 1995; 245:172–178.
155. Sluzewska A, Rybakowski J, Bosmans E, Sobieska M, Berghmans R, Maes M, Wiktorowicz K. Indicators of immune activation in major depression. Psychiatry Res 1996; 64:161–167.
156. Song C, Dinan T, Leonard BE. Changes in Immunoglobulin, complement, and acute phase protein levels in depressed patients and normal controls. J Affect Disord 1994; 30:283–288.
157. Ur E, White PD, Grossman A. Hypothesis: cytokines may be activated to cause depressive illness and chronic fatigue syndrome. Eur Arch Psychiatry Clin Neurosci 1992; 241:317–322.

158. Ader R, Felten DL, Cohen N, eds. Psychoneuroimmunology. New York: Academic Press, 1990.
159. Bellinger DL, Lorton D, Romano T. Neuropeptide innervation of lymphoid organs. Ann NY Acad Sci 1990; 594:17–33.
160. Berczi I. The influence of pituitary adrenal axis on the immune system. In: Berczi I, ed. Pituitary Function and Immunity. Boca Raton, FL: CRC Press, 1986: 133–160.
161. Blalock EJ. Relationships between neuroendocrine hormones and lymphokines. Lymphokines 1984; 9:1–13.
162. Epstein RH. Neuroendocrine-immune interactions. N Engl J Med 1993; 329: 1246–1253.
163. Felten DL, Felten SY, Bellinger DL. Noradrenergic sympathetic neural interactions with the immune system: structure and function. Immunol Rev 1987; 100: 255–260.
164. Livnat S, Felten SY, Carlson SL. Involvement of peripheral and central catecholamine systems in neural-immune interactions. J Neuroimmunol 1985; 10:5–30.
165. Lasckow JW, Mulcahey JJ, Han JH, Owens MJ, Stipetic MD, Breitman D, Nemeroff CB. Interleukin-1 alpha induces corticotropin-releasing factor secretion and synthesis from NPLC-KC cells through various second messenger pathways. Synapse 1994; 18:354–358.
166. Tsagarakis S, Gillies G, Rees LH, Besser GM, Grossman A. Interleukin-1 directly stimulates the release of corticotropin releasing factor from rat hypothalamus. Neuroendocrinology 1989; 49:98–101.
167. Denicoff KD, Durkin TM, Lotze MT, Quinlan PE, Davis CL, Litwak SJ, Rosenbert SA, Ribinow DR. The neuroendocrine effects of interleukin-2 treatment. J Clin Endocrinol Metab 1986; 63:1292–1299.
168. Irwin MR, Britton KT, Vale W. Central corticotropin releasing factor suppresses natural killer cell activity. Brain Behav Immun 1987; 1:81–87.
169. Staubaugh H, Irwin M. Central corticotropin-releasing hormone reduces cellular immunity. Brain Behav Immun 1992; 6:11–17.
170. Seidel A, Arolt V, Hunstiger M, Riuk L, Behnisch A, Kirchner H. Cytokine production and serum proteins in depression. Scand J Immunol 1995; 41:534–538.
171. Anderson JL. The immune system and major depression. Adv Neuroimmunol 1996; 6:119–129.
172. Ben-Eliyahu S, Yirmiya R, Liebeskind JC. Stress increases metastatic spread of a mammary tumor in rats: evidence for mediation by the immune system. Brain Behav Immun 1991; 5:193–205.
173. Brenner GH, Cohen N, Ader R. Increased pulmonary metastases in mice following handling. Life Sci 1990; 47:1813–1819.
174. Page GG, Ben-Eliyahu S, Yirmiya R. Morphine attenuates surgery-induced enhancement of metastatic colonization in rats. Pain 1993; 54:21–28.
175. Esterling BA, Kiecolt-Glaser JK, Glaser R. Psychosocial modulation of cytokine-induced natural killer cell activity in older adults. Psychosom Med 1996; 58: 264–272.

176. Mathe G. Depression, stressful events, and the risk of cancer. Biomed Pharmacother 1996; 50:1–2.
177. Haig RA. Management of depression in patients with advanced cancer. Med J Aust 1992; 156:499–503.
178. Stoudemire A, Moran M, Fogel B. Psychotropic drug use in the medically ill. Psychosomatics 1990; 31:377–391.
179. Stoudemire A. New antidepressant drugs and the treatment of depression in the medically ill patient. Psychiatr Clin North Am 1996; 19:495–514.
180. Nemeroff CB, DeVane CL, Pollock BG. New antidepressants and the cytochrome P450 system. Am J Psychiatry 1996; 153:311–320.
181. Breitbart W, Mermelstein H. Pemoline: an alternative psychostimulant for the management of depressive disorders in cancer patients. Psychosomatics 1992; 33:352–356.
182. Olin J, Masand P. Psychostimulants for depression in hospitalized cancer patients. Psychosomatics 1996; 37:57–62.
183. Fernandez F, Adams F. Methylphenidate treatment of patients with head and neck cancer. Head Neck 1986; 8:296–300.
184. Kraus MF, Burch EA. Methylphenidate hydrochloride as an antidepressant. South Med J 1992; 85:985–991.
185. Natenshon AL. Clinical evaluation of ritalin. Dis Nerv Syst 1956; 17:392–396.
186. Stiebel V, Kemp K. Long term methylphenidate use in the medically ill patient with organic mood syndrome. Psychosomatics 1990; 31:454–456.
187. Abrams R. Electroconvulsive Therapy. New York: Oxford University Press, 1992.
188. Kalinowsky LB, Hoch PH. Shock Treatments and Other Somatic Procedures in Psychiatry. New York: Grune & Stratton, 1946.
189. Thompson JW, Blaine JD. Use of ECT in the United States in 1975 and 1980. Am J Psychiatry 1987; 144:557–562.
190. Janicak PG, Davis JM, Gibbons RD. Efficacy of ECT: a meta-analysis. Am J Psychiatry 1985; 142:297–302.
191. Scovern AW, Kilman PR. Status of ECT: a review of the outcome literature. Psychol Bull 1980; 87:260–303.
192. Siris SG, Glassman AH, Stetner F. ECT and psychotropic medication in the treatment of depression and schizophrenia. In: Abrams R, Essman WB, eds. Electroconvulsive Therapy: Biological Foundations and Clinical Applications. New York: Spectrum Publications, 1982:91–111.
193. Addonizio G, Susman VL. ECT as a treatment alternative for patients with symptoms of neuroleptic malignant syndrome. J Clin Psychiatry 1987; 48:102–105.
194. Greenberg LB. Electroconvulsive therapy in treating neuroleptic malignant syndrome. Convuls Ther 1986; 2:61–62.
195. Hughes JR. ECT during and after the neuroleptic malignant syndrome: case report. J Clin Psychiatry 1986; 47:42–43.
196. Pearlman CA. Neuroleptic malignant syndrome: a review of the literature. J Clin Psychopharmacol 1986; 6:257–273.
197. Andersen K, Balldin J, Gottfries CG. A double-blind evaluation of electroconvul-

sive therapy in Parkinson's disease with "on-off" phenomena. Acta Neurol Scand 1987; 76:191–199.
198. Post PM, Putman F, Uhde TW, Weiss SR. Electroconvulsive therapy as an anticonvulsant. Implications for its mechanism of action in affective illness. Ann NY Acad Sci 1986; 462:376–388.
199. Sackeim HA, Devanand DP, Prudic J. Stimulus intensity, seizure threshold, and seizure duration: impact on the efficacy and safety of electroconvulsive therapy. Psychiatr Clin North Am 1991; 14:803–843.
200. American Psychiatric Association. The Practice of ECT: Recommendations for Treatment, Training, and Privileging. Washington, DC: American Psychiatric Press, 1990.
201. Sackeim HA, Devanand DP, Nobler MS. Electroconvulsive therapy. In: Bloom FE, Kupfer DJ, eds. Psychopharmacology: The Generation of Progress. New York: Raven Press, 1995:1123–1141.
202. Stoudemire A. Expanding psychopharmacologic treatment options for the depressed medical patient. Psychosomatics 1995; 36(Suppl):19–26.
203. Alter CL, Fleishman SB, Kornblith AB, Holland JC, Biano D, Levenson R, Vinciguerra V, Rai KR. Supportive telephone intervention for patients receiving chemotherapy. Psychosomatics 1996; 37:425–431.
204. Bloom JR. Social support systems and cancer: a conceptual overview. In: Cohen J, Cullen J, Martin RL, eds. Psychosocial Aspects of Cancer. New York: Raven Press, 1982:129–149.
205. Cunningham AJ, Edmonds CV. Group psychological therapy for cancer patients: a point of view and discussion of the hierarchy of options. Int J Psychiatry Med 1996; 26:51–82.
206. Fawzy FI, Wellisch D, Yager J. Psychiatric liaison to the bone marrow transplant project. In: Hollingsworth OE, Pasnau RO, eds. The Family in Mourning. New York: Grune & Stratton, 1977:181–189.
207. Gordon WA, Friedenbergs I, Diller L, et al. Efficacy of psychosocial intervention with cancer patients. J Consult Clin Psychol 1980; 48:743–759.
208. Holland JC, Rowland JH. Psychiatric, psychosocial, and behavioral interventions in the treatment of cancer: an historical perspective. In: Weiss SM, Herd JA, Fox BH, eds. Perspectives on Behavioral Medicine. Orlando, FL: Academic Press, 1981:235–260.
209. Kaufman E, Micha VG. A model for psychotherapy with the good prognosis cancer patient. Psychosomatics 1987; 28:540–548.
210. Kay JM, Schindler BA. Hypnosis on a consult-liaison service. Gen Hosp Psychiatry 1990; 12:379–383.
211. Levitan AA. The use of hypnosis with cancer patients. Psychiatr Med 1992; 10: 119–131.
212. Massie MJ. Depression. In: Holland JC, Rowland JH, eds. Handbook of Psychooncology. New York: Oxford University Press, 1989:283–290.
213. Yalom ID, Greaves C. Group therapy with the terminally ill. Am J Psychiatry 1977; 134:396–400.
214. Spiegel D, Bloom JR, Yalom I. Group support for patients with metastatic cancer. Arch Gen Psychiatry 1981; 38:527–533.

215. Spiegel D, Bloom JR, Kraemer HC, Gottheil E. Effect of psychosocial treatment on survival of patients with metastatic breast cancer. Lancet 1989; 2:888–891.
216. Richardson J, Sheldon D, Krailo M, Levine A. The effect of compliance with treatment on survival among patients with hematologic malignancies. J Clin Oncol 1990; 8:356–364.
217. Spiegel D. Psychosocial aspects of cancer. Curr Opin Psychiatry 1991; 4:889–897.
218. Forester B, Kornfeld DS, Fleiss JL, Thompson S. Group psychotherapy during radiotherapy: effects on emotional and physical distress. Am J Psychiatry 1993; 150:1700–1706.
219. Fawzy FI, Kemeny ME, Fawzy NW, et al. A structured psychiatric intervention for cancer patients: II. Changes over time in immunological measures. Arch Gen Psychiatry 1990; 47:729–735.
220. Lipsey JR, Spencer WC, Rabins PV, Robinson RG. Phenomenological comparison of poststroke depression and functional depression. Am J Psychiatry 1986; 143:527–529.
221. Eastwood MR, Rifat SL, Nobbs H, Ruderman J. Mood disorder following cerebrovascular accident. Br J Psychiatry 1989; 154:195–200.
222. Robinson RG, Coyle JY, Starr LB, Price TR. A two-year longitudinal study of mood disorders following stroke: prevalence and duration at 6 months follow-up. Br J Psychiatry 1984; 144:256–262.
223. Astrom M, Adolfsson R, Apslund K. Major depression in stroke patients. Stroke 1993; 24:976–982.
224. Sharpe M, Hawton K, House A, Nolyneux A, Sandercock P, Bamford J, Warlow C. Mood disorders in long-term survivors of stroke: associations with brain lesion and volume. Psychol Med 1990; 20:815–828.
225. Parikh M, Robinson RG, Lipsey JR. The impact of post-stroke depression on recovery in activities of daily living over a 2-year follow-up. Arch Neurol 1990; 47:785–790.
226. Angeleri F, Angeleri VA, Foschi N, Fiaquinto S, Nolfe G, Saginario A, Signorino M. Depression after stroke: an investigation through catamnesis. J Clin Psychiatry 1997; 58:261–265.
227. Angeleri F, Angeleri VA, Foschi N. The influence of depression, social activity, and family stress on functional outcome after stroke. Stroke 1993; 24:1478–1483.
228. Sharpe M, Hawton K, Seagroatt V. Depressive disorders in long-term survivors of stroke: associations with demographic and social factors, functional status, and brain lesion volume. Br J Psychiatry 1994; 164:380–386.
229. Lazarus LW, Moberg PJ, Langsley PR, Lingam VR. Methylphenidate and nortriptyline in the treatment of poststroke depression: a retrospective comparison. Arch Phys Med Rehabil 1994; 75:403–406.
230. Crisostomo EA, Duncan MA, Propst M. Evidence that amphetamine with physical therapy promotes recovery of motor function in stroke patients. Ann Neurol 1988; 23:94–97.
231. Robertson MM. Affect and mood in epilepsy: an overview with a focus on depression. Acta Neurol Scand 1992; 86:127–132.

232. Mendez MF, Doss RC, Taylor JL, Salguero P. Depression in epilepsy: relationship to seizures and anti-convulsant therapy. J Nerv Ment Dis 1993; 181:447–448.
233. Robertson MM, Trimble MR, Townsend HRA. The phenomenology of depression in epilepsy. Epilepsia 1987; 28:364–372.
234. Seidenberg M, Hermann B, Noe A, Wyler AR. Depression in temporal lobe epilepsy: interaction between laterality of lesion and Wisconsin Card Sort performance. Neuropsychiatry Neuropsychol Behav Neurol 1995; 8:81–87.
235. Altshuler LL, Devinsky O, Post RM, Theodore W. Depression, anxiety, and temporal lobe epilepsy: laterality of focus and symptoms. Arch Neurol 1990; 47:284–288.
236. Palisa SS, Harper MA. Mood disorders in epilepsy: a survey of psychiatric patients. Presented at the Annual Meeting of the Royal College of Psychiatrists. University of Southampton, UK, July 8–10, 1986.
237. Kramer LD, Fralin C, Berman NG, Locke GE. Relationship of seizure frequency and interictal depression. Epilepsia 1987; 28:629.
238. Herman BP, Wyler AR. Depression, locus of control, and the effects of epilepsy surgery. Epilepsia 1989; 30:332–338.
239. Ojeman LM, Friel PN, Trejo WJ, Dudley DL. Effect of doxepin on seizure frequency in depressed epileptic patients. Neurology 1983; 33:646–648.
240. Whitlock FA, Siskind MM. Depression as a major symptom of multiple sclerosis. J Neurol Neurosurg Psychiatry 1980; 43:861–865.
241. Young AC, Saunders J, Ponsford JR. Mental changes as an early feature of multiple sclerosis. J Neurol Neurosurg Psychiatry 1976; 39:1008–1013.
242. Goodstein RK, Ferrel RB. Multiple sclerosis presenting as depressive illness. Dis Nerv System 1997; 38:127–131.
243. Salloway S, Price LH, Charney DS, Shapiro M. Multiple sclerosis presenting as major depression: a diagnosis suggested by MRI scan but not CT scan. J Clin Psychiatry 1988; 49:364–366.
244. Dalos NP, Rabins PV, Brooks BR, O'Donnell P. Disease activity and emotional state in multiple sclerosis. Ann Neurol 1983; 13:573–577.
245. Feinstein A, Ron M, Thompson A. A serial study of psychometric and magnetic resonance imaging changes in multiple sclerosis. Brain 1993; 116:569–602.
246. Honer WG, Hurwitz T, Li DKB, Palmer M, Paty DW. Temporal lobe involvement in multiple sclerosis patients with psychiatric disorders. Arch Neurol 1987; 44:187–190.
247. Campbell M, Fleming JA, Li D. Sleep disturbance, depression and lesion site in patients with multiple sclerosis. Arch Neurol 1992; 49:641–643.
248. Starkstein SE, Sabe L, Vaquez S. Neuropsychological, psychiatric, and cerebral blood flow findings in vascular dementia and Alzheimer's disease. Stroke 1996; 27:408–414.
249. Mayeux R. Depression in the patient with Parkinson's disease. J Clin Psychiatry 1990; 51(Suppl 7):20–23.
250. Taylor AE, Saint-Cyr JA, Lang AE, Kenny FT. Parkinson's disease and depression: a critical re-evaluation. Brain 1986; 109:279–292.

251. Levin BE, Llabre MM, Weiner WJ. Parkinson's disease and depression: psychometric properties of the Beck Depression Inventory. J Neurol Neurosurg Psychiatry 1988; 51:1401–1404.
252. Huber SJ, Freidenberg DL, Paulson GW, Shuttleworth EC, Christy JA. The pattern of depressive symptoms varies with progression of Parkinson's disease. J Neurol Neurosurg Psychiatry 1990; 53:275–278.
253. Wise MG, Taylor SE. Anxiety and mood disorders in medically ill patients. J Clin Psychiatry 1990; 51(Supple 1):27–32.
254. Starkstein SE, Preziosi TJ, Forrester AW, Robinson RG. Specificity of affective and autonomic symptoms of depression in Parkinson's disease. J Neurol Neurosurg Psychiatry 1990; 53:869–873.
255. Cummings JL. Depression and Parkinson's disease: a review. Am J Psychiatry 1992; 149:443–452.
256. Faber R. Electroconvulsive therapy in Parkinson's disease. In: Koller WC, Paulson G, eds. Therapy of Parkinson's Disease. New York: Raven Press, 1995:533–537.
257. Viinamaki H, Niskanen L, Uusitupa M. Mental well-being in people with non-insulin-dependent diabetes. Acta Psychiatr Scand 1995; 92:392–397.
258. Wells KB, Golding JM, Burnam MA. Psychiatric disorder in a sample of the general population with and without chronic medical conditions. Am J Psychiatry 1988; 145:976–981.
259. Gavard JA, Lustman PJ, Clouse RE. Prevalence of depression in adults with diabetes—an epidemiological evaluation. Diabetes Care 1993; 16:1167–1178.
260. Lustman PJ, Harper GW, Griffith LS. Use of the Diagnostic Interview Schedule in patients with diabetes mellitus. J Nerv Ment Dis 1986; 174:743–746.
261. Mazze RS, Lucido D, Shanoon H. Psychological and social correlates of glycemic control. Diabetes Care 1984; 7:360–366.
262. McGill JB, Lustman PJ, Griffith LS, Freedland RE, Gavard JA, Clouse RE. Relationship of depression to compliance with self-monitoring of glucose. Diabetes 1992; 41(Suppl 1):84.
263. Lustman PJ, Clouse RE, Griffith LS, Carney RM, Freedland KE. Screening for depression in diabetes using the Beck Depression Inventory. Psychosom Med 1997; 59:24–31.
264. Goodnick PJ, Henry JH, Buki VMV. Treatment of depression in patients with diabetes mellitus. J Clin Psychiatry 1995; 56:128–136.
265. Paykel ES, Mueller PS, De La Vergne PM. Amitryptiline, weight gain, and carbohydrate cravings: a side effect. Br J Psychiatry 1973; 123:501–507.
266. Lustman PJ, Griffith LS, Clouse RE. Effects of nortriptyline on depression and glycemic control in diabetes: results of a double-blind, placebo-controlled study. Psychosom Med 1997; 59:241–250.
267. Aleyassine H, Lee SH. Inhibition of insulin release by substrates and inhibitors of monoamine oxidase. Am J Physiol 1972; 222:565–569.
268. Feldman JM. Inhibition of pancreatic islet monoamine oxidase by adrenergic antagonists and ethanol. Endocr Res 1975; 2:503–520.
269. Bressler R, Johnson D. New pharmacological approaches to therapy of NIDDM. Diabetes Care 1992; 15:793–805.

270. Cooper AJ, Keddie KMG. Hypotensive collapse and hypoglycemia after mebanazine, a monoamine oxidase inhibitor. Lancet 1964; 1:1133–1135.
271. Furman BL. The hypoglycemic effect of 5-hydroxytryptophan. Br J Pharmacol 1974; 50:575–580.
272. Wilson GA, Furman BL. Effects of inhibitors of 5-hydroxytryptamine uptake on plasma glucose and their interactions with 5-hydroxytryptophan in producing hypoglycemia in mice. Eur J Pharmacol 1982; 78:263–270.
273. Van Loon BJP, Radder JK, Frolich M. Fluoxetine increases insulin action in obese nondiabetic and in obese non-insulin-dependent diabetic individuals. Int J Obes Relat Metab Disord 1992; 16:79–85.
274. Gray DS, Fujioka K, Devine W, Bray GA. Fluoxetine treatment of the obese diabetic. Int J Obes Relat Metab Disord 1992; 16:193–198.
275. Connolly VM, Gallagher A, Kesson CM. A study of fluoxetine in obese elderly patients with type 2 diabetes. Diabet Med 1995; 12:416–418.
276. O'Kane M, Wiles PG, Wales JK. Fluoxetine in the treatment of obese type 2 diabetic patients. Diabet Med 1994; 11:105–110.
277. Vinci GG, Fasullo S. Paroxetine treatment of painful diabetic neuropathy. Biol Psychiatry 1997; 42(Suppl):160.
278. Cowdry RW, Wehr TA, Ziz AP. Thyroid abnormalities associated with rapid-cycling bipolar illness. Arch Gen Psychiatry 1983; 40:414–420.
279. Loosen PT. Thyroid function in affective disorders and alcoholism. Endocrinol Metab Clin North Am 1988; 17:55–82.
280. Loosen PT, Chambliss R, DeBold CR. Psychiatric phenomenology in Cushing's disease. Pharmacopsychiatry 1992; 25:192–198.
281. Mazet PH, Simon D, Luton JP. Syndrome de Cushing: symptomatologie psychique et personnalité de 50 malades. Nouv Presse Med 1981; 10:2565–2570.
282. Sonino N, Fava GA, Belluardo P. Course of depression in Cushing's syndrome: response to treatment and comparison with Graves' disease. Horm Res 1993; 39: 202–206.
283. Kornstein SE, Gardner DF. Endocrine disorders. In: Stoudemire A, Fogel B, eds. Psychiatric Care of the Medical Patient. New York: Oxford University Press, 1993.
284. Abbas A, Styra R. Valproate prophylaxis against steroid induced psychosis. Can J Psychiatry 1994; 39:188–189.
285. Falk WE, Mahnke MW, Pozkanzer DC. Lithium prophylaxis of corticotropin-induced psychosis. JAMA 1979; 241:1011–1012.
286. Hall RCW, Popkin MK, Stickney SD. Presentation of the steroid psychosis. J Nerv Ment Dis 1979; 167:229–236.
287. Mastrogiacomo I, Fava M, Fava GA. Correlations between psychological symptoms in hyperprolactinemic amenorrhea. Neuroendocrinol Lett 1983; 5:117–122.
288. Buckman MT, Kellner R. Reduction of distress in hyperprolactinemia with bromocriptine. Am J Psychiatry 1985; 142:242–244.
289. Koppelman MCS, Parry BL, Hamilton JA. Effect of bromocriptine on affect and libido in hyperprolactinemia. Am J Psychiatry 1987; 144:1037–1041.
290. Carney RM, Rich MW, TeVelde A, Saini J, Clark K, Freedland KE. The rela-

tionship between heart rate, heart rate variability and depression in patients with coronary artery disease. J Psychosom Res 1988; 32:159–164.
291. Schleifer SJ, Macari-Hinson MM, Coyle DA. The nature and course of depression following myocardial infarction. Arch Intern Med 1989; 149:1785–1789.
292. Freedland KE, Carney RM, Lustman PJ, Rich MV, Jaffe AS. Major depression in coronary artery disease patients with vs. without a prior history of depression. Psychosom Med 1992; 54:416–421.
293. Anda R, Williamson D, Jones D. Depressed affect, hopeless, and the risk of ischemic heart disease in a cohort of US adults. Epidemiology 1993; 4:285–294.
294. Frasure-Smith N, Lesperance F, Talajic M. Depression and 18-month prognosis following myocardial infarction. Circulation 1995; 91:999–1005.
295. Roose SP, Glassman AH, Dalack GW. Depression, heart disease, and tricyclic antidepressants. J Clin Psychiatry 1989; 50:12–16.
296. Krittayaphong R, Cascio WE, Light KC, Sheffield D. Heart rate variability in patients with coronary artery disease: differences in patients with higher and lower depression scores. Psychosom Med 1997; 59:231–235.
297. Pollock BG, Laghrissi-Thode F, Wagner WR, Finkel M, Johnson PC. Increased platelet factor 4 and β-thromboglobulin in depressed patients with ischemic heart disease. Scientific Abstracts of the 34th Annual Meeting of the American College of Neuropsychopharmacology, San Juan, PR, 1995, abstract 121.
298. Musselman DL, Tomer A, Manatunga AK. Exaggerated platelet reactivity in major depression. Am J Psychiatry 1996; 153:1313–1317.
299. Glassman AH, Roose SP, Bigger JT. The safety of tricyclic antidepressants in cardiac patients: risk-benefit reconsidered. JAMA 1993; 269:2673–2675.
300. Janowsky D, Curtis G, Zisook S. Trazodone-aggravated ventricular arrhythmias. J Clin Psychopharmacol 1983; 3:372–376.
301. Maj M. Psychiatric aspects of HIV-1 infection and AIDS. Psychol Med 1990; 20:547–563.
302. Grant I, Atkinson JH. The evolution of neurobehavioral complications of HIV infection. Psychol Med 1990; 20:747–754.
303. Perkins DO, Stern RA, Golden RN, Murphy C, Naftolowitz D, Evans DL. Mood disorders in HIV infection: prevalence and risk factors in a nonepicenter of the AIDS epidemic. Am J Psychiatry 1994; 151:233–236.
304. Price RW, Brew B, Sidtis J. The brain in AIDS: central nervous system HIV-1 infections and AIDS dementia complex. Science 1988; 239:586–592.
305. Rabkin JG, Rabkin R, Harrison W. Effect of imipramine of mood and enumerative measures of immune status in depressed patients with HIV illness. Am J Psychiatry 1994; 151:516–523.
306. Manning D, Jacobsberg L, Erhart S. The efficacy of imipramine in the treatment of HIV-related depression. Abstracts of the VI International Conference on AIDS, San Francisco, 1990, abstract ThB 32.
307. Levine S, Anderson D, Bystritsky A. A report of eight HIV-seropositive patients with major depression responding to fluoxetine. J AIDS 1990; 3:1074–1077.
308. Rabkin JG, Wagner G, Rabkin R. Sertraline effects on mood and immune status in patients with major depression and HIV illness: an open trial. J Clin Psychiatry 1994; 55:433–439.

309. Fernandez F, Levy JK, Samley HR, Pirozzolo Fj, Lachar D, Crowley J, Adams S, Ross B, Ruiz P. Effects of methylphenidate in HIV-related depression: a comparative trial with desipramine. Int J Psychiatry 1995; 25:53–67.
310. Janicak PG. Psychopharmacotherapy in the HIV-infected patient. Psychiatric Ann 1995; 25:609–613.
311. Sahai J. Risks and synergies from drug interactions. AIDS 1996; 10(Suppl 1): S21–S25.
312. Merry C, Barry MG, Mulcahy F, Ryan M, Heavey J, Tjia JF, Gibbons SE, Breckenridge AM, Back DJ. Saquinavir pharmacokinetics alone and in combination with ritonavir in HIV-infected patients. AIDS 1997; 11:29–33.
313. Chiba M, Hensleigh M, Lin JH. Hepatic and intestinal metabolism of indinavir, an HIV protease inhibitor, in rat and human microsomes. Biochem Pharmacol 1997; 53:1187–1195.
314. Cheng CL, Smith DE, Carver PL, Cox SR, Watkins PB, Blake DS, Kauffman CA, Meyer KM, Amidon GL, Stetson PL. Steady-state pharmacokinetics of delavirdine in HIV-positive patients: effect on erythromycin breath test. Clin Pharmacol Ther 1997; 61:531–543.
315. Kumar GN, Rodrigues AD, Buko AM, Denissen JF. Cytochrome P450-mediated metabolism of the HIV-1 protease inhibitor ritonavir (ABT-538) in human liver microsomes. J Pharmacol Exp Ther 1996; 277:423–431.
316. Iatsimirskaia E, Tulebaev S, Storohik E, Utkin I, Smith D, Gerber N, Koudriakova T. Metabolism of rifabutin in human enterocyte and liver microsomes: kinetic parameters, identification of enzyme systems, and drug interactions with macrolides and antifungal agents. Clin Pharmacol Ther 1997; 61:554–562.
317. Grange JM, Winstanley PA, Davies PD. Clinically significant drug interactions with antitubercular agents. Drug Safety 1994; 11:242–251.
318. Middleboe T, Oveson L, Mortensen El, Beck P. Depressive symptoms in cancer patients undergoing chemotherapy: a psychometric analysis. Psychother Psychosom 1994; 61:171–177.
319. Silberfarb PM, Philibert D, Levine PM. Psychosocial aspects of neoplastic disease. II. Affective and cognitive effects of chemotherapy in cancer patients. Am J Psychiatry 1980; 137:597–601.
320. Evans DL, McCartney LF, Haggerty JJ. Treatment of depression in cancer patients is associated with better life adaptation: a pilot study. Psychosom Med 1988; 50:72–76.
321. Van Heeringen K, Zivkov M. Pharmacological treatment of depression in cancer patients. Br J Psychiatry 1996; 169:440–443.
322. Nemeroff CB, DeVane CL, Pollock BG, Newer antidepressants and the cytochrome P450 system. Am J Psychiatry 1996; 153:311–320.
323. Stoudemire A. New antidepressant drugs and the treatment of depression in the medically ill patient. Psychiatr Clin North Am 1996; 19:495–514.
324. Chabot GG. Factors involved in clinical pharmacology variability in oncology: review. Anticancer Res 1994; 14:2269–2272.
325. Kivisto KT, Kroemer HK, Eichelbaum M. The role of human cytochrome P450 enzymes in the metabolism of anticancer agents: implications for drug interactions. Br J Clin Pharmacol 1995; 40:523–530.

4

Comorbidity of Depressive Illnesses and Personality Disorders

THOMAS J. DOYLE and MING T. TSUANG
Harvard Medical School
Boston, Massachusetts

MICHAEL J. LYONS
Boston University
Boston, Massachusetts

> It seems necessary to give a brief reference to some features of character, not already enumerated in connection with the clinical features, which need brief mention. Hoch and others have emphasized the frequency with which a gloomy, pessimistic, worrying disposition is found in those patients. . . . Variability of mood was found. . . . There were patients who had always been rather suspicious . . . seclusive, shy, and unsociable.
>
> The inadequacy of this affixing of epithets is so great that it was proposed to abstain from it in favor of the more plastic delineation of the reactions of the personality, but as it has some bearing . . . it has been included.
>
> —"Melancholia: A Clinical Survey of Depressive States," Aubrey J. Lewis

I. INTRODUCTION

The relationship between personality and depression has been discussed in the clinical and research literature for many years, as evidenced by the above excerpt from Lewis's 1934 (1) seminal paper on depressive states (2,3). Prior to the publication of DSM-III (4), with its multiaxial nomenclature enabling distinct but comorbid diagnoses of disorders of both mood and personality, personality pathology was considered primarily in terms of personality trait effects on the vulnerability to, severity of, and course of depressive disorders (3,5,6). As in the above quote from Lewis, descriptions of personality in depressive illness historically have tended to appear in terms of the "reactions" of a patient's personality to depressive illness. Lewis found that knowing "where personality ends and the illness begins" was "a point calling for skillful casuistry, if it were worth deciding at all" (7).

This tendency to give less attention to personality pathology is understandable; many authors have asserted that the distinction between personality and mood is arbitrary. Also, treatment of depressive disorders tends to focus on the distress caused by depressive symptoms, leaving less time for a detailed exploration of comorbid personality disorders. Research reports in this area have been difficult to interpret. Although measures of personality *traits* (e.g., the Maudsley Personality Inventory) have existed for some time, systematic measures and categorization of personality *disorders* have appeared only within the past two decades, primarily since the publication of DSM-III (8–10).

Reports on the comorbidity of personality disorders and depression published since DSM-III provide evidence that depressed and dysthymic patients with personality disorders may have qualitatively distinct forms of depression and thus different treatment response patterns compared to patients without personality disorder comorbidity (11,12). The characteristics of these comorbid patients include greater frequency of previous episodes of depression and higher levels of distress and depressive symptomatology (10,13,14). There are also indications that clinicians' treatment choices for depressed patients with comorbid personality disorders may differ from those of patients with major depression alone (11,15,16).

While the pre-DSM-III literature in this area tends to address theoretical questions related to clinical observations of effects of personality traits on depressive illness (17), we will focus on the post-DSM-III literature, which has produced a wealth of information on the comorbidity of depression and personality disorders based on systematic assessments. The tables included here are intended to provide a concise guide to the extensive literature in this area. Among the 32 articles summarized in Table 1, the percentage of depressed patients interviewed with a semistructured personality disorder instrument who received a personality disorder diagnosis ranges from 16% to 93%, with a median of 47%. The median percentage of personality disorder comorbidity in samples with an index illness of dysthymia (Table 2) is 56%, with a range of 34–90%. These percentages include studies of inpatients and outpatients.

In this chapter, first we describe and summarize substantive comorbidity findings in the context of pre- and post-DSM-III time frames and grouped by family, i.e., epidemiological, and treatment, i.e., clinical, studies. We then address the broad conceptual, empirical and methodological, and modeling issues relevant to comorbidity, including discussion of depression and personality from the psychodynamic and interpersonal (18), methodological, diagnostic (19,20), and treatment (11) perspectives. Finally, we explore future directions in treatment and research.

The historical constant in our discussion is depression; many of the illness' DSM-IV signs and symptoms can be broadly correlated with ancient constructs of melancholia (7). Thus, there is a common language to clinical and research reports on depression. Early studies of dysthymia using DSM-III criteria found that up to 95% of patients with dysthymia also met criteria for major depression (21). These nosological redundancies led to revision of the criteria for dysthymia such that clinicians can differentiate between early- (before age 21) and late-onset dysthymia and distinguish dysthymia's more prolonged and insidious onset from major depression (22,23). Clarification of the criteria for dysthymia has resulted in a surge of publications exploring comorbidity in this disorder, and we will confine our discussion of dysthymia to these reports (23–26).

Research on personality pathology, on the other hand, especially as it affects a patient with an Axis I diagnosis of depression, has suffered until recently from mixed language and a general lack of attention in terms of empirical and epidemiological studies. The majority of pre-DSM-III articles in this area tend to speculate on the effects of personality pathology on depression but are often difficult to interpret (18) because they are unable systematically to differentiate between personality and depressive pathology. Post-DSM-III articles in this area, on the other hand, have generally been based on studies with rigorous selection and diagnostic criteria, use of control populations, and interview instruments with demonstrated interrater reliability.

II. BACKGROUND AND DEFINITION OF TERMS

The *Diagnostic and Statistical Manual of Mental Disorders*, fourth edition, groups major depressive disorders and dysthymia with the bipolar disorders under the rubric "mood disorders," with mood defined as prolonged emotion encompassing the entire psychic life (27). Depression and dysthymia are distinguished from the bipolar disorders in that there is an absence of one or more episodes of mania or hypomania. Major depressive disorder is characterized by "one or more major depressive episodes (i.e., at least two weeks of depressed mood or loss of interest accompanied by at least four additional symptoms of depression)." The lifetime risk of major depression in community samples is between 10 and 25% for women and 5 and 12% for men (28). Dysthymic disorder is characterized by "at least two years of depressed mood for more days than not, accompanied by additional depressive symptoms that do not meet criteria for a major depressive episode." According to DSM-IV, lifetime prevalence of dysthymia with or without superimposed major depression is 6%.

Personality *traits* are described by DSM-IV as "enduring patterns of perceiving, relating to, and thinking about the environment and oneself that are exhib-

Table 1 Prevalence of Personality Disorders in Populations with an Index Illness of Major Depression

Author	Population	Instrument and criteria	Prevalence of personality disorder	Comments/limitations
Agbayewa (1996)	Depressed inpatients over a 10-year period	Retrospective comparison chart review by psychiatrists for DSM-III and DSM-III-R Axis I; "best estimate approach" for chart diagnosis of Axis II	40% of the younger patients (mean age 40.2) met criteria for at least one PD; 27% of the elderly patients (mean age 71.6) met criteria for at least one PD	In the younger group, borderline PD was most frequent diagnosis after PD NOS; obsessive-compulsive and dependent PD's were the most common diagnoses in the elderly group
Casey et al. (1996)	40 inpatients with a diagnosis of major depression receiving ECT treatment	DSM-III-R Axis I instrument not specified; Personality Assessment Form (PAS) for ICD-10	45% of patients met criteria for at least one PD: Paranoid: 2.5% Schizoid: 2.5% Histrionic: 2.5% Explosive: 2.5% Asthenic: 5% Avoidant: 7.5% Anancastic: 10% Passive-dependent: 7.5% Sensitive-aggressive: 2.5% Dysthymic: 2.5%	Personality assessed after discharge from hospital; no impact of personality on short-term symptomatic recovery or on readmission to hospital during the follow-up period; obsessionality contributed to good outcome

Pepper et al. (1995)	45 outpatients with episodic major depression	SCID for DSM-III-R Axis I; PDE-R for DSM-III-R Axis II	18% of patients met criteria for at least one PD: Paranoid: 2% Schizotypal: 0% Schizoid: 0% Histrionic: 0% Narcissistic: 0% Borderline: 0% Antisocial: 0% Dependent: 2% Avoidant: 4% Obsessive-compulsive: 0% Passive-aggressive: 0% Self-defeating: 0% NOS: 11%	Large, clearly defined cohort, structured diagnostic interviews, and independent assessments of patients and informants
Patience et al. (1995)	113 patients with major depression	Clinical diagnosis of Axis I by DSM-III; PAS for DSM-III Axis II	26% of patients met criteria for at least one PD	
Oldham et al. (1995)	200 inpatients and outpatients with various Axis I disorders	SCID (nonpatient version) for DSM-III-R Axis I; SCID-II and PDE for DSM-III-R Axis II	78% of applicants for inpatient treatment of a DSM-III-R Axis I mood disorder (includes major depression, bipolar disorder, cyclothymia, and dysthymia) met criteria for at least one PD; 16% of applicants for psychoanalysis for the same group of mood disorders met criteria for at least one PD	Borderline personality disorder co-occurred significantly with all Axis I categories but mood disorders; this finding argues against the notion of borderline personality disorder as a subsyndromal form of depression; however, patients with mood disorder pathology did have elevated levels of borderline traits

(continued)

Table 1 Continued

Author	Population	Instrument and criteria	Prevalence of personality disorder	Comments/limitations
Golomb et al. (1995)	316 depressed outpatients (aged 18–65) enrolled in three clinical treatment trials	SCID-P for DSM-III-R Axis I; PDQ-R and SCID-II for DSM-III-R Axis II	Prevalence of PD assessed with the PDQ-R was 92% in the younger (18–41) group; and 91% in the older (42–65) group; PD prevalence assessed by the SCID-II was 55% in the younger group and 57% in the older group; comorbid prevalences as measured by the SCID-II:[a] Paranoid: 33% Schizotypal: 2% Schizoid: 4% Histrionic: 2% Narcissistic: 25% Borderline: 33% Antisocial: 6% Dependent: 23% Avoidant: 40% Obsessive-compulsive: 61% Passive-aggressive: 19%	Neither age group was more likely to meet criteria for a comorbid personality disorder as measured by the SCID-II; using the PDQ-R, the younger age group was significantly more likely to meet criteria for comorbid avoidant personality disorder; no association between age and comorbid personality disorder when Axis I diagnosis was controlled for
Kunik et al. (1994)	547 elderly inpatients grouped by DSM-III-R Axis I diagnoses	Consensus Axis I and Axis II diagnoses by research team according to DSM-III-R	24% of depressed patients met criteria for at least one PD	

Mulder et al. (1994)	104 depressed patients and 40 control subjects "recruited from a variety of sources"	SCID for DSM-III-R Axis I; SCID-PQ and SCID II for DSM-III-R Axis II	53% of patients met criteria for at least one PD:	
			Paranoid:	3%
			Schizotypal:	1%
			Schizoid:	0%
			Histrionic:	1%
			Narcissistic:	2%
			Borderline:	10%
			Antisocial:	4%
			Dependent:	4%
			Avoidant:	15%
			Obsessive-compulsive:	6%
			Passive-aggressive:	<1%
			Self-defeating:	7%
Fava et al. (1994)	83 outpatients with major depression	PDQ-R for DSM-III-R; subset ($n = 53$) assessed by clinician for DSM-III-R Axis II cluster B (only) with SCID-II	93% of patients met criteria for at least one PD diagnosis:	
			Cluster A:	76%
			Cluster B:	67%
			Cluster C:	67%

(continued)

Table 1 Continued

Author	Population	Instrument and criteria	Prevalence of personality disorder	Comments/limitations
Vine et al. (1994)	64 elderly (age ≥ 60) outpatients treated for depression	Axis II diagnosis at time of admission from patient records according to DSM-III-R; follow-up included SCID-II and SCID-II PQ for DSM-III-R Axis II	33% of patients met criteria for at least one PD at admission; 36% met criteria at follow-up: Paranoid: 0% Schizotypal: 0% Schizoid: 0% Histrionic: 3% Narcissistic: 10% Borderline: 0% Antisocial: 0% Dependent: 14% Avoidant: 0% Obsessive-compulsive: 6% Passive-aggressive: 0%	Presence of a personality disorder, particularly a cluster B PD, was associated with chronic outcome of depression and impaired social support; personality is a significant factor in the outcome of depression in the elderly
Andreoli et al. (1993)	31 patients assigned to outpatient crisis intervention for depressive symptoms	Psychiatrist assessment of DSM-III-R Axis I and Axis II (PD subtypes not assessed)	54% of patients met criteria for at least one PD	Presence of PD predicted a poorer 2-year outcome; PD subjects with better working alliance and increased insight at termination of crisis intervention had increased compliance with long-term psychiatric treatment and better 2-year outcome

Diguer et al. (1993)	25 outpatients with major depression	SADS-C for DSM-III-R Axis I; PAF for DSM-III-R Axis II	48% of patients met criteria for at least one PD	Depressed patients with comorbid PD diagnosis had more severe psychiatric disturbance at intake, termination of therapy, and at follow-up; although all patients improved and maintained their gains at follow-up, those with a comorbid PD diagnosis did not improve as much as those without a PD
Flick et al. (1993)	352 outpatients with anxiety and depression	SCID for DSM-III-R Axis I and SCID PQ followed by SCID II for DSM-III-R Axis II	61% of patients with depression met criteria for at least one PD	Major depression subjects did not differ from remainder of sample in frequency of occurrence of PDs; subjects with a PD had more severe symptoms of anxiety and depression than those without a PD
Marin et al. (1993)	68 consecutive evaluations in an outpatient clinic and inpatient psychiatric service	SCID for DSM-III-R Axis I and PDE for DSM-III-R Axis II	42% of depressed patients met criteria for at least one PD: Paranoid: 5% Schizotypal: 0% Schizoid: 0% Histrionic: 5% Narcissistic: 0%	Data suggest that dysthymics and episodic major depressives have comparable overall rates of personality disorders but quantitatively differ from each other on the distribution of personality pathology

(continued)

Table 1 Continued

Author	Population	Instrument and criteria	Prevalence of personality disorder	Comments/limitations
			Borderline: 11% Antisocial: 0% Dependent: 0% Avoidant: 5% Obsessive-compulsive: 0% Passive-aggressive: 0% NOS: 16%	
Stuart et al. (1992)	59 outpatients with acute unipolar depression	Semistructured initial evaluation for DSM-III-R Axis I; PDE for DSM-III-R Axis II	24% of patients met criteria for at least one PD at intake: Paranoid: 4% Schizotypal: 0% Schizoid: 0% Histrionic: 2% Narcissistic: 0% Borderline: 2% Antisocial: 9% Dependent: 7% Masochistic: 5% Avoidant: 2% Obsessive-compulsive: 2% Passive-aggressive: 0% NOS: 0%	Authors conclude that there may be a sizeable minority of acutely depressed outpatients who manifest state-dependent false-positive PD diagnoses that convey no useful information concerning illness correlates and prognosis

Sanderson et al. (1992)	292 consecutive outpatients with mutually exclusive diagnoses of major depression, dysthymia, and double depression	SCID-P for DSM-III-R Axis I; SCID-II for DSM-III-R Axis II	50% of patients met criteria for at least one PD: Paranoid: 2% Schizotypal: <1% Schizoid: 0% Histrionic: 4% Narcissistic: 3% Borderline: 4% Antisocial: 2% Dependent: 15% Avoidant: 12% Obsessive-compulsive: 9% Passive-aggressive: 7% NOS: 8%	Patients with dysthymia did not have a higher rate of personality disorders than patients with major depression
Maier et al. (1992)	Family study with 109 control probands matched to 555 consecutively admitted inpatients with affective or schizophrenic disorders	SADS-LA for DSM-III Axis I; SCID-II for DSM-III-R Axis II	23% of subjects with unipolar MDD met criteria for at least one PD: Cluster A: 15.4% Cluster B: 33.3% Cluster C: 19.2%	Tested hypothesis that Axis I disorders and personality disorders are not occurring independently; the community sample in this study showed that associations between affective disorders and borderline PD and between anxiety disorders and avoidant PD were significant

(*continued*)

Table 1 Continued

Author	Population	Instrument and criteria	Prevalence of personality disorder	Comments/limitations
Jackson et al. (1991)	30 inpatients with unipolar affective disorder	SCID-P for DSM-III-R Axis I; SID-P for DSM-III Axis II	Overall prevalence for depressed patients with at least one PD not given: Paranoid: 13% Schizotypal: 23% Schizoid: 0% Histrionic: 33% Narcissistic: 3% Borderline: 53% Antisocial: 0% Dependent: 40% Avoidant: 33% Obsessive-compulsive: 13% Passive-aggressive: 17%	
Alnaes et al. (1991)	289 consecutive outpatients, 97 of whom were diagnosed with unipolar major depression	SCID-I for DSM-III Axis I; SID-P for DSM-III Axis II	85% of depressed patients met criteria for at least one PD: Paranoid: 8% Schizotypal: 6% Schizoid: 1% Histrionic: 16% Narcissistic: 2% Borderline: 16% Antisocial: 0% Dependent: 54% Avoidant: 62% Compulsive: 21%	

Casey et al. (1990)	"Patients who presented to a general practitioner and were recognized as having a primary psychiatric abnormality"	Present State Examination (PSE) for ICD-9; PAS for ICD-98	19% of patients with an ICD-9 diagnosis of neurotic depression were diagnosed with at least one PD	
Fogel et al. (1990)	2322 inpatients with diagnosis of major depression	Chart review for ICD-9 diagnoses of major depression and personality disorders	16% of patients met criteria for at least one PD	
O'Boyle et al. (1990)	20 inpatients with major depression	SCID-P for DSM-III-R Axis I disorders; SCID II and PDE for DSM-III-R Axis II	55% of patients met criteria for at least one PD. Interinstrument agreement diagnoses: Paranoid: 40% Schizotypal: 15% Schizoid: 0% Histrionic: 15% Narcissistic: 0% Borderline: 30% Antisocial: 0% Dependent: 25% Avoidant: 20% Compulsive: 15% Passive-aggressive: 10% Self-defeating: 10%	Diagnostic agreement between instruments for any disorder was fair (kappa = 0.38); depressive state did not consistently affect categorical diagnoses, although dimensional scores were higher during depressive episode

(continued)

Table 1 Continued

Author	Population	Instrument and criteria	Prevalence of personality disorder	Comments/limitations
Zimmerman et al. (1989)	797 first-degree relatives of normal controls and patients with a variety of psychiatric disorders	DIS for DSM-III Axis I disorders; SID-P for DSM-III Axis II	47% of relatives with major depression met criteria for at least one PD: Paranoid: 2% Schizotypal: 13% Schizoid: 0% Histrionic: 10% Narcissistic: 0% Borderline: 7% Antisocial: 8% Dependent: 3% Avoidant: 7% Obsessive-compulsive: 4% Passive-aggressive: 9%	
Thompson et al. (1988)	79 elderly (age ≥ 60) depressed outpatients	SADS-C for RDC diagnosis of MDD; SIDP for DSM-III Axis II	33% met PD criteria "when usual self"; 66% met PD criteria during episode Principal diagnoses: self : episode: Paranoid: 0% : 4% Schizotypal: 0% : 0% Schizoid: 1% : 1% Histrionic: 0% : 0% Narcissistic: 1% : 0% Borderline: 3% : 4% Antisocial: 0% : 0% Dependent: 8% : 17% Avoidant: 8% : 21%	Interviewed subjects 12–24 months after treatment and asked them to rate each PD criteria with instructions to describe personality: 1. "When you are your usual self"; 2. "During a depressive episode"

			Obsessive-compulsive: 5% : 4% Passive-aggressive: 4% : 4% Mixed: 3% : 16%	
Zimmerman et al. (1988)	66 depressed inpatients	SCID-I for DSM-III Axis I disorders; SID-P for DSM-III Axis II	36% met criteria for at least one PD based on patient report only; 65% met criteria based on patient and informant report: Consensus prevalences: Paranoid: 6% Schizotypal: 5% Schizoid: 3% Histrionic: 26% Narcissistic: 8% Borderline: 24% Antisocial: 15% Dependent: 15% Avoidant: 3% Compulsive: 11% Passive-aggressive: 17% Mixed: 12%	
Black et al. (1988)	228 patients with major depressive disorder	Chart diagnosis made using DSM-III criteria for Axis II; at baseline, patient charts were divided into PD+ and PD– groups.	50% of patients met criteria for at least one PD Paranoid: 1% Schizotypal: 1% Schizoid: 8% Histrionic: 16% Narcissistic: 0%	Used "naturalistic design" based on chart review of patients over 10-year period

(continued)

Table 1 Continued

Author	Population	Instrument and criteria	Prevalence of personality disorder	Comments/limitations
			Borderline: 26% Antisocial: 22% Dependent: 18% Avoidant: 5% Compulsive: 1% Passive-aggressive: 8% Mixed: 8% NOS: 4%	
Pilkonis et al. (1988)	119 treatment-responsive patients with recurrent unipolar depression; patients were experiencing at least their third episode of major, unipolar depression	SADS for DSM-III Axis I; Hirschfeld-Klerman Personality Battery (self-report) and PAF for DSM-III Axis II	48% of patients met criteria for at least one PD: Avoidant: 30% Compulsive: 19% Dependent: 16% (others not given)	A discriminant function analysis using personality variables alone was able to distinguish (with 65% accuracy) between patients who responded normally to treatment and those who responded more slowly
Shea et al. (1987)	249 outpatients with major depression	SADS for DSM-III Axis I; PAF for DSM-III Axis II	35% of patients met criteria for at least one PD: Paranoid: 5% Schizotypal: <1% Schizoid: 0% Histrionic: 4% Narcissistic: <1% Borderline: 2% Antisocial: 0%	PD patients had more frequent and more chronic periods of depression, were more likely to be diagnosed as endogenous by the RDC criteria, and reported higher distress levels on multiple dimensions of general symptomatology

			Dependent: 6% Avoidant: 13% Compulsive: 13% Passive-aggressive: 1%	
Kocsis et al. (1986)	26 outpatients with major depression	Diagnoses based on "semistructured interview by research psychiatrists" for DSM-III Axis I and Axis II	40% of patients met criteria for at least one PD	
Koenigsberg et al. (1985)	2462 medical center patients (in- and out-) evaluated by psychiatric residents over 18-month period	Diagnoses based on chart review for DSM-III Axis I and Axis II	23% of depressed patients met criteria for at least one PD	Interrater reliability not available. Ratings based on chart review; Axis I florid symptoms may have taken treatment priority
Pfohl et al. (1984)	78 inpatients with major depression	"Structured interview" for RDC endogenous depression; SID-P for DSM-III Axis II	53% of patients met criteria for at least one PD	Patients with comorbid PDs showed less improvement by discharge, poorer response to antidepressant medication, and decreased treatment response at 6 months

(continued)

Table 1 Continued

Author	Population	Instrument and criteria	Prevalence of personality disorder	Comments/limitations
Charney et al. (1981)	64 nonmelancholic unipolar depressed patients	Retrospective chart review for DSM-III major depression; personality disorder assessed independently by two psychiatrists using DSM-III definitions	61% of patients met criteria for at least one PD	Personality disorder was significantly more common in unipolar nonmelancholic depressed patients (61%) than in unipolar melancholic (14%) or bipolar depressed patients (23%); personality disorder did not affect symptom manifestation but was related to earlier onset of depressive illness and worse outcome within the unipolar nonmelancholic group

[a]Overall prevalence of personality disorders given may be less than percentage totals of individual PDs because patients may have met criteria for more than one PD or PD cluster.

ited in a wide range of social and personal contexts" (28). DSM-IV defines personality *disorders* as inflexible and maladaptive personality *traits* that cause either significant functional impairment or subjective distress. The personality disorders are grouped in three clusters: (A) paranoid, schizoid, and schizotypal disorders, characterized by odd or eccentric behavior; (B) histrionic, narcissistic, antisocial, and borderline disorders, characterized by dramatic, erratic, or emotional behavior; and (C) avoidant, dependant, and obsessive-compulsive disorders, characterized by anxious or fearful behavior. DSM-IV also includes three "experimental" disorders: self-defeating, depressive, and negativistic. DSM-III and DSM-III-R included passive-aggressive personality disorder in cluster C, but this was eliminated (29). Personality disorders have an estimated prevalence of 10% in epidemiological samples (29).

The personality disorders are coded on Axis II in the DSM-IV nomenclature, with this caveat: "The personality traits that define these disorders must also be distinguishable from characteristics that emerge in response to specific situational stressors or more transient mental states (e.g., Mood or Anxiety Disorders, Substance Intoxication). The clinician should assess the stability of personality traits over time and across different situations" (28). In other words, the diagnosis of personality disorders should not be made if the characteristics occur only during episodes of an Axis I disorder (29).

Comorbidity, as defined in general medicine, is "any distinct additional clinical entity that has existed or that may occur during the clinical course of a patient who has the index disease under study" (11,30). Psychiatric comorbidity has received considerable attention in recent years, especially in light of the findings of the National Comorbidity Survey (31), which concluded that the prevalence of psychiatric comorbidity is higher than previously thought. The survey further found that the observed comorbidity is concentrated in approximately one-sixth of the population with a history of three or more comorbid disorders. There is a difference between comorbidity as defined by general medicine and the psychiatric comorbidity we are examining. For example, there is a clear difference in the "comorbid" status of a patient with leukemia who contracts a bacterial infection and a patient with major depressive disorder comorbid with dependent personality disorder. In psychiatry, making clear-cut distinctions regarding etiology and diagnoses can be difficult. There is some nosological overlap, for example, between a depressed patient's depressive and dependent pathology. This overlap stems from the lack of definitive evidence concerning the etiology of these disorders and may result in substantially distorted assessments (11). Klerman noted this issue (32) by pointing out that DSM-III-R's "multiaxial system is 'agnostic' with respect to any implications of a causative relationship for specific conditions listed in Axis I and II" (11). We will explore these interrelated issues of the definition and classification of depressive disorders and personality disorders in detail.

Table 2 Prevalence of Personality Disorders in Populations with an Index Illness of Dysthymia

Author	Population	Instrument and criteria	Prevalence	Comments/limitations
Shelton et al. (1997)	410 outpatients with dysthymia, primary type, early onset without concurrent MDD	SCID-P for DSM-III-R Axis I; SCID II for DSM-III-R Axis II	68% of patients met criteria for at least one PD: Cluster A: 11% Cluster B: 12% Cluster C: 47% Dependent: 8% Avoidant: 25% Obsessive-compulsive: 23% Passive-aggressive: 9% Self-defeating: 11% (Others not given)	Dysthymic patients in this sample were found to be significantly undertreated; comorbid personality disorder increased the likelihood of prior psychotherapy (71% vs. 50%) while having no effect on past pharmacotherapy
Pepper et al. (1995)	97 outpatients with early-onset dysthymia	SCID for DSM-III-R Axis I; PDE-R for DSM-III-R Axis II	60% of patients met criteria for at least one PD: Paranoid: 11% Schizotypal: 4% Schizoid: 2% Histrionic: 14% Narcissistic: 4% Borderline: 24% Antisocial: 4% Dependent: 9% Avoidant: 16% Obsessive-compulsive: 4% Passive-aggressive: 2% Self-defeating: 10% NOS: 9%	Contrary to SCID instructions, the dysthymia section was not skipped for patients who had experienced major depressive episodes for more than 50% of the past 2 years; clearly defined cohort, structured diagnostic interviews, and independent assessments of patients and informants

Flick et al. (1993)	352 outpatients with anxiety and depressive disorders	SCID for DSM-III-R Axis I and SCID PQ followed by SCID II for DSM-III-R Axis II	71% of patients met criteria for at least one PD	Subjects with dysthymia were more likely than the rest of the sample to have a PD
Marin et al. (1993)	68 out- and inpatients with dysthymia but without concurrent MDD	SCID for DSM-III-R Axis I; PDE for DSM-III-R Axis II	40% of patients met criteria for at least one PD: Paranoid: 4% Schizotypal: 0% Schizoid: 0% Histrionic: 0% Narcissistic: 0% Borderline: 0% Antisocial: 0% Dependent: 8% Avoidant: 12% Obsessive-compulsive: 4% Passive-aggressive: 4% NOS: 24%	Authors speculate that high rates of anxious cluster diagnoses in the dysthymic group may reflect diagnostic overlap between dysthymia and cluster C personality disorders
Sanderson et al. (1992)	292 consecutive outpatients with mutually exclusive diagnoses of major depression, dysthymia, and double depression	SCID-P for DSM-III-R Axis I; SCID-II for DSM-III-R Axis II	52% of patients with dysthymia met criteria for at least one PD: Paranoid: 3% Schizotypal: 2% Schizoid: 0% Histrionic: 2% Narcissistic: 6% Borderline: 8% Antisocial: 2% Dependent: 8% Avoidant: 22% Obsessive-compulsive: 13% Passive-aggressive: 3% NOS: 6%	Among patients who received a personality disorder diagnosis, those with dysthymic disorder had a significantly higher incidence of two personality disorders than those with major depression or double depression

(continued)

Table 2 Continued

Author	Population	Instrument and criteria	Prevalence	Comments/limitations
Markowitz et al. (1992)	34 outpatients with dysthymia	SCID-P for DSM-III Axis I; SCID-II for DSM-III Axis II	85% of patients met criteria for at least one PD: Paranoid: 3% Schizotypal: 12% Schizoid: 0% Histrionic: 12% Narcissistic: 6% Borderline: 24% Antisocial: 0% Dependent: 21% Avoidant: 32% Obsessive-compulsive: 6% Passive-aggressive: 0% Self-defeating: 35% NOS: 18%	High PD comorbidity hypothesized to reflect either oversensitivity of the SCID-II or possibility that dysthymics may be diagnosed on Axis II under guise of self-defeating, avoidant, and perhaps borderline and dependent PDs; data are reported to contradict assertion of some that dysthymia generally postdates anxiety disorders
Alnaes et al. (1991)	289 consecutive outpatients, 18 of whom were diagnosed with dysthymia	SCID-I for DSM-III Axis I; SID-P for DSM-III Axis II	90% of dysthymic patients met criteria for at least one PD: Paranoid: 2% Schizotypal: 11% Schizoid: 2% Histrionic: 4% Narcissistic: 6% Borderline: 15% Antisocial: 0% Dependent: 53% Avoidant: 68% Compulsive: 26% Passive-aggressive: 11%	Small sample size may limit findings

Tyrer et al. (1990)	65 patients with dysthymic disorder	Comprehensive Psychopathological Rating Scale (CPRS) for DSM-III Axis I; PAS for DSM-III Axis II	51% of patients met criteria for at least one PD	Patients with PD comorbidity responded less well to treatment; PD category did not appear to influence symptoms
Kocsis et al. (1986)	39 outpatients with dysthymia	Diagnoses based on "semistructured interview by research psychiatrists" for DSM-III Axis I and Axis II	47% of patients met criteria for at least one PD: Paranoid: 0% Schizotypal: 8% Schizoid: 0% Histrionic: 0% Narcissistic: 8% Borderline: 0% Antisocial: 0% Dependent: 23% Avoidant: 10% Obsessive-compulsive: 5% Passive-aggressive: 0%	95% of chronic depressives (dysthymics) fulfilled DSM-III criteria for major depressive disorder in addition to their dysthymic disorder, and 59% also met criteria for melancholia
Koenigsberg et al. (1985)	2462 medical center patients evaluated by psychiatric residents over 18-month period	DSM-III Axis I and Axis II diagnoses made by chart review	34% of dysthymic patients met criteria for at least one PD	Approximately half of the dysthymic disorder patients with Axis II diagnoses were classified in the mixed-atypical-other PD category and about 20% were classified in each of the borderline and dependent personality disorder categories

III. SUBSTANTIVE FINDINGS

A. Comorbid Prevalence Studies Using Family Samples

1. *Pre-DSM-III*

We are not aware of any data concerning the epidemiological prevalence of comorbidity of depression and personality disorders prior to DSM-III.

2. *Post-DSM-III*

Comorbidity studies of the "true," i.e., epidemiological, prevalence of depression and personality disorders have been rare. In one of the first nonpatient studies to examine comorbidity of various Axis I disorders with Axis II personality disorders, Zimmerman and Coryell (33) found that among a group of first-degree relatives of normal controls and patients with a variety of psychiatric disorders, 47% of the individuals with major depression also met criteria for at least one personality disorder. The most frequent personality disorder diagnoses were histrionic, borderline, and avoidant, and the most infrequently diagnosed disorders were paranoid, schizoid, and narcissistic disorders. In the same study, 48% of individuals with dysthymia met criteria for at least one personality disorder (33).

In an attempt to provide an estimate of comorbidity in a community sample, Maier et al (34) studied lifetime personality disorder diagnoses in families of randomly recruited control probands and found that 23% of subjects with a DSM-III diagnosis of depression met criteria for at least one DSM-III-R personality disorder. The discrepancy between these studies (47% vs. 23% comorbid prevalence) might be explained by the lower base rate of individual disorders in Maier's sample (34). An alternative explanation may lie in the different instruments used in these studies. Zimmerman and Coryell used the Structured Interview for Diagnosing Personality Disorders (SID-P) by telephone interview. Maier et al., on the other hand, utilized the SCID-II for Axis II assessment and all interviews were conducted in person.

One interesting study found in a family medical practice setting that primary-care patients who were not diagnosed with a personality disorder but were at high risk for personality disorder based on a SCID-II screening interview had a higher risk for depression or alcohol abuse and lower functional status (35). In particular, patients at high risk for schizoid, borderline, and dependent personality disorders had the highest risk of depression, and patients who were at high risk for narcissistic, schizotypal, antisocial, and obsessive-compulsive disorders had the fewest depressive symptoms (35).

B. Comorbid Prevalence in Patient Samples

1. *Pre-DSM-III*

Several early studies analyzed the relationship between personality and depression by identifying aspects of personality that may serve as predictors of depression or as modifiers of depressive symptomatology. Some of these reports (5,6,8), but not all (36,37), show that the depressive state increases levels of neuroticism and decreases levels of extraversion (38). In a mid-1960s study of 35 depressed female inpatients, Lazare and Klerman described the clinical features of patients with significant "hysterical" personality profiles, including "demanding, dependent, seductive, histrionic, and egocentric" traits. Among patients with hysterical personalities, they found a trend for less improvement with electroconvulsive therapy (ECT). Two earlier studies also noted poor response of hysterical patients to ECT (39–41). In a follow-up study of 150 women who had undergone treatment for depression, the most important factor for prediction of a long-term negative outcome after treatment was the Neuroticism Scale of the Maudsley Personality Inventory (3). The conclusions of some of these early studies may have been affected by a lack of systematic personality assessments and diagnostic correlates. This situation changed with the publication of DSM-III in 1980.

2. *Post-DSM-III*

The advent of DSM-III and its multiaxial diagnostic system opened the door to a more detailed exploration of the relationship between personality disorders and depression. In spite of the clarification of terms and categorical distinctions that DSM-III provided, the comorbidity literature includes mixed and occasionally conflicting results (42). However, a common finding of recent studies, including several that utilize DSM-III-R or DSM-IV criteria, supports the suggestions of earlier work, namely that comorbid personality disorder has an adverse effect on the outcome of treatment for major depressive disorders (43) and that patients with a personality disorder tend to have higher levels of depressive symptomatology (13). Furthermore, one treatment study (44) showed that discriminant function analysis using personality variables alone distinguished (with 65% accuracy) between depressed patients who responded normally to treatment and those who responded more slowly. Several studies have shown that recovery from depression in patients with personality disorders is slower, particularly as measured in terms of social recovery (45,46), although there have been conflicting results (12,47). As measured by rehospitalization, some researchers have found that personality does not predict relapse (9,16), whereas others have found that personality disorder patients have a higher rate of rehospitalization (15,48).

In a longitudinal twin study of major depressive disorder and personality in women, Kendler et al. found that there was a substantial relationship between neuroticism and liability to major depression, supporting pre-DSM-III findings (38). Tyrer et al. (49) found that patients with dysthymia and cormorbid personality disorders responded less well to treatment. However, poor outcome was also found among dysthymic patients without personality disorder comorbidity. The authors concluded that the chronic course of dysthymic patients overall contributed to these results (49).

These reports are among those that contributed to early suggestions that a history of personality problems or maladaptive personality traits was a predictor of a poor prognosis in patients with depression. A hypothesis advanced by Akiskal et al. (20) for poorer treatment prognosis is that patients with comorbid depression and personality disorders have a different, less biologically based disorder. Support for this view comes from studies demonstrating that patients with depressive and personality disorders are less likely to show the biological abnormality of dexamethasone nonsuppression (9,11,15,50), although there are indications that the dexamethasone test is subject to a variety of confounding influences (51).

Given these predictions of poor outcome in patients with comorbid depressive and personality disorders, one might ask if there are any mitigating or protective factors that improve treatment outcome in this group. Andreoli's study of "crisis intervention" treatment of depressed outpatients found that the presence of personality disorder at intake predicted a poorer 2-year outcome. But within this comorbid group, the authors found the establishment of a better treatment alliance increased compliance with long-term treatment and resulted in an improved 2-year outcome. Early identification and management of personality abnormalities in comorbid patients was thus hypothesized to be an important element in effective treatment of these patients' depressive disorders, as was a longer treatment course (11,52).

Also, it has been found that depressed patients with small social networks are less likely to recover than patients with larger social networks (53). Tyrer et al. (54) found that among patients with various Axis I disorders (more than 50% of which were depressive disorders), social networks were smaller among patients with comorbid personality disorders. More research is required to establish whether reduced social networks in patients with depression and personality disorders are a cause or consequence of either disorder and thus how this factor may be integrated into psychotherapy (54,55).

The broad characteristics of comorbidity of personality disorders and depressive disorders may be quite variable when examined at the level of individual personality disorders. We will further summarize substantive comorbidity findings with the cluster A, B, and C disorders before we move on to their conceptual underpinnings and related empirical issues.

C. Comorbidity with Cluster A Personality Disorders

The cluster A personality disorders, characterized by odd or eccentric behavior, have been found to be comorbid with depression less frequently than (9) or as frequently as clusters B and C. Among the depression articles reviewed in Table 1, the median prevalence of paranoid personality disorder among depressed individuals is 5% (range 0–40%), the median prevalence of schizotypal personality disorder is 1% (range 0–23%), and the median prevalence of schizoid personality disorder is 0% (range 0–8%). The generally low incidence of schizotypal personality disorder comorbidity may be a result of exclusionary criteria applied by most researchers to individuals with schizophrenia-spectrum symptoms (10). Also, comparison of the effect of cluster A personality disorders on the outcome of treatment for major depression has occasionally not been possible because of inadequate numbers of cases within the cluster (56).

Among the dysthymia articles reviewed in Table 2, the median prevalence of paranoid personality disorder among individuals with dysthymia is 3% (range 0–11%), the median prevalence of schizotypal personality disorder is 6% (range 0–12%), and the median prevalence of schizoid personality disorder is 0% (range 0–2%).

Peselow et al. (57) found that cluster A and C personality traits assessed during a depressive episode tended to decrease after successful clinical treatment, although cluster A and B categorical diagnoses were unchanged, regardless of recovery. The authors speculated that the difference between traits before and after recovery may have been due to an inability of raters to distinguish withdrawal associated with depression from the aloofness and coldness associated with schizoid personality disorder. That is, personality pathology appeared to diminish when it may actually have been an expression of depression (57). In the NIMH Collaborative Study of Personality Disorders and Treatment Outcome of Depression, Shea et al. (58) found that although patients with personality disorders as a group had a significantly worse outcome in social functioning and were significantly more likely to have residual depressive symptoms, outcome was similar for patients in each of the three personality disorder clusters. With regard to clusters A and B, however, these results are difficult to generalize because the study excluded subjects with schizotypal features and antisocial personality disorder (58).

A study of the influences of temperament and childhood environment on comorbidity of personality disorders found that depressed patients with a low reward dependence score on the Tridimensional Personality Questionnaire (TPQ) (59) were more likely to have a personality disorder, especially in cluster A. The reward dependence construct is defined as a heritable influence on the maintenance or continuation of behaviors manifested by sentimentality, persistence, social attachment, and dependence on approval by others (59). Cloninger et al., who developed the TPQ, reported an association between lower reward dependence scores (i.e., less sentimental, fewer social attachments) and immature character development (60). However, a number of studies found no significant association of cluster A personality disorders with outcome of treatment for depression (2). Benjamin (61) suggested that individuals with schizoid (and paranoid and antisocial) personality disorders tend to be resistant to depression because they are not dependent, self-critical, or sensitive to rejection.

Sato et al. (62), on the other hand, found that presence of a cluster A personality disorder was associated with a poorer outcome of treatment for depression, even in patients receiving adequate antidepressant treatment. This adverse outcome was hypothesized to result from the combined effect that the social anhedonia, withdrawal, and flat affect that characterize schizoid and schizotypal personality disorders might have on diminished social support and hence a poorer outcome. However, because of Sato's small sample size, examination of the specific personality disorders within the clusters was not possible (62).

We now turn to the cluster B and C personality disorders, which have generally been found to have higher rates of comorbidity with depressive disorders and have received significant clinical and research attention.

D. Comorbidity with Cluster B Personality Disorders

In Table 1, the median prevalence of histrionic personality disorder among depressed patients is 4% (range 0–33%), the median prevalence of narcissistic personality disorder is 1% (range 0–25%), the median prevalence for borderline personality disorder is 10% (range 0–53%), and the median prevalence for antisocial personality disorder is 1% (range 0–22%).

Among studies of dysthymia in Table 2, the median prevalence of histrionic personality disorder is 3% (range 0–14%), the median prevalence of narcissistic personality disorder is 6% (range 0–8%), the median prevalence of borderline personality disorder is 11.5% (range 0–24%), and the median prevalence of antisocial personality disorder is 0% (range 0–4%).

Within cluster B, borderline personality disorder has received the most attention based in part on the suggestion that it is a subsyndromal form of depression (63) and because it is the most frequently reported personality disorder diagnosis among depressed inpatients (64,65). The flamboyant, aggressive, or self-destructive behavior characteristic of patients with cluster B disorders might explain their increased prevalence in inpatient settings.

In a study comparing patients with borderline personality disorder with groups of subjects with antisocial personality and bipolar II illness, Perry (66) found that lifetime prevalence of DSM-III major depression was high in all groups. Ninety-three percent of subjects with antisocial personality disorder and 87% of subjects with a diagnosis of borderline personality disorder reported a history of DSM-III major depression (66).

Pope et al. followed patients with borderline personality disorder over time and found that those with comorbid affective disorders had a better outcome and were more likely to have positive response to pharmacological treatment (67). However, another similar study with a longer follow-up period found few significant differences between borderline patients with or without depression (68). The latter study did find that borderline personality disorder comorbidity is associated with earlier onset of major depression, a fairly consistent result (15,68).

The comorbidity of antisocial personality disorders and depression has received less attention than the other disorders in cluster B, partly because antisocial personality traits have been an exclusion criterion for a number of studies (58,69). Clayton and Lewis found that the frequency of depression in patients with antisocial personality disorder who made outpatient emergency room visits ranged from 28% to 63% (70). There are sparse data on the impact of depressive symptoms on the outcome of treatment for personality disorders, but there is some evidence that depressive symptoms may be a favorable indicator for treatment of patients with a primary diagnosis of antisocial personality disorder or borderline personality disorder (11). Woody et al (71), for example, found that treatment response of opiate-dependent men with antisocial personality disorder and symptoms of depression showed significant improvement on measures of psychiatric symptoms, employment, drug use, and illegal activities. Antisocial patients without depression showed little improvement (11,71).

In a study comparing response to fluoxetine treatment among a group of outpatients with major depression, Fava et al. (69) found that patients who lost a cluster A or cluster C diagnosis after treatment experienced a more significant drop in depressive symptoms than patients who kept cluster A and C diagnoses. However, loss or maintenance of a cluster B personality disorder among depressed patients was not associated with significant changes in severity of depressive symptoms, leading the authors to hypothesize that depressed patients with a cluster B diagnosis experience alterations in pathological behavior patterns independent of associated symptoms of depression (69).

Oldham et al. (72) found that borderline personality disorder co-occurred significantly with all Axis I categories except mood disorders. In their study of Axis I and II comorbidity in 200 in- and outpatients, they found that mood disorders co-occurred significantly with avoidant personality disorder (cluster C) but not with cluster A or B (72). Mulder et al. found that more depressed patients in their sample had more cluster C than cluster B personality disorders (59).

What is the explanation for such diverse findings? One answer may lie in the variation in interview methods utilized to distinguish borderline symptoms from depressive symptoms. Depression seen in borderline personality disorder patients has been described as characterized by feelings of loneliness, emptiness, boredom, inner sense of badness, and deprivation (73). This contrasts with the depression of a mood disorder, which more often involves feelings of remorse, guilt, and failure in self-esteem. A significant characteristic of mood in borderline personality disorder is the degree to which affectivity tends to be reactive (74). This aspect of the disorder is incorporated in the DSM-IV description of the typical affect of borderline patients. For example, individuals with borderline personality disorder are likely to become depressed in response to a perceived object loss. Benjamin has suggested that individuals with borderline personality disorder and with dependent, histrionic, and passive-aggressive personality disorders may also be more likely to become depressed because they share the trait of dependency (61).

Another explanation for the heterogeneity of these results emerges from a handful of pharmacological treatment studies that indicate that the qualitative distinctions among different facets of the cluster B personality disorders may be the expression of biologically distinct subtypes of depression (11). For example, Liebowitz et al.'s (75) controlled treatment study of atypical depression (major depression or dysthymia with reactive mood and other atypical symptoms) found that phenelzine was superior for outcome on borderline and labile personality traits, interpersonal sensitivity, and "touchiness" (11,75; see Table 3). Detailed analysis of treatment response of subjects with borderline pathology to specific pharmacological treatment demonstrated that phenelzine treatment was significantly superior for treatment of patients with atypical depression and four or more borderline symptoms (76). More research across heterogeneous patient samples is necessary to verify the hypothesis that differential response to pharmacological treatment indicates a link to distinct biological substrates.

Recent reports on the comorbidity of dysthymia indicate that early-onset dysthymia may be associated with higher rates of cluster B personality disorder comorbidity than have been found for major depression (25). Markowitz et al. found that dysthymic patients were significantly more likely than patients with other Axis I conditions (more than 50% of which were depression) to have borderline personality disorder (23). These findings were not replicated in another study by Marin et al. (26) comparing prevalence of personality disorder among dysthymic and depressed patients. Marin et al. found that major depression patients were more likely to meet criteria for a cluster B personality disorder whereas dysthymic patients were more likely to receive a cluster C diagnosis (26).

E. Comorbidity with Cluster C Personality Disorders

As mentioned above, the personality disorder most frequently diagnosed among depressed *inpatients* is borderline personality disorder. Among *outpatient* samples, the most frequent personality disorder diagnoses are obsessive-compulsive and avoidant personality disorders, followed by dependent personality disorder (10,12,44).

Among the depression articles reviewed in Table 1 (which include both inpatient and outpatient samples), the median prevalence of dependent personality disorder in depressed subjects is 14.5% (range 0–54%), the median prevalence of avoidant personality disorder is 8% (range 0–62%), the median prevalence of obsessive-compulsive personality disorder is 9.5% (range 0–61%), and the median prevalence of passive-aggressive personality disorder is 5.5% (range 0–19%).

Among the dysthymia articles reviewed in Table 2, the median prevalence of dependent personality disorder is 9% (range 8–53%), the median prevalence of avoidant personality disorder is 22% (range 10–68%), the median prevalence of obsessive-compulsive personality disorder is 6% (range 4–26%), and the median prevalence of passive-aggressive personality disorder is 3% (range 0–11%).

Many studies have found significantly elevated rates of co-occurrence of mood disorders with avoidant and dependent personality disorders (45,72, 77,78). The increased prevalence of the cluster C personality disorders in depressed outpatients might be expected given the anxiety, introversion, and avoidance that characterize this cluster.

Hardy et al. (12) found significant differences in treatment response among a group of depressed patients stratified by severity of depression and presence or absence of a cluster C personality disorder. Twenty-four percent of the sample received a diagnosis of one or more cluster C personality disorders; this group began treatment with more severe symptomatology (12). Patients completed sessions of either cognitive-behavioral or psychodynamic-interpersonal therapy, and personality-disordered patients had significantly poorer outcomes than non-personality-disordered patients in psychodynamic-interpersonal therapy but not in cognitive-behavioral therapy. The authors noted that this finding supports conjecture by Shea et al. (58) that depressed patients with comorbid personality disorders respond more favorably to the structure of cognitive and behavioral treatment (12). The results of Hardy's study did not replicate previous findings that cluster C patients respond more slowly to treatment (44,79). Nor did it show, as others have suggested, (80,81) that longer-term treatment is more effective for depressed patients with a cluster C diagnosis (12).

Reich (84) and others (82,83) have found that those with a more severe clinical state of depression have higher dependence scores; as such, the finding appears to be an artifact of measurement of clinical state rather than an indication of a direct relationship between depression and dependent personality disorder (84; see Table 4).

Casey et al. (16) studied depressed patients with and without personality disorders who were receiving ECT treatment. Their results showed that personality had no effect on short-term symptomatic recovery from depression or readmission rates during a 12-month follow-up period. They did find that high ratings of obsessionality contributed to a positive treatment response, confirming an earlier report (16,85). In terms of vulnerability to depression among the cluster C personality disorders, Benjamin (61) suggested that "persons with avoidant personality disorder are vulnerable to depression because of their tendency to

Table 3 Prevalence of Personality Disorders in Populations with an Index Illness of Another Depressive Disorder

Author	Population	Instrument and criteria	Prevalence	Comments/limitations
Sanderson et al. (1992)	292 consecutive outpatients with mutually exclusive diagnoses of major depression, dysthymia, and double depression	SCID-P for DSM-III-R Axis I; SCID-II for DSM-III-R Axis II	69% of patients with double depression met criteria for at least one PD: Paranoid: 0% Schizotypal: 3% Schizoid: 0% Histrionic: 0% Narcissistic: 3% Borderline: 16% Antisocial: 3% Dependent: 19% Avoidant: 16% Obsessive-compulsive: 9% Passive-aggressive: 3% NOS: 9%	

Maier et al. (1992)	Family study with 109 control probands matched to 555 consecutively admitted inpatients with affective or schizophrenic disorders	SADS-LA for DSM III Axis I; SCID-II for DSM-III-R Axis II	Overall PD prevalence in subjects with "other affective disorder," i.e., minor, intermittent depression, hypomania, not given. Cluster A: 39% Cluster B: 44% Cluster C: 42%	Tested hypothesis that Axis I disorders and personality disorders are not occurring independently; the community sample in this study showed that associations between affective disorders and borderline PD and between anxiety disorders and avoidant PD were significant
Koenigsberg et al. (1985)	2462 medical center patients evaluated by psychiatric residents over 18-month period	DSM III Axis I and Axis II diagnoses made by chart review	38% of atypical depressive patients met criteria for at least one PD	Of the atypical depressive disorder patients with Axis II diagnoses, one-third had borderline personality disorder, 20% schizotypal disorder, 20% passive-aggressive disorder, 20% mixed-atypical disorder, and 7% dependent personality disorder

Table 4 Prevalence of Depression and/or Dysthymia in Samples with Personality Disorders

Author	Population	Criteria and instrument	Prevalence	Comments/limitations
Reich et al. (1996)	Male outpatients with a diagnosis of dependent PD	Structured Interview for DSM-III-R Axis I; PDE for Axis II	42% of patients with dependent PD met criteria for major depression; 8% met criteria for dysthymia	There was significantly more social phobia among patients with dependent PD, and significantly increased amounts of borderline and histrionic PD traits; the findings contrast with other studies, which found a significant relationship between dependence and major depressive disorder
Maier et al. (1992)	Family study with 109 control probands matched to 555 consecutively admitted inpatients with affective or schizophrenic disorders	SADS-LA for DSM-III Axis I; SCID-II for DSM-III-R Axis II	Rate of major depression among probands with PDs from the following clusters: Cluster A: 15% Cluster B: 33% Cluster C: 19%	
Perry (1985)	82 subjects from outpatient clinics, recruitment for symptomatic volunteers, and court probation department	DIS for Axes I and II and Borderline Personality Scale	87% of borderline PD subjects met criteria for lifetime occurrence of a major depressive disorder	Chronic depression demonstrated a specific relationship to borderline psychopathology

feel rejected and to be self-critical. Persons with obsessive–compulsive personality disorders are vulnerable because they are easily reduced to self-criticism if they are not in control and 'perfect' " (61). There is also some evidence that dependent personality disorder increases the risk of depression, as well as alcohol dependence and obesity (35,86).

Several studies have found significant rates of comorbidity of cluster C personality disorders and dysthymia (24–26,77,87). Marin et al. (26) found that dysthymics were significantly more likely than depressed patients to meet criteria for avoidant, dependent, and self-defeating personality disorders. These authors speculated that their observations may have been due to overlap in criteria between the cluster C disorders and dysthymia, including items assessing social withdrawal and self-esteem (26).

F. Age and Personality Disorder Comorbidity

Findings concerning the relationship between age and personality disorder in depressed patients, like much of the comorbidity literature, include conflicting data. Fogel and Westlake's (88) retrospective study of inpatients with major depression found that patients older than 65 had a lower rate of Axis II disorders, regardless of sex or comorbid medical illness, than patients under age 65, leading the authors to infer that personality disorders decline with increasing age. In the 65-or-older group, obsessive-compulsive personality disorder accounted for 46% of all Axis II diagnoses (88). Kunik et al. (89) found no association between age and comorbid personality disorder in elderly patients when Axis I diagnosis was controlled for. These studies did not utilize standardized assessment instruments (89).

Golomb et al., using standardized assessment instruments, found that the frequency of personality disorders in depressed outpatients did not significantly change with age (90). Similar data have been published by Abrams et al., who found that early-onset depression among elderly patients was associated with more lifetime personality pathology than late-onset elderly depression (91). The authors concluded that late-onset geriatric depression represents a disorder distinct from the comorbid depression and personality disorder seen in young adult patients and early-onset geriatric depressives.

Among a sample of elderly depressed patients, Vine and Steingart (92) found that personality was a significant factor in the outcome of depression in the elderly. In particular, a cluster B diagnosis was associated with a chronic outcome of depression and with impaired social support (92). Thompson et al. (93), on the other hand, found an increase in dependent and avoidant traits in patients with late-life depression (93). Black et al. (15) and Agbayewa (94) found that cluster C personality disorders were the most common among elderly depressed patients. In Thompson's sample, elderly patients without a personality disorder were significantly more likely to respond to treatment for depression. Within the group of patients with comorbid personality disorders, patients with a dependent or avoidant personality disorder responded more favorably to treatment, and those with compulsive or passive-aggressive comorbidity responded less well (93). All studies of geriatric comorbidity of depression and personality disorders stress the importance of continued longitudinal research to confirm their conclusions.

G. Sex and Personality Disorder Comorbidity

DSM-IV reports that antisocial personality disorder is diagnosed more frequently in men, while borderline, histrionic, and dependent personality disorders are diagnosed more frequently in women (28). Alneas and Torgerson found that among a group of outpatients with various Axis I disorders (over 50% of which were depressive disorders), obsessive-compulsive, passive-aggressive, schizotypal, paranoid, and narcissistic personality disorders tended to occur more frequently in men (95).

One report, by Golomb et al., addressing generalized sex differences in personality disorders chose to control for Axis I comorbidity by studying a group of patients with a primary diagnosis of major depression (96). They found that men were significantly more likely than women to meet criteria for narcissistic, antisocial, and obsessive-compulsive personality disorders when measured by the Personality Diagnostic Questionnaire–Revised (PDQ-R). Assessment by the Structured Clinical Interview for Personality Disorders–II (SCID-II) showed that men were significantly more likely than women to meet criteria for narcissistic and obsessive-compulsive personality disorders. However, the authors found that neither the PDQ-R nor the SCID-II indicated a higher prevalence of any personality disorder in women. Their results, as well as the findings of another study (65), appear to contradict previous findings that borderline personality disorder is more common among women (97,98).

IV. CONCEPTUAL ISSUES

DSM-IV excludes the diagnosis of a personality disorder when it occurs exclusively in the context of an Axis I disorder. This rule is an attempt to distinguish reliably between mood states and personality traits, i.e., between transient emotional states and enduring patterns of perceiving and relating to the environment and oneself. In many ways, the conceptualization of comorbidity of depression and personality disorder touches at the heart of psychiatric nosology and is directly related to assessment techniques and instruments. We will address two broad questions: (1) How has the post-DSM-III classification of depressive disorders on Axis I and personality disorders on Axis II been justified? (2) What evidence exists for *depressive personality disorder* (included in the DSM-IV "experimental section"), and how does the depressive personality disorder construct affect conceptions of the comorbidity of depression and personality disorders?

Classification of the mood disorders on Axis I and the personality disorders on Axis II has been supported by early theories positing that Axis I disorders are biogenetic in origin and Axis II personality disorders are developmental in origin (99). Many authors have since argued that there are biogenetic links between Axes I and II (100). For example, schizotypal personality disorder is thought to lie on a biogenetic continuum with schizophrenia, and avoidant personality disorder is thought to be related to Axis I anxiety disorders (27). Gunderson et al. have suggested that some of the more severe personality disorders, such as schizotypal, paranoid, and borderline, might be clinical syndromes with discrete etiological pathways, while the less severe personality disorders, such as obsessive-compulsive, avoidant, and dependent, are extremes of normally occurring traits (29,101).

Livesley et al. have argued that the DSM-III assignment of the personality disorders to Axis II was pragmatic rather than scientific, and indeed DSM-III justified the separation to ensure that less florid (i.e., personality) disorders would be given diagnostic attention along with the Axis I disorders (4,102). There has been a great deal of debate over the categorization of the personality disorders instituted by DSM-III. Some authors have argued in favor of a dimensional approach to personality disorders (102), suggesting that a mechanism of assessing personality traits as well as disorders be created on Axis I as a means of ensuring that personality traits are considered within the context of Axis I disorders. In practice, these authors asserted, personality traits that may affect treatment decisions are rarely coded. Furthermore, they concluded that a personality disorder diagnosis is often addressed only when justifying pessimism about anticipated treatment response or when withholding a particular course of treatment (102).

It is unlikely that the personality disorder classification system will be shifted from a categorical to a dimensional system in the foreseeable future unless it is demonstrated that personality disorders should be described dimensionally. Research on the pathophysiology of depression and personality disorders might, for example, demonstrate that genetic factors related to affective dysregulation in borderline personality disorder distinguish it as a variant of Axis I depressive disorders such that a dimensional interpretation of borderline traits would be preferable (103,104). Many authors have chosen to address the issue of categorical versus dimensional approaches by publishing both types of data. This approach enables a more sensitive presentation of traits that might otherwise be missed by a categorical diagnosis.

The construct of an Axis II depressive personality disorder has gained attention, especially since its inclusion in the experimental section of DSM-IV. Hirschfeld has published extensively on the relationship of mood disorders to personality disorders, and in particular on the relationship between depressive personality disorder and depression. He suggested that evidence is still inconclusive to support the hypothesis that depressive disorders such as major depression, dysthymia, and recurrent brief depression are distinct entities. In the case of depressive personality disorder, Hirschfeld argued that the defining characteristics of depressive personality disorder are cognitive- rather than affective-oriented, including aspects of pessimism, low self-esteem, self-criticalness, and guilt that are persistent across situations and over time (105). He also described the substantial evidence that has accumulated to warrant placing this diagnostic entity on Axis II (27).

An earlier historical review of the depressive personality by Phillips et al. (106) also advocated a categorical treatment of depressive personality disorder. They asserted that some affective and personality disorders exist on a continuum, with variants along a spectrum. The notion of a depressive personality disorder was proposed to be a categorical description of one of these variants—one that might otherwise be described as "characterological" depression (106).

This distinction between depressive personality disorder and dysthymia, major depression, and the other personality disorders has been supported by depressive personality disorders' observed early onset, stability across time and social situations, and tendency for less medication-induced change than dysthymia or depression (106). Akiskal has published extensively on the so-called "characterologic depressions," which he subdivided into the character-spectrum and subaffective dysthymic disorders. Akiskal posited that subaffective dysthymic disorder (later defined as depressive personality disorder) was a drug-responsive, attenuated form of affective disorder that should be placed on Axis II (20,107). Akiskal reasoned that this "subaffective" disorder should be shifted to Axis II because is is defined by an early onset and has features that are trait- rather than state-related. Phillips et al.'s (106) detailed review of depressive personality groups Akiskal's second subtype, the character-spectrum disorders, with "Winokur's depressive-spectrum disease (108,109), Klein and Davis's hysteroid dysphoria (110), Blatt's anaclitic depression (111), and Pfohl et al.'s description of patients with depression and personality disorder (9)." The character-spectrum disorders were judged to be a mixture too heterogeneous to classify on either Axis I or Axis II (106).

Data from the DSM-IV mood disorder field trials showed that the diagnosis of dysthymia does not appear to capture many individuals with lifelong depressive traits, and conversely, that many individuals diagnosed with dysthymia would not meet criteria for depressive personality disorder (112). Continued research on the diagnostic stability of depressive personality disorder and associated familial aggregation may demonstrate whether it can be considered "the personality disorder of the mood disorders," combining personality and "subaffective" traits into a formal Axis II category in future editions of the DSM.

V. EMPIRICAL AND METHODOLOGICAL ISSUES

Related to conceptual issues of the categorical/dimensional approach to personality disorders, including depressive personality disorder, is the "trait-state" problem in personality assessment. A number of reports have appeared over the years that clearly indicate that depressive states may distort personality assessments. First, we turn briefly to findings of earlier studies, which tended to employ questionnaires. We then discuss more recent issues relevant to studies that have utilized semistructured interviews.

The majority of early studies of the personality attributes of depressed patients utilized self-report measures, including the Maudsley Personality Inventory, the MMPI, and the Guilford-Zimmerman Temperament Survey, among others. Several of these reports indicated that assessment of personality traits such as emotional strength, interpersonal dependency, neuroticism, and extraversion are colored by depressive states, even when instructions are modified to try to prevent a state effect (5,8,113).

Liebowitz et al. (114), for example, found significant differences between depressed outpatients and controls on the extraversion and neuroticism scales of the Maudsley Personality Inventory. However, when mood was controlled for, the observed differences disappeared. This led the authors to speculate that the subjects' mood contaminated their personality assessment, in spite of the fact that subjects were given instructions to describe their usual (i.e., nondepressed) selves (114).

Hirschfeld et al. (8) replicated some of these findings in their personality assessment study of recovered depressed patients 1 year after their illness. Measures of emotional strength, interpersonal dependency, and extraversion were strongly influenced by the depressed state. Self-reported assessments of activity level, rigidity, and dominance were not changed after recovery (8). Reich et al. (78) compared personality differences in depressed and panic patients in their ill and recovered states. State was found to have a significant effect on self-reported personality—both groups appeared to have greater interpersonal dependency and less emotional strength than controls. Interestingly, no differences between the panic and depressed groups were observed on any of the measures (78).

As a general rule, self-report measures that assess DSM-III-R personality disorder traits have been found to be more sensitive, but less specific, than semistructured interviews. Golomb et al. (96) found that 91.5% of a group of depressed outpatients met criteria for at least one personality disorder when assessed by the PDQ. When the same sample was assessed with the SCID-II, 56% met criteria for at least one personality disorder. Other studies have found similar patterns of higher personality disorder prevalence with self-report tests (78,115).

Since the publication of DSM-III, semistructured personality disorder interviews with demonstrated reliability have become the assessment instruments of choice. They include the SCID-II (116), the Personality Disorder Examination (PDE) (117), the Structured Interview for DSM-IV Personality (SID-P) (118), and the Diagnostic Interview for Personality Disorders, Revised (119). In a sense, these instruments are written with issues of comorbidity in mind; they enable the clinician to probe and rate responses according to whether they indicate features of personality or of Axis I conditions. There are still some suggestions that interview measures are less sensitive to depressive state effects than self-report measures (120).

To test empirically whether a structured, clinician-administered personality interview could effectively distinguish between mental state and personality traits, Loranger et al. (64) interviewed 84 patients diagnosed with a variety of Axis I disorders. Roughly one-half of the sample met criteria for major depression. Using the PDE, they found no evidence that anxiety or depression affected global personality disorder diagnosis or criteria associated with most individual disorders (64).

These findings are contradicted by Stuart et al. (121), who found that among a sample of acutely depressed outpatients, pretreatment personality disorders diagnoses were not typically confirmed after effective cognitive-behavioral therapy. In contrast to Loranger et al.'s study, Stuart et al. used systematic criteria to assess recovery, specified their follow-up assessment time period, and included only depressed patients. They concluded that a significant number of outpatients may be given false positive personality disorder diagnoses, which may result in inadequate or less aggressive pharmacological treatment (121). An earlier study (122) also found that the number of personality disorders diagnosed in depressed patients decreased after treatment.

There are some indications that trait and state influences may vary across the personality disorder clusters. Results from a treatment study of depressed outpatients by Peselow et al. (57) led them to hypothesize that cluster A and C personality traits may indeed be intertwined with depressive features and thus subject to state influences. In their study, cluster B disorders, on the other hand, were observed not to differ between patients who did and did not recover from depression. The investigators speculated that cluster B symptoms may be associated with true personality traits and are thus less likely to be influenced by depressive state (57). A comparison study by O'Boyle and Self showed that dimensional scores of patients assessed with the PDE and SCID-II tended to be higher in the depressed state, although depression did not consistently alter categorical diagnoses (123).

These data indicate that depressive states negatively affect patients' abilities to differentiate between trait and state on self-report and semistructured personality assessments. Given this problem, the next question for clinicians and researchers is methodological; if personality cannot be adequately assessed during a depressive episode, it must be assessed when an individual is not in a depressive episode and followed over time.

An ambitious, longitudinal study along these lines conducted by Hirschfeld et al. (124) examined first-degree relatives of patients with affective disorders. They found that among older (31–41 years) subjects, premorbid personality traits of decreased emotional strength, increased interpersonal dependency, and increased thoughtfulness were associated with a subsequent first onset of depression. However, this same report noted that expected differences were not found that would indicate that dependency and introversion might be associated with an onset of depression. Furthermore, the authors concluded with a caveat that what were assessed as personality predispositions might in fact have been the prodromal phases of subsyndromal depressive states (124). One of the few other longitudinal studies of a similar design (125) found that mild depressive symptoms considered in relation to general measures of neuroticism predicted subsequent depressive episodes. But this study also found that the risk was not specific to major depression, leading the authors to argue that depressive trait measures may only be a nonspecific predictor of future psychiatric illness (125).

Longitudinal studies that follow individuals through their entire lives and utilize structured personality disorder assessments are the only means of knowing with a greater degree of certainty which personality traits predispose to depressive illness, which are associated only with episodes of illness, and which represent "scarring" effects of prior depressive episodes. Such an ambitious effort would enable clinicians to know when personality traits might indicate that a personality disorder is operating independent of a depressive illness and when such traits are simply an artifact of the depressive state (126).

VI. MODELS OF COMORBIDITY

If we step back for a moment from the diagnostic details of depressive and personality disorders and take a broader view, we can see that any method used to test depressive and personality disorder comorbidity interactions must include developmental, environmental, and biogenetic factors. Methodological issues, of course, go hand-in-hand with the models being tested. Some of the models described below are presented heuristically; they await empirical testing for validation. Others have been or are currently in use in longitudinal studies.

Klein et al. (127) have published extensively on models of depression and personality. Included among Klein and colleagues' theories of the interaction between mood and personality is the common-cause model, which assumes that there is a "core liability" underlying personality disorders and depression and that each disorder is caused by independent processes. It is difficult to test this model because problems may arise in separating the timing and interaction of proposed causal factors.

A subclinical or "spectrum" model involves the assumption that personality disorders and depression have identical underlying processes but differential expression; i.e., one disorder manifests another. Vulnerability models, on the other hand, focus on predisposing personality factors that can lead to depression or vice versa (127).

Pathoplasty models presume that there are distinct etiologies for depression and personality but that features of both disorders interact and can exacerbate each other's presentation. A common pathway, then, leads from the disorders, producing a personality disorder with depressive features or depressed mood with some personality disturbance. Yet another model is the complication or "scar" model, which assumes that the etiologies of personality and depressive disorders are distinct, but that residual symptoms of each illness can result in continued alteration of mood or personality (127).

Klein et al. have integrated many aspects of Axis I and Axis II disorders—biogenetic factors, family environment, and social background, among others—into a complex "biopsychosocial-development" model. Temporal aspects play a key moderating role in this model, which is further broken down into first- and subsequent-onset subgroups (127).

Commenting on this large-scale model, Barnett suggested that focused research programs might be most effective in their endeavors by first concentrating on the small elements that such an all-inclusive model comprises. He recommended study of the construct validity of variables, demonstrations of the nomological networks of the constructs of personality and depression, and empirical tests of the underlying processes of these disorders as a means of "building up" to a more inclusive model (128).

We have made a point of emphasizing the importance of longitudinal studies in the study of the comorbidity of depressive and personality disorders. Junker and Pilkonis (129) make a number of specific recommendations for such studies. They are worth quoting: "1) Focus on a limited number of global constructs; 2) Focus on longitudinal and developmental understanding, and remain close to the clinical phenomena of interest; 3) Exploit the possibilities of sound exploratory data analysis; 4) Consider a "two-step" approach to structural modeling;

5) Use standardized assessment instruments and consider ways to aggregate data." Kendler et al.'s (38) data analysis in their longitudinal study of personality and depression in women, for example, utilized rigorous sampling, questionnaire and interview instruments, and included five regression analyses, defined as "descriptive, causal, prodromal, state, and scar."

VII. SUMMARY AND FUTURE DIRECTIONS

Clearly, to paraphrase Lewis, skillful casuistry is needed to discern where personality ends and a depressive illness begins. However, this type of casuistry alone is insufficient for clinical and epidemiological research. As we have seen, a significant number of patients with depression and dysthymia have comorbid personality disorders. Sometimes, these disorders are an artifact of the individual's depressed state. We have briefly described two examples (124,125) of work that used longitudinal methodology as a means of obtaining a clearer picture of the interaction of affect and personality. There are also indications that individuals at high risk for personality disorders have a higher risk for depression (35).

However, almost all of the data reviewed here come from treated samples. This is a serious limitation for generalizing observed rates of comorbidity. It will be important to test samples that are representative of the general population because an association observed solely in clinical populations could reflect the influence of having two disorders on the probability of seeking treatment, rather than a true association. The influence of treatment seeking on the probability of observing a spurious association between two variables is known as Berkson's bias (130).

The combined distress caused by depressive and personality disorders warrants continued epidemiological and clinical research. Improved understanding of the pathophysiological processes involved will promote improved understanding of the true nature of the observed comorbidity. Studies of dysthymia and depressive personality disorder, in particular, will help complete the picture of how depressive disorders and personality disorders are interrelated. There are many unanswered questions in this emerging area of psychiatry, and many promising avenues of research that will contribute to improved patient care in mental health and primary care settings.

REFERENCES

1. Lewis AJ. Melancholia: a clinical survey of depressive states. J Ment Sci 1934; 80:277–378.
2. Patience DA, McGuire RJ, Scott AIF, Freeman CPL. The Edinburgh primary care

depression study: personality disorder and outcome. Br J Psychiatry 1995; 167: 324–330.
3. Weissman MM, Prusoff BA, Klerman GL. Personality and the prediction of long-term outcome of depression. Am J Psychiatry 1978; 135:797–800.
4. American Psychiatric Association. Diagnostic and Statistical Manual and Mental Disorders, 3rd ed. Washington, DC: American Psychiatric Association Press, 1980.
5. Coppen A, Metcalfe M. Effect of a depressive illness on MPI scores. Br J Psychiatry 1965; 111:236–239.
6. Kerr TA, Schapira K, Roth M, Garside RF. The relationship between the Maudsley Personality Inventory and the course of affective disorders. Br J Psychiatry 1970; 116:11–19.
7. Lewis AJ. Melancholia: a historical review. J Ment Sci 1934; 80:1–42.
8. Hirschfeld RMA, Klerman GL, Clayton PJ, Keller MB, McDonald-Scott P, Larkin BH. Assessing personality: effects of the depressive state on trait measurement. Am J Psychiatry 1983; 140:695–699.
9. Pfohl B, Stangl D, Zimmerman M. The implications of DSM-III personality disorders for patients with major depression. J Affect Disord 1984; 7:309–318.
10. Shea MT, Glass DR, Pilkonis PA, Watkins J, Docherty JP. Frequency and implications of personality disorders in a sample of depressed outpatients. J. Personal Disord 1987; 1:27–42.
11. Shea MT, Widiger TA, Klein MH. Comorbidity of personality disorders and depression: implications for treatment. J Consult Clin Psychol 1992; 60:857–868.
12. Hardy GE, Barkham M, Shapiro D, Stiles WB, Rees A, Reynolds S. Impact of cluster C personality disorders on outcomes of contrasting brief psychotherapies for depression. J Consult Clin Psychol 1995; 63:997–1004.
13. Diguer L, Barber JP, Luborsky L. Three concomitants: personality disorders, psychiatric severity, and outcome of dynamic psychotherapy of major depression. Am J Psychiatry 1993; 150:1246–1248.
14. Flick SN, Roy-Byrne PP, Cowley DS, Shores MM, Dunner DL. DSM-III-R personality disorders in a mood and anxiety disorders clinic: prevalence, comorbidity, and clinical correlates. J Affect Disord 1993; 27:71–79.
15. Black DW, Bell S, Hulbert J, Nasrallah A. The importance of Axis II in patients with major depression. A controlled study. J Affect Disord 1988; 14:115–122.
16. Casey PR, Meagher D, Butler E. Personality, functioning, and recovery from major depression. J Nerv Ment Dis 1996; 184:240–245.
17. Hirschfeld RMA. Commentary on Widiger. In: Klein MH, Kupfer DJ, Shea MT, eds. Personality and Depression. New York: Guilford Press, 1993:127–132.
18. Chodoff P. The depressive personality: a critical review. Arch Gen Psychiatry 1972; 73:666–673.
19. Docherty JP, Fiester SJ, Shea T. Syndrome diagnosis and personality disorder. Psychol Assoc Annu Rev 1986; 5:315–355.
20. Akiskal HS, Jirschfeld RMA, Yerevanian BI. The relationship of personality to affective disorders: a critical review. Arch Gen Psychiatry 1983; 40:801–810.

21. Kocsis J, Voss C, Mann J, Frances A. Chronic depression: demographic and clinical characteristics. Psychopharmacol Bull 1986; 22:192–195.
22. Kocsis JH, Frances AJ. A critical discussion of DSM-III dysthymic disorder. Am J Psychiatry 1987; 144:1534–1542.
23. Markowtiz JC, Moran ME, Kocsis JH, Frances AJ. Prevalence and comorbidity of dysthymic disorder among psychiatric outpatients. J Affect Dis 1992; 24:63–71.
24. Klein DN, Riso LP, Donaldson SK, Schwartz JE, Anderson RL, Ouimette PC, Lizardi H, Aronson TA. Family study of early-onset dysthymia. Arch Gen Psychiatry 1995; 52:487–496.
25. Pepper CM, Klein DN, Anderson RL, Riso LP, Ouimette PC, Lizardi H. DSM-III-R Axis II comorbidity in dysthymia and major depression. Am J Psychiatry 1995; 152:239–247.
26. Marin DM, Kocsis JH, Frances AJ, Klerman GL. Personality disorders in dysthymia. J Personal Disord 1993; 7:223–231.
27. Hirschfeld RMA. Major depression, dysthymia, and depressive personality disorder. Br J Psychiatry 1994; 165:23–50.
28. American Psychiatric Association. Diagnostic and Statistical Manual of Mental Disorders, 4th ed. Washington, DC: American Psychiatric Association Press, 1994.
29. Lyons MJ. Epidemiology of personality disorders. In: Tsuang MT, Tohen M, Zahner G, eds. Textbook in Psychiatric Epidemiology. New York: Wiley-Liss, 1995:407–436.
30. Feinstein AR. The pre-therapeutic classification of comorbidity in chronic disease. J Chronic Dis 1970; 23:455–468.
31. Kessler RC, McGonagle KA, Zhao S, Nelson CB, Hughes M, Eshleman S, Wittchen HU, Kendler KS. Lifetime and 12-month prevalence of DSM-III-R psychiatric disorders in the United States: results from the National Comorbidity Survey. Arch Gen Psychiatry 1994; 51:8–19.
32. Klerman GL. Approaches to the phenomena of comorbidity. In: Master JD, Cloninger RC, eds. Comorbidity of Mood and Anxiety Disorders. Washington, DC: American Psychiatric Press, 1990:13–37.
33. Zimmerman M, Coryell W. DSM-III personality disorder diagnoses in a nonpatient sample. Arch Gen Psychiatry 1989; 46:682–689.
34. Maier W, Lichtermann D, Klingler T, Heun R, Hallmayer J. Prevalences of personality disorders (DSM-III-R) in the community. J. Personal Disord 1992; 6: 187–196.
35. Hueston HJ, Mainous AG III, Schilling R. Patients with personality disorders: functional status, health care utilization, and satisfaction with care. J Fam Pract 1996; 42:54–60.
36. Bartholomew AA, Marley E. The temporal reliability of the Maudsley Personality Inventory. J Ment Sci 1959; 105:238–240.
37. Mezey AG, Cohen SI, Knight EJ. Personality assessment under varying physiological and psychological conditions. J Psychosom Res 1963; 7:237–240.
38. Kendler KS, Neale MC, Kessler RC, Heath AC, Eaves LJ. A longitudinal twin

study of personality and major depression in women. Arch Gen Psychiatry 1993; 50:853–862.
39. Lazare A, Klerman GL. Hysteria and depression. Am J Psychiatry 1968; 124: May (Suppl):48–56.
40. Grinker RR, Sr., Miller J, Sabshin M, Nunn R, Nunnally JC. The Phenomena of Depression. New York: Harper & Row, 1961.
41. Friedman AS, Cowitz B, Cohen HW, Granick S. Syndromes and themes of psychotic depression. Arch Gen Psychiatry 1963; 9:504–509.
42. Corruble E, Ginestet D, Guelfi JD. Comorbidity of personality disorders and unipolar major depression: a review. J Affect Disord 1996; 37:157–170.
43. Reich JH, Vasile RG. Effect of personality disorders on the treatment outcome of Axis I conditions: an update. J Nerv Ment Dis 1993; 181:475–484.
44. Pilkonis PA, Frank E. Personality pathology in recurrent depression: nature, prevalence and relationship to treatment response. Am J Psychiatry 1988; 145:435–441.
45. Casey PR, Butler E. The effects of personality on response to ECT in major depression. J Personal Disord 1995; 9:134–142.
46. Paykel ES, Weissman MM. Social adjustment and depression. A longitudinal study. Arch Gen Psychiatry 1973; 28:659–663.
47. Reich JH, Green AI. Effect of personality disorders on outcome for treatment. J Nerv Ment Dis 1991; 179:74–82.
48. Zimmerman M, Coryell W, Pfohl B, Cornethal C, Stangl D. ECT response in depressed patients with and without a DSM-III personality disorder. Am J Psychiatry 1986; 143:1030–1032.
49. Tyrer P, Seivewright N, Ferguson B, Murphy S, Darling C, Brothwell J, Kingdon D, Johnson AL. The Nottingham study of neurotic disorder: relationship between personality status and symptoms. Psychol Med 1990; 20:423–431.
50. Siever LJ, Coccaro EF, Klar H, Losonczy MF, Silverman JF, Davis KL. Biological markers in borderline and related personality disorders. In: Shagrass C, Josiassen RG, Wagner BH, Weiss KJ, Stoff D, Simpson GM, eds. Biological Psychiatry: Proceedings of the Fourth World Congress of Biological Psychiatry. New York: Elsevier Science, 1986:566–568.
51. Kupfer D, Thase M. Laboratory studies and validity of psychiatric diagnosis: has there been progress? In: Robins L, Barrett J, eds. The Validity of Psychiatric Diagnosis. New York: Raven Press, 1989:177–200.
52. Andreoli A, Frances A, Gex-Fabry M, Aapro N, Gerin P, Dazord A. Crisis intervention in depressed patients with and without DSM-III-R personality disorders. J Nerv Ment Dis 1993; 181:732–737.
53. Brugha TS, Bebbington, PE, MacCarthy B, Sturt E, Wykes T, Potter J. Gender, social support and recovery from depressive disorders: a prospective clinical study. Psychol Med 1990; 20:147–157.
54. Tyrer P, Merson S, Onyett S, Johnson T. The effect of personality disorder on clinical outcome, social networks and adjustment: a controlled clinical trial of psychiatric emergencies. Psychol Med 1994; 24:731–740.
55. Conte HR, Plutchik R, Picard S, Karasu TB. Can personality traits predict psychotherapy outcome? Comp Psychiatry 1991; 32:66–72.

56. Pfohl B, Coryell W, Zimmerman M, Stangl D. Prognostic validity of self-report and interview measures of personality disorder in depressed inpatients. J Clin Psychiatry 1987; 48:468–472.
57. Peselow ED, Sanfilipo MP, Fieve RR, Gulbenkian G. Personality traits during depression and after clinical recovery. Br J Psychiatry 1994; 164:349–354.
58. Shea MT, Pilkonis PA, Beckham E, Collins JF, Elkin I, Sotsky SM, Docherty JP. Personality disorder and treatment outcome in the NIMH treatment of depression collaborative research program. Am J Psychiatry 1990; 147:711–718.
59. Mulder RT, Joyce PR, Cloninger CR. Temperament and early environment influence comorbidity and personality disorders in major depression. Comp Psychiatry 1994; 35:225–233.
60. Cloninger CR, Svrakic DM, Przybeck TR. A psychobiological model of temperament and character. Arch Gen Psychiatry 1993; 50:975–990.
61. Benjamin LS. Commentary on Widiger. In: Klein MH, Kupfer DJ, Shea MT, eds. Personality and Depression. New York: Guilford Press, 1993:119–126.
62. Sato T, Sakado K, Sato S, Morikawa T. Cluster A personality disorder: a marker of worse treatment outcome of major depression? Psychiatry Res 1994; 53:153–159.
63. Akiskal HS. Subaffective disorders: dysthymic, cyclothymic and bipolar II disorders in the "borderline" realm. Psychiatr Clin North Am 1981; 4:25–46.
64. Loranger AW, Lenzeweger MF, Gartner AF, Susman VL, Herzig J, Zammit GK, Gartner JD, Abrams RC, Young RC. Trait-state artifacts and the diagnosis of personality disorders. Arch Gen Psychiatry 1991; 48:720–728.
65. Jackson HJ, Whiteside HL, Bates GW, Bell R, Rudd RP, Edwards J. Diagnosing personality disorders in psychiatric inpatients. Acta Psychiatr Scand 1991; 83: 206–213.
66. Perry JC. Depression in borderline personality disorder: lifetime prevalence at interview and longitudinal course of symptoms. Am J Psychiatry 1985; 142: 15–21.
67. Pope HG, Jonas JM, Hudson JI, Cohen BM, Gunderson JG. The validity of DSM-III borderline personality disorder: a phenomenologic, family history, treatment response, and long-term follow-up study. Arch Gen Psychiatry 1983; 40:23–30.
68. McGlashan TH. Borderline personality disorder and unipolar affective disorder. J Nerv Men Dis 1987; 175:467–473.
69. Fava M, Bouffides E, Pava JA, McCarthy MK, Steingard RJ, Rosenbaum JF. Personality disorder comorbidity with major depression and response to fluoxetine treatment. Psychother Psychosom 1994; 62:160–167.
70. Clayton PJ, Lewis CI. The significance of secondary depression. J Affect Disord 1981; 3:25–35.
71. Woody GE, McLellan T, Luborsky L, O'Brien CP. Sociopathy and psychotherapy outcome. Arch Gen Psychiatry 1985; 42:1081–1086.
72. Oldham JM, Skodol AE, Kellman HD, Hyler SE, Doidge N, Rosnick L, Gallaher PE, Comorbidity of Axis I and Axis II disorders. Am J Psychiatry 1995; 152: 571–578.

73. Gunderson J, Elliot G. The interface between borderline personality disorder and affective disorder. Am J Psychiatry 1985; 142:277–288.
74. Gunderson J. Diagnostic controversies. In: Tasman A, Riba MB, eds. Review of Psychiatry, vol 11. Washington, DC: American Psychiatric Press, 1992:9–24.
75. Liebowitz MR, Quitkin FM, Stewart JW, McGrath PJ, Harrison WM, Markowitz JS, Rabkin JG, Tricamo E, Goetz DM, Klein DF. Antidepressant specificity in aytpical depression. Arch Gen Psychiatry 1988; 45:129–137.
76. Parsons B, Quitkin FM, McGrath PJ, Stewart JW, Tricamo E, Ocepek-Welikson K, Harrison W, Rabkin JG, Wager SG, Nunes E. Phenelzine, imipramine, and placebo in borderline patients meeting criteria for atypical depression. Psychopharmacol Bull 19889; 25:524–534.
77. Sanderson WC, Wetzler S, Beck AT, Betz F. Prevalence of personality disorders in patients with major depression and dysthymia. Psychiatr Res 1992; 42:93–99.
78. Reich J, Noyes R, Hirschfeld R, Coryell W, O'Gorman T. State and personality in depressed and panic patients. Am J Psychiatry 1987; 144:181–187.
79. Frank E, Kupfer DJ, Jacob M, Jarrett D. Personality features and response to acute treatment in recurrent depression. J Personal Disord 1987; 1:14–26.
80. Stein DJ, Young JE, eds. Cognitive Science and Clinical Disorders. London: Academic Press, 1992.
81. Beck AT, Freeman A. Cognitive Therapy of Personality Disorders. New York: Guilford Press, 1990.
82. Klein DN, Harding K, Taylor EB, Dickstein S. Dependency and self-criticism in depression: evaluation in a clinical population. J Abnorm Psychol 1988; 97: 399–404.
83. Overholser JC, Kabakoff R, Norman WH. The assessment of personality characteristics in depressed and dependent psychiatric inpatients. J Personal Assess 1989; 53:40–50.
84. Reich J. The morbidity of DSM-III-R dependent personality disorder. J Nerv Ment Dis 1996; 184:22–26.
85. Sargent W, Slater E. Physical Treatments in Psychiatry. Edinburgh: Churchill Livingstone, 1944.
86. Greenberg RP, Bornstein RF. The dependent personality. I. Risk for psychological disorders. J Personal Disord 1988; 2:136–144.
87. Shelton RC, Davidson J, Yonkers KA, Koran L, Thase ME, Pearlstein T, Halbreich U. The undertreatment of dysthymia. J Clin Psychiatry 1997; 58:59–65.
88. Fogel BS, Westlake R. Personality disorder diagnoses and age in patients with major depression. J Clin Psychiatry 1990; 51:232–235.
89. Kunik ME, Mulsant BH, Rifai AH, Sweet RA, Paternak R, Zubenko GS. Diagnostic rate of comorbid personality disorder in elderly psychiatric inpatients. Am J Psychiatry 1994; 151:603–605.
90. Golomb M, Fava M, Abraham M, Rosenbaum JF. The relationship between age and personality disorders in depressed outpatients. J Nerv Ment Dis 1995; 183: 43–44.

91. Abrams RC, Rosendahl E, Card C, Alexopoulos GS. Personality disorder correlates of late and early onset depression. J Am Geriatr Soc 1994; 42:727–731.
92. Vine RG, Steingart AB. Personality disorder in the elderly depressed. Can J Psychiatry 1994; 39:392–398.
93. Thompson LW, Gallagher D, Czirr R. Personality disorder and outcome in the treatment of late-life depression. J Geriatr Psychiatry 1988; 133–146.
94. Agbayewa MO. Occurrence and effects of personality disorders in depression: are they the same in the old and young? Can J Psychiatry 1996; 41:223–226.
95. Alnaes R, Torgerson S. DSM-III personality disorders among patients with major depression, anxiety disorders, and mixed conditions. J Nerv Ment Dis 1990; 178: 693–698.
96. Golomb M, Fava M, Abraham M, Rosenbaum JF. Gender differences in personality disorders. Am J Psychiatry 1995; 152:579–582.
97. Sheehy M, Goldsmith L, Charles E. A comparative study of borderline patients in a psychiatric outpatient clinic. Am J Psychiatry 1980; 137:1374–1379.
98. Zanarini MC, Gunderson JG, Frankenburg FR. Axis I phenomenology of borderline personality disorder. Compr Psychiatry 1989; 30:149–156.
99. Marin DB, DeMeo M, Frances AJ, et al. Biological models and treatments for personality disorders. Psychiatr Ann 1989; 18:143–146.
100. Wetzel RD, Cloninger CR, Hong B, et al. Personality as a subclinical expression of the affective disorders. Comp Psychiatry 1980; 21:197–205.
101. Gunderson JG, Links PS, Reich JH. Competing models of personality disorders. J Personal Disord 1991; 5:60–68.
102. Livesley WJ, Schroeder ML, Jackson DN, Jang KL. Categorical distinctions in the study of personality disorder: implications for classification. J Abnorm Psychol 1994; 103:6–17.
103. Manning DW, Frances AJ. Combined Pharmacotherapy and Psychotherapy for Depression. Washington, DC: American Psychiatric Press, 1990.
104. Widiger TA, Shea MT. The differentiation of Axis I and Axis II disorders. J Abnorm Psychol 1991; 100:399–406.
105. Hirscheld RMA, Shea MT, Gunderson JG, Phillips KA. Proposal for a depressive personality disorder. Unpublished manuscript, DSM-IV Work Group on Personality Disorder, 1989.
106. Phillips KA, Gunderson JG, Hirschfeld RMA, Smith LE. A review of the depressive personality. Am J Psychiatry 1990; 147:830–837.
107. Akiskal HS. Validating affective personality types. In: Robins L, Barret J, eds. The Validity of Psychiatric Diagnosis. New York: Raven Press, 1989:217–227.
108. Winokur G. Depression spectrum disease: description and family study. Compr Psychiatry 1972; 13:3–8.
109. Winokur G. Unipolar depression: is it divisible into autonomous subtypes? Arch Gen Psychiatry 1979; 36:47–52.
110. Klein DF, Davis JM. The diagnosis of affective disorders. In: Klein DF, Davis JM, eds. Diagnosis and Treatment of Psychiatric Disorders. Baltimore: Williams & Wilkins, 1969.

111. Blatt SJ. Levels of object representation in anaclitic and introspective depression. Psychoanal Stud Child 1974; 29:107–157.
112. Shea MT, Hirschfeld RMA. Chronic mood disorder and depressive personality. Psychiatr Clin North America 1996; 19:103–120.
113. Bianchi GN, Fergusson DM. The effect of mental state on EPI scores. Br J Psychiatry 1977; 131:306–309.
114. Liebowitz MR, Stallone F, Dunner DL, Fieve RF. Personality features of patients with primary affective disorder. Acta Psychiatr Scand 1979; 60:214–224.
115. Wetzel S, Kahn R, Cahn W, van Praag HM, Asnis G. Psychological test characteristics of depressed and panic patients. Psychiatry Res 1990; 31:179–192.
116. Spitzer RL, Williams JBW, Gibbon M. Structured Clinical Interview for DSM-III-R Personality Disorders. New York: Biometrics Research Department, New York State Psychiatric Institute, 1987.
117. Loranger AW. Personality Disorders Examination. Yonkers, NY: DV Communications, 1988.
118. Phohl B, Stangl DA, Zimmerman M, Bowers W, Corenthal C. A structured interview for the DSM-III personality disorders: a preliminary report. Arch Gen Psychiatry 1982; 42:591–596.
119. Zanarini MC, Frankenburg FR, Chauncey DL, Gunderson JG. The diagnostic interview for personality disorders: interrater and test-retest reliability. Compr Psychiatry 1987; 28:467–480.
120. Zimmerman M, Pfohl B, Coryell WH, Cornethal C, Stangl D. Major depression and personality disorder. J Affect Disord 1991; 22:199–210.
121. Stuart S, Simons AD, Thase ME, Pilkonis P. Are personality assessments valid in acute major depression? J Affect Disord 1992; 24:281–290.
122. Joffe RT, Regan JJ. Personality and depression. J Psychiatr Res 1988; 22:279–286.
123. O'Boyle M, Self D. A comparison of two interviews of DSM-III-R personality disorders. Psychiatry Res 1990; 32:85–92.
124. Hirschfeld RMA, Klerman GL, Lavori P, Keller MB, Griffith P, Coryell W. Premorbid personality assessments of first onset of major depression. Arch Gen Psychiatry 1989; 46:345–350.
125. Zonderman A, Herbst J, Schmidt C, Costa R, McRae R. Depressive symptoms as a non-specific, graded risk for psychiatric diagnosis. J Abnorm Psychol 1993; 102:544–552.
126. Widiger TA. Personality and depression: assessment issues. In: Klein MH, Kupfer DJ, Shea MT, eds. Personality and Depression. New York: Guilford Press, 1993: 77–118.
127. Klein MH, Wonderlich S, Shea MT. Models of relationships between personality and depression: toward a framework for theory and research. In: Klein MH, Kupfer DJ, Shea MT, eds. Personality and Depression. New York: Guilford Press, 1993:1–54.
128. Barnett PA, Commentary on Klein et al. In Klein MH, Kupfer DJ, Shea MT, eds. Personality and Depression. New York: Guilford Press, 1993:68–76.
129. Junker BW, Pilkonis PA. Personality and depression: modeling and measurement

issues. In: Klein MH, Kupfer DJ, Shea MT, eds. Personality and Depression. New York: Guilford Press, 1993:133–170.

130. Berkson J. Limitations of the application of fourfold table analysis to hospital data. Biomet Bull 1946; 2:47–53.

5

The Comorbidity of Depression and Medical Illness in the Elderly

ANDREW SATLIN
Harvard Medical School
Boston, Massachusetts

I. INTRODUCTION

In elderly persons, both depression and medical illness are very common. As a result, their co-occurrence would be great even by chance alone. However, the comorbidity of these disorders encompasses far more than their mere coincidence. A special relationship between depression and medical illness in the elderly is suggested by studies comparing the rates of chronic physical illnesses and nonpsychotropic medication use among patients with major depression and other psychiatric illnesses such as schizophrenia and Alzheimer's disease (AD). In one such study, overall comorbidity was highest in the major depression group, with 48% having three or more concurrent physical illnesses, compared to 13% in the schizophrenia group and 15% in the AD group (1). Nonpsychotropic drug prescription also was highest in the major depression group. According to the results of a logistic regression, major depression predicted the presence of concomitant physical illnesses; a diagnosis of major depression was associated with an OR of 9.7 for having three or more concurrent physical illnesses, compared to patients with AD. Another study found that medical comorbidity was twice as high in patients with depression as in patients with schizophrenia (2). Because of this close relationship between depression and medical illness, the study of the interactions between them offers important insights into psychiatric nosology, diagnosis, natural history, and treatment. In this chapter, we will review the mutual interactions of depressive illness and medical illness as they occur in patients in the later years of life.

II. EPIDEMIOLOGY AND RISK FACTORS

A. Rates of Depression in the Medically Ill

The rate of comorbid depression in patients with medical illness varies with the population studied, the medical illnesses and other risk factors in the population, the method of assessment, the criteria for diagnosis, and other patient-related factors. Among adult outpatients attending medical clinics, rates range from 6.6% for major depression (3), to roughly 15% for scoring above the cutoff on the Center for Epidemiologic Studies Depression (CES-D) Scale (3,4), to 20–25% for self-rated depression on the Zung Self-Rating Depression Scale (5,6). Elderly patients hospitalized with medical illness generally have higher rates, although more variability is found because of the range of medical pathology and differences in the timing of the assessment. Using research diagnostic criteria (RDC) diagnoses, one study found 6% of patients to have major depression, and an additional 9.3% to have minor or intermittent depression (7). However, other studies have found rates of major depression to be about 13%, with minor depression in an additional 20–30% (8,9). One study of a VA population found the rate of major depression to be 45%, although many of these cases were mild, with a mean Hamilton Depression Rating Scale (HAM-D) score among the depressed patients of only 14.9 (10).

Among different diagnostic groups, the highest rates of comorbid depression are found in patients with coronary artery disease (CAD). Outpatients assessed around the time of angiography have rates of major depression in the range of 15–20% (11–13), and rates are similar in patients hospitalized with myocardial infarction (14–16). In a large community survey in Finland, the mean depression score and the prevalence of clinical depression were higher in patients with cardiovascular diseases than in other persons (17). However, uncomplicated hypertension was not associated with depression, and another study of VA patients seen in an outpatient geriatric psychiatry clinic found that depression was associated with only a slightly higher prevalence of hypertension (2). Cancer patients also have high rates of depression. A review of studies of patients with cancer suggests that among those who are hospitalized with significant levels of physical impairment, at least 25% are likely to meet criteria for major depression or adjustment disorder with depressed mood (18). Advanced stages of cancer and cancer in the pancreas were associated with the highest risk for depressive symptoms. In a study of patients attending a general medical clinic, the group with major depression had a higher percentage of patients with malignancy (3).

A number of other medical illnesses may be associated with comorbid depression. In a study of hospitalized elderly medical and neurological patients, the illnesses most likely to be predictive of depression were renal disease and neurological illness (19). In a sample of nearly 2000 subjects including controls, spouses, and first-degree relatives of patients with depression, the rates of 17 physical illnesses, especially frequent and severe migraine or cluster headaches, diabetes, and stomach ulcer, were higher among the group with major depressive disorder (20). The only medical illness specifically related to the development of major depression in a study of 471 elderly VA inpatients was respiratory disease (8). Similarly, among 917 elderly men with chronic medical illnesses requiring long-term management at a VA primary-care clinic, only chronic obstructive lung disease was differentially associated with high depression scores (6).

B. Other Risk Factors

A more consistent finding than the association of any specific medical diagnosis with the development of depression is the association of depression with the overall burden of medical illness, measured either as illness severity, number of medical diagnoses, or functional disability. In a study of hospitalized elderly medical patients, the severity of depression was strongly correlated with a number of health variables, including physician-rated global illness severity, number of medical problems, cognitive status, functional status, and number of medications (19). The most powerful predictor of depression was the physician-rated global measure of physical illness severity, which accounted for 14% of the variance in HAM-D score. Other studies also have found an association between depression and the severity of medical illness, measured as overall medical burden using the Cumulative Illness Rating Scale (CIRS) (21); tumor status, extent of malignant illness, months since diagnosis, and prognosis (22); the effect of the medical illness on functional disability (8); difficulties with activities of daily living (9); and disability defined as inability to return to work (6). Among a sample of 283 patients admitted to cardiac care units for myocardial infarction (MI), depression was associated with the presence of additional noncardiac medical illness, but was not associated with the severity of the cardiac disease (15). The association of depression and poor functioning with other medical comorbidity suggests that depression and its sequelae are most associated with the overall burden of medical illness. In a follow-up study of about 200 medical clinic outpatients over a 33-month period, the number of new medical diagnoses during the interval was the strongest predictor of the development of depression in patients initially not depressed (5). Thus, the development of a new physical illness was a stronger risk factor than the existence of one or more chronic illnesses. A greater number of diagnoses also was associated with being depressed at both time points, suggesting that there is an association between the number of coexisting medical diagnoses and the chronicity of depression (5).

The burden of medical illness often combines with other stresses to cause depression. Unanticipated, age-inappropriate adverse life events are powerful predictors of the development of depression, compared to the effects of stressful life events that are expected in later life. Among 917 men over the age of 60 with chronic medical illnesses requiring long-term medical management at a VA primary-care clinic, depression was associated with marital separation or divorce and with inability to work because of medical disability, but widowhood and voluntary retirement were less common in the depressed group (6). The results suggest a strong association between depression and disability, defined as inability to work, and are consistent with a model in which unanticipated consequences of aging and medical illness are more frequent risk factors for depression and thus more common sources of comorbidity. Depression in post-MI patients has also been associated with more stressful life events in the year prior to the MI, and with lower self-esteem and sense of being in control of one's life (15). In a survey of over 4000 patients who had seen a general medical provider in the last 6 months, the strongest predictor of developing a diagnosis of depressive disorder in the following year was feelings of guilt (23). Other predictive factors were low income, female sex, and unmarried status.

C. Depression in the Medically Ill as Reactive Depression

The association of comorbid depression with the overall burden of medical illness, functional disability, and the presence of additive psychosocial stressors suggests that much of this comorbid depression might be described as reactive to these factors. A number of investigators have found that depression in the medically ill patient often has features thought to be common in reactive depressions. Some believe that these depressions are more often milder ("subsyndromal") and more transient than depressions not associated with medical illness (9,24,25). Other studies have found evidence that the depression associated with medical illness is a psychological reaction to the illness. In a study of 215 randomly selected cancer patients who were new admissions to inpatient or outpatient cancer centers, only 6% had major affective disorders, but another 12% had adjustment disorder with depressed mood. The high rate of adjustment disorders suggests that treatment of the underlying condition, together with psychological interventions, may be helpful in most patients with cancer and a depressive disorder (22). Among older men admitted to a VA hospital, the most important factor mediating the presence of depression was the overall severity of the medical illness and the effect it had on functional disability (8). These findings are consistent with the hypothesis that depression associated with medical illness is largely related to the psychological effects of the loss of function and threat to existence that accompany the medical disorder. A greater effect of medical illness on the appearance of depression in the elderly may then be due to the greater functional effect and threat to life that medical illness often represents in this age group.

In another study of 150 medical inpatients in the week after admission, it appeared that 65% of the depressives had their illness largely as a consequence of the physical illness, generally as a result of the psychological implications of the disability and threat to life (26). Compared to depressives admitted to psychiatric services, the medically ill depressives had fewer previous depressions, also suggesting that the depression reflects the effect of the medical illness rather than an underlying vulnerability to psychiatric illness. A lower biological vulnerability also was suggested by lower rates of family history of depression in these patients (27). Medically ill depressives also tend to have less suicidality and guilt (9,26–28). In this respect, they are similar to patients with intense grief, who also seem to represent a gray area between the normal and the abnormal (26). Finally, the reactive nature of the depression in medically ill patients may sometimes result in better outcomes, possibly related to treatment of the underlying medical condition (25,27,29).

Although these studies appear to suggest that depression in the medically ill patient is likely to be psychologically based, other evidence suggests that some depressions associated with medical illness may be more closely related to primary psychiatric disorders, or may even have a biological basis. In a study of hospitalized elderly medical and neurological patients, there was a history of previous psychiatric illness in 43% of the patients with major depression, compared to only 19% of those without major depression (19). Preexisting anxiety or major depression also predicted the development of a depressive diagnosis among medical outpatients (23), and alcoholism may increase the risk among cancer patients (18). An interaction between overall medical burden and biological factors in the increased risk of depression among elderly medical patients is suggested by a study of 28 subjects with late-life depression who were compared with 29 healthy control subjects for the severity of medical illness and for magnetic resonance imaging findings of atrophy and high-intensity signals (21). Subjects with depression had more atrophy than controls, greater medical burden, and more severe ratings of high-intensity signals in the periventricular and deep white matter areas. However, a logistic regression indicated that only atrophy and medical burden were independent and significant predictors of the presence of depression. High-intensity signals suggestive of cerebrovascular disease were not significant in this analysis, and there also was no difference between the contribution of cerebrovascular risk factors or cardiovascular disease and the contribution of all other illnesses to the development of depression. These findings suggest that atrophy may predispose the elderly brain to depression, but that general illness burden, rather than disease specifically affecting the brain, is sufficient to precipitate a depressive illness (21).

III. HEALTH EFFECTS OF COMORBID DEPRESSION IN THE MEDICALLY ILL

A. Medical Morbidity

Evidence suggests that even if the depression associated with medical illness has a reactive component, the added health burden associated with depression in the elderly is great, and the effects of comorbid depression and medical illness are additive. Patients with comorbid depression and medical disorders are especially likely to present to physicians for this reason (30). In a sample of 11,242 adult outpatients receiving medical care who where screened as part of the Medical Outcomes Study, depression was associated with impairments in physical, social, and role functioning and in current health, bed days, and bodily pain that were comparable to those from chronic medical conditions such as hypertension, diabetes, arthritis, back, lung, or gastrointestinal problems. Current health was found to be significantly worse for patients with depressive symptoms than for patients with all of the medical conditions studied with the exception of angina and current advanced CAD. Among an inpatient psychiatric population admitted for depression, the largest single contributor to functional level was disability due to psychiatric illness (31). Medical illness contributed to disability in the more basic functional tasks (e.g., toileting, dressing) among older patients, but explained only one-third as much variance as psychiatric illness. Neither the overall severity of the depression or of the medical illness was predictive. Pain has been found to be more frequent and severe among depressed patients, even when controlling for physical illness, although some of the association may be due to the effect of depression on activity level (32,33). Thus, the impact of depression on health and functioning is generally as great as the impact of medical illness.

When depression and medical illness occur together, the impairment is greater than with either alone. A number of studies have examined the effects of comorbid depression on the disability, cost and length of treatment, course, prognosis, and mortality associated with medical illness. Depression is an especially strong predictor of poor outcome in patients with cardiovascular illness. In one study of 52 patients with significant CAD on cardiac catheterization, the 17% who were classified as having major depression prior to angiography had a significantly greater rate of major cardiac events during a year of follow-up (13). The presence of major depression remained the strongest independent risk factor for these events even when severity of CAD, left ventricular ejection fraction, and the presence of smoking were included in a multiple regression analysis. Other studies have found higher rates of angina (14), lower rates of returning to work (14,15), and higher rates of smoking (11,14,24) among depressed patients with CAD and those in the immediate post-MI period. This latter finding suggests that depression predicts poor compliance with prescribed rehabilitation or life-style modifications after a myocardial infarction, which could contribute to poorer outcomes. Patients with noncardiac illness and depression also are found to have less favorable outcomes. For example, among 219 patients with a mean age of 78.5 years who were followed up at 2, 6, and 12 months after surgical treatment for a fractured hip, those with persistently elevated depressive symptoms had significantly lower rates of walking independently and of returning to prefracture levels in other physical function parameters, even when controlling for age, prefracture physical condition, and postfracture cognitive status (29).

B. Health Care Utilization

Poor outcomes are also reflected in greater utilization of medical resources. Several studies have found longer lengths of hospital stay in patients with depression than in patients with matched medical diagnoses or comparable physical impairment but without depression (34–36). In a 4-year follow-up to one of these studies, patients with more depression on the index admission had significantly greater hospital utilization during the follow-up period, even when other factors were controlled (37). Both the readmission rate and the number of days spent in the hospital were more than twice as high in patients with depression at the index admission. These higher rates of medical utilization are associated with increased costs of care. A 4-year prospective follow-up study of 2558 HMO Medicare enrollees (mean age 73) found that the 14% with baseline CES-D scores above the depressive cutoff of 16 had higher median costs for medical care over the follow-up period (4). The association of higher costs with depression persisted after controlling for age, sex, race, the severity of chronic medical illness, and whether or not patients were participating in an intervention of preventive health services. The model estimated a 1.9% cost increase for each point of increase on the CES-D. There was a higher use of services in all categories of medical care, including inpatient admissions, outpatient visits, laboratory tests, emergency department visits, number of prescriptions, number of ancillary visits, and number of optometry visits. Thus, general utilization of medical services, and higher costs, are comorbid conditions among elderly patients with depression (4).

C. Mortality

Comorbid depression in elderly medical patients is also associated with higher mortality, much of which is due to cardiovascular disease. As long ago as 1937, Malzberg found that the death rate was 6.8 times greater in melancholic female patients than in the general population, and 6 times greater in melancholic male patients (38). Cardiac disease accounted for almost 40% of all the deaths in patients with affective disorder, which was 8 times the corresponding rate for the general population. In a sample of 3007 subjects aged 55 and over who were surveyed as part of the epidemiological catchment area (ECA) project in New Haven, follow-up over a period of 15 months revealed that patients with affective disorders were 4.3 times as likely to die than those without affective disorders, even when controlling for age, sex, physical health status, cognitive impairment, and other psychiatric status (39). The increase in mortality was entirely among the group with major depression. Thus, the increased risk of death associated with major depression appeared to be independent of the possible effects of depression on the development, severity, or treatment of physical health problems. Among 62 patients with major depression who were treated as inpatients at a mean age of 70 and then followed for 1 year, the mortality rate was 2.6 times that expected after adjusting for age (40). Six of the eight deaths were related to cardiovascular illness, and the presence of cardiovascular disease at discharge was the only significant predictor of death. Other studies have also found increased mortality in depressed patients with cardiovascular disease (16,17) and in patients with cancer (41).

Although increased cardiovascular mortality in depressed patients may reflect poor compliance with treatment or less aggressive attempts by physicians to treat depression in patients with severe cardiac disease, biological factors may also have a role. During Holter monitoring of 103 patients with CAD documented by elective angiography, ventricular tachycardia was more frequent among the depressed patients than among those without depression, with a relative risk of 8.2 (12). The association persisted after adjusting for sex, current cigarette smoking, and use of beta-blockers and nitrates. These findings suggest a biological vulnerability of depressed patients to adverse consequences of cardiac disease, which may be due to increased sympathetic tone leading to ventricular tachycardia and even ventricular fibrillation and the possibility of sudden death. Other effects might include a lowering of the ventricular vulnerable period threshold due to psychological stress, leading to a greater likelihood of fatal ventricular fibrillation; more frequent baseline premature ventricular contractions; and a decrease in parasympathetic tone (24). Lower parasympathetic tone may be reflected in lower heart rate variability, which has been found in patients with major depression. This in turn may lower the threshold for ventricular fibrillation and predispose to sudden cardiovascular death (24). Other authors who have noted increased cardiovascular mortality in depressed patients suggest that these patients have greater susceptibility to other illnesses because of the agitation, malnutrition, and poor hygiene associated with the depression (42).

D. Effects of Comorbidity on Depression

The prognosis for the depression in patients with comorbid depression and medical illness also is less favorable. In a comparison of 37 patients with major depression only who were admitted to an acute-care psychiatric hospital and 41 patients whose major depression was comorbid with another psychiatric and/or medical condition, all of whom were followed for 12 months, about half as many patients with comorbid conditions as those with pure depression recovered (43). At 1-year follow-up of 555 patients with current major depression, patients with a lifetime history of myocardial infarction had worse outcomes on five of six comparisons, including more frequent episodes of depression and more depressive symptoms (44). This poorer prognosis persisted over a second year of follow-up. The study did not address the reasons for the association with poorer outcome, which may be due to persistent limitations in functioning due to chronic CAD, or to reluctance on the part of physicians to treat depression in patients with a history of MI (44). In a large national VA survey of late-middle-aged and older patients admitted to mental health units, the number of medical diagnoses was associated with longer episodes of inpatient care (45).

Viewed more comprehensively, the effects of medical illness and depression on each other in elderly patients are complex and bidirectional. A longitudinal study of the prevalence of both somatic and psychiatric disorders (depression and/or anxiety) was part of a large epidemiological survey of the general population in a county in Canada performed in 1952 with follow-up in 1968 (46). In the follow-up, there were 618 survivors from the original sample of 1003. Overall, the prevalence of depressive and anxiety disorders was 12.5% in 1952 and 12.7% at follow-up, and at both times the rate of somatic disorders was about 25%. There were identical odds ratios of 2.2 for both the likelihood of developing a psychiatric illness at follow-up given the presence of a somatic illness at baseline, and the likelihood of developing a somatic illness at follow-up given the presence of a psychiatric illness at baseline. The fact that neither direction of influence was stronger than the other suggests that "generalized vulnerability" to illness may be a more valuable concept. In other words, there are differences among individuals in general susceptibility to illness, but those individuals who have the largest number of illness episodes also have the broadest range of illness types (46).

We have already seen that two common factors mediating between the effects of depression and medical illness are functional impairment in activities of daily living and somatic pain. Another possible link is psychic pain, especially anxiety. In an early review of the studies seeking associations between psychological and social factors and the development of coronary disease, the conclusion was that anxiety, neuroticism, and other painful affects were associated with coronary disease, and in particular with angina more so than with myocardial infarction (47). In a large survey from the ECA study, persons with affective, anxiety, and substance use disorders had a greater prevalence of multiple lifetime chronic medical conditions than persons without a psychiatric disorder (48). However, the associations between the presence of affective disorder and specific medical conditions were weakened after controlling for concurrent anxiety disorders. Thus, anxiety may be the common factor among patients with depression and physical illness, and may be the primary psychiatric component in patients with such comorbid conditions (48).

IV. IDENTIFICATION OF DEPRESSION IN THE MEDICALLY ILL

A. Patient Self-Report of Symptoms

The identification of a depressive disorder in a medically ill patient can be influenced by many factors. Although the added functional disability due to the combination of depression and medical illness often leads patients to seek more frequent medical attention, there are mixed findings in the literature regarding whether elderly patients are more or less likely to report depressive symptoms. Two studies suggest underreporting by elderly patients. To assess the hypothesis that older depressed patients are less likely to report symptoms than younger depressives, 97 subjects admitted with major depression were evaluated using the HAM-D and self-rated Beck Depression Inventory (BDI) (49). HAM-D and BDI scores were significantly correlated. However, older age correlated with lower scores on the self-rated BDI, despite the lack of any correlation of age with scores on the HAM-D. Even when adjusted for HAM-D scores, older patients had significantly lower scores on the BDI. When the HAM-D and BDI were divided into instruments that included only somatic/neurovegetative or psychological/affective symptoms, the effect of age was significant only for the subtotals that included the psychological/affective symptoms (49). In other words, as patients aged they were less likely to self-report affective and psychological symptoms of depression, even when these symptoms could be elicited by clinicians evaluating the patients using the HAM-D, but they continued to report somatic/neurovegetative symptoms. In another study of patients 60 years and older admitted to the medical and neurology services of a VA hospital, 45% were found to have major depression. Patient self-ratings using the Zung Self-Rating Depression Scale identified only 58% of these depressions, missing many of the mild cases (10). Perhaps the lower sensitivity suggests that older patients tend to underreport their symptoms on a self-rating instrument.

Two other studies, however, tend to contradict the finding that elderly patients are less likely to report symptoms. In one study of 618 patients attending a general medical clinic, 6.6% were found to meet criteria for a major depressive episode. Fewer than half of the patients with major depression had any indication of this diagnosis in their charts. However, there was no difference between diagnosed and undiagnosed depressive patients in the severity of self-report of depressive symptoms on the initial screening evaluation, suggesting that it is misinterpretation of symptoms, rather than underreporting of them, that prevents the diagnosis from being made (3). In another study of 598 nursing home and congregate housing residents, there were strong associations between diagnoses of depression and experienced pain intensity, with greater pain reported by those with more severe depressive diagnoses (32). Patients with major depression were more sensitive to pain that had a possible physical cause than were patients with either minor depression or no depression. This finding suggests that the presence of depression may increase either the patient's sensitivity to the pain caused by an existing somatic disorder, or the patient's willingness to report it. If true, this finding would seem to contradict the finding that elderly patients are less likely to report symptoms, even when depressed. However, it suggests that they may be more likely to report somatic symptoms, but less likely to report depressed mood or to attribute somatic sensations to depression (32).

The whole question of whether elderly patients are more or less likely to "report" depressive symptoms, of course, presupposes that the depression identified by clinicians using the *Diagnostic and Statistical Manual* (DSM) criteria has universal symptoms that characterize patients of all ages, and that if elderly patients do not report these symptoms it must be due to a failure of self-report. However, studies such as the ones above cannot rule out the possibility that older patients have a different subjective experience of depression and actually do not feel depressed mood even when objective observers note depressed affect (note that the first item on the HAM-D is called depressed mood but allows a rater to score the item based on observation of depressed affect). Although this possibility may not be relevant to diagnosis when a comprehensive evaluation is performed by a skilled clinician, it may be very relevant for attempts to screen populations at risk for depression using self-rating instruments. In general, the studies described above suggest that such screening should be weighted toward the identification of somatic symptoms rather than psychological or affective ones. Such a conclusion is somewhat counterintuitive in the medically ill elderly population, because one might suspect that somatic depressive symptoms are more likely to be confounded by the presence of medical illness. However, some evidence contradicts that suspicion. Data from the Durham VA Mental Health Survey indicate that although hospitalized elderly have more severe medical illness, among those with major depression younger and older patients had the same frequency of somatic complaints. Overall, somatic symptoms were as predictive of the presence of major depression in the elderly patients as in the younger patients (50). In another study that found somatic symptoms to be common in medically ill patients with depression, the somatic symptoms tended to cluster with depressed mood, further suggesting that somatic symptoms are important predictors of depressive disorders (9).

B. Effects of Medical Illness on the Presentation of Depression

Another possible reason for different self-reports of depression in elderly patients with medical illness is that age or the medical condition may influence the presentation of the depression. The effect of age is seen in the fact that substance abuse and personality disorder are less frequently contributing factors to depression in older persons, while there is a greater association with systemic medical conditions such as arthritis, sensory dysfunction, diabetes, ischemic heart disease, hypertension, stroke, and neurodegenerative diseases. The association with these conditions may influence the presentation of depression, which may be a final, common pathway for the manifestation of a variety of diseases. We do not understand how these diseases influence the expression of disordered mood, but the effect may be analogous to the way in which medical changes with age influence the presentation of common conditions such as angina and pneumonia. For example, some investigators have reported that elderly depressives with medical illness may have less guilt or suicidal ideation, but more cognitive impairment (51).

The strongest evidence for a direct effect of a medical illness on the presentation of depression can be found in studies of patients with dementia. A study of 1304 elderly subjects with and without dementia rated on the HAM-D found that a factor analysis could identify two clusters of symptoms: a mood factor including dysphoria, sleep disturbance, appetite disturbance, feelings of guilt and suicidal thoughts; and a motivational disturbance that included loss of interest, difficulty with concentration, psychomotor change, and loss of energy. Although motivational symptoms were found to increase linearly with declines in cognitive function, mood symptoms had a quadratic relationship to cognition, with first an increase as cognitive function declined, and than a decrease as dementia became more severe (52). Thus, these findings suggest that patients with different degrees of cognitive function or different stages of dementia may have different presentations of depression, and may need to be evaluated differently. Other investigators have suggested that atypical presentations of depression, characterized by agitation and functional change, may be especially common in patients in the later stages of dementia (53).

C. Diagnostic Criteria

In diagnosing a depressive syndrome in a medically ill patient, the clinician must determine whether the syndrome is due to a primary depressive disorder or to the medical condition. Starting with DSM-III, established diagnostic criteria have recognized that a disturbance of mood may be due to organic factors. In DSM-III, "organic affective syndrome" was defined as having the same phenomenology as a major depressive episode, and was diagnosed if evidence could be found for a specific organic factor that was judged to be etiologically related to the disturbance. DSM-III-R changed the term to "organic mood syndrome," but the criteria and differentiation from major depressive episode were the same. The latest revision of the diagnostic manual, DSM-IV, abandons the "organic" terminology and instead lists criteria for a "mood disorder due to a general medical condition." In contrast to the previous criteria for an organic disorder, which required any etiological relationship between the organic factor and the mood disturbance, the criteria for mood disorder due to a general medical condition require that the mood disturbance be the direct physiological consequence of the medical disorder. Although the intent appears to be to limit the diagnosis of this condition to episodes of illness in which a clear physiological link can be established, the manual acknowledges that "there are no infallible guidelines for determining whether the relationship between the mood disturbance and the general medical condition is etiological." It is suggested that temporal associations between the medical condition and the mood disorder, and the presence of features that are atypical of primary mood disorders, may be considered in making this determination. If the mood disturbance is thought to be a maladaptive psychological reaction to the stress of having the general medical condition, then "adjustment disorder with depressed mood" would be diagnosed.

It is clear that these definitions allow for a considerable degree of ambiguity in diagnosis. A typical depressive syndrome in a medically ill patient may represent a primary psychiatric disorder, a true symptom of the medical disorder, a secondary or functional reaction to the impairment associated with the medical disorder, or a coincidental occurrence, but it is often difficult to distinguish among these possibilities (54). In practice, subjectivity, bias toward identifying medical causes, or sheer persistence in searching for them may determine whether a medical cause for depression will be found. In one study of 50 community-dwelling subjects diagnosed with RDC depression after identification through a screening process (i.e., not self-referred or identified by their physicians as depressed), 26 were judged to have a medical cause associated with at least some of their depressive symptoms, and in nine the depression was felt to be "definitely" associated with a specific medical cause (physical illness or medication use) (55). Despite regular contact with physicians, neither the depression nor the possibility of its medical cause had been previously identified, and treatment was almost entirely with a variety of symptom-oriented medications including hormones, sedatives, hypnotics, and analgesics. The authors concluded that the determination of whether a medical illness is the probable cause of a depressive disorder is highly subjective (55).

D. Inclusive, Exclusive, and Substitutive Symptom Assessment

Although the diagnosis of a depressive disorder as primary or due to a general medical condition can be ambiguous, the clinician facing this dilemma is at least aware that a depression is present. A more serious clinical problem is the failure to recognize that the patient has a depression at all because of the presence of a medical disorder. This problem may arise if symptoms that may be part of a depressive disorder are ascribed to the medical illness, and thus are not counted toward making a depression diagnosis. Omitting these somatic symptoms when diagnosing depression results in requiring a stricter definition of depression among medical patients than patients without medical illness, and risks missing cases of depression. On the other hand, the consequence of including somatic symptoms in diagnosing depression in patients with medical illnesses such as cancer is that there may be an increase in the false positive rate of diagnosis (56). Overdiagnosis may lead to unnecessary treatment, or the medical significance of some symptoms may be missed if they are attributed to depression. The decision about whether to count somatic symptoms or not is thus a choice between what is called an inclusive approach, where all symptoms count, regardless of presumed cause, and the etiological approach as described in the DSM-IV, where symptoms are not counted if the clinician feels they are "clearly and fully accounted for by the physiological effects" of medical illness.

There is some evidence that use of the inclusive and etiological approaches may have similar results in practice: one study of elderly patients admitted to the medical services of a university teaching hospital and diagnosed using an inclusive approach (9) found similar rates of depressive disorders to those found in another study by the same group using an etiological approach to symptoms among elderly veterans admitted to the medical services of a VA hospital (8). However, the potential pitfalls associated with using an inclusive approach are seen in the results of a study of internists' recoding of individual items on the HAM-D as rated by psychiatrists (57). Items were recoded as very probably, possibly, or not probably related to somatic illness or medication use. Overall, more than half of the positive scores were questioned by internists for eight of the 21 items of the HAM-D. Even for a psychological item such as depressed mood, one-third of positive responses were considered possibly related to a somatic cause, presumably medication use in most cases. None of these positive scores for depressed mood, however, were considered very probably due to a somatic cause. Somatic causes were most often considered the cause of items such as general somatic symptoms (e.g., fatigue), somatic anxiety, and loss of interest or work impairment. Somatic causes were considered most unlikely for guilt, suicidality, diurnal variation, and paranoia, and were not ever considered as causes of loss of insight, depersonalization, and obsessive-compulsive symptoms. These findings suggest that the HAM-D might overestimate depression in the somatically ill, and that some items are more susceptible to ambiguity than others (57).

One solution that might rescue the inclusive approach would be to exclude these ambiguous items from use in the medically ill population, or to give additional weight to those items considered more unambiguously related to depression (especially those that are less ambiguously related to depression than to other psychiatric illnesses, such as diurnal variation, guilt, and suicidality, in that order). However, eliminating the somatic symptoms altogether results in poorer classification because of decreased sensitivity (7). Another solution is Endicott's suggestion of substituting alternative associated symptoms for the somatic symptoms required for a diagnosis of major depression. Instead of poor appetite or weight loss; insomnia or hypersomnia; loss of energy; and decreased ability to think or concentrate, she suggests substituting fearfulness or depressed appearance in face or body posture; social withdrawal or decreased talkativeness; brooding, self-pity, or pessimism; and lack of reactivity to good news or funny situations (56). The substitutive approach is supported by the work of Cavanaugh et al., who found that decreased energy was a poor discriminator of depression in medically ill patients, and "indecisiveness" was a good one (58).

To test the usefulness of the Endicott criteria for diagnosing major depression in patients with multiple somatic symptoms, 150 elderly medical inpatients were give schedule for affective disorders and schizophrenia (SADS) interviews and then diagnosed using the standard criteria and also using the substitutive symptom criteria proposed by Endicott (7). The correlation between the somatic symptoms and the alternative symptoms substituted for them was low; nevertheless, 96% of the patients were classified the same way using both sets of criteria, indicating that the nonsomatic criteria are equally sensitive and specific to depressive disorders in this population. Since substitution of the nonsomatic symptoms did not lead to additional patients being diagnosed, the results suggest that use of the standard criteria does not result in missed diagnoses. However, in this study somatic symptoms were counted using an inclusive approach. If an etiological approach were used, and many of the somatic symptoms were not counted because they were felt to be possibly related to medical illness, then the rates of diagnosis of depression using the standard criteria probably would have been lower. If so, then use of the substitutive symptom criteria approach would probably yield a higher sensitivity of identifying depression (7).

The usefulness of a combined etiological and substitutive diagnostic approach was tested in another study. Pairs of raters used either an inclusive approach or an etiological approach; in addition, both approaches were tested using three different criterion lists of symptoms: the standard list, an exclusive list that eliminated fatigue and anorexia/weight loss, and a substitutive list that replaced fatigue, anorexia/weight loss, psychomotor retardation, and impaired concentration with irritability, tearfulness, social withdrawal, and feeling punished (59). Thus, six different approaches were compared. In addition, interviewers made unstructured diagnoses of depression based on their overall impression of the patient. The authors hypothesized that using a strict inclusive approach would result in higher interrater reliability for the diagnosis of major and minor depression than the DSM-IV etiological approach, and that interrater agreement on the etiology of individual symptoms would be poor. The results suggested that neither hypothesis was correct. There were high rates of agreement for the diagnosis of depression, especially major depression, regardless of the diagnostic approach, and most symptoms had either 100% or at least over 80% agreement for etiology, despite the lack of reliability training for the raters. The only symptoms for which raters tended to disagree on etiology were weight loss, fatigue or loss of energy, loss of sexual interest, and social withdrawal. Thus, when a structured psychiatric interview is used to diagnose depression in hospitalized medically ill patients, an inclusive approach to counting symptoms has no advantage over the DSM-IV approach. However, given the lack of agreement over symptoms of fatigue, psychomotor retardation, and sexual interest, these symptoms should probably be given less weight when the etiological approach required by DSM-IV is used (59).

A reasonable conclusion from the results of all of these studies is that when skilled clinicians comprehensively evaluate elderly medically ill patients for the presence of depression, the etiological approach to symptom counting required by DSM-IV does not result in many missed cases of depression, and probably helps to avoid overdiagnosis. On the other hand, an inclusive approach that permits the identification of multiple somatic complaints may be more useful for screening such populations for possible depression. Despite general support for these conclusions, other caveats must be mentioned. First, of course, there are no good definitions of a skilled clinician or a comprehensive evaluation. In the study cited above comparing structured diagnostic approaches, interviewers also made unstructured diagnoses of depression based on their overall impression of the patient (59). Agreement among these raters, even on the diagnosis of major depression, was very low (kappas of agreement around 0.40). At the least, this finding suggests that raters who base their general impression on an etiological interpretation of symptoms will often fail to diagnose a major depression. Perhaps the very use of a structured approach tends to collapse the distinction between an inclusive and an etiological counting of symptoms, leading clinicians to bias their assessment of etiology in favor of the symptoms being due to depressive disorder rather than medical illness (59). Thus, the usefulness of the etiological approach may require that clinicians consider each symptom individually as part of a structured assessment.

A second caveat is that the decision about whether to count a symptom is based not only on its presumed relationship to a possible depressive disorder, but also on its severity. Several studies have examined the effect of using different thresholds for symptom severity. In one, 130 subjects with terminal cancer (mean age 71.5 years) were rated for depression using both the RDC and the Endicott criteria. In addition, two different symptom severity thresholds were evaluated, separated by single points on the SADS scores for the depressed mood item and the loss of interest item (60). Both the Endicott and RDC criteria identified similar rates of depression, but the use of low versus high thresholds resulted in rates that varied by as much as twofold. In the study cited above in which internists recoded symptoms initially identified by psychiatrists, another interesting finding was that items were less likely to be recoded by internists when psychiatrists rated their severity as greater (57). Thus, the selection of symptom severity as a diagnostic indicator is more important than whether one uses or avoids potentially confounded somatic symptoms in making a diagnosis.

The decision about how severe symptoms must be before they are counted toward a diagnosis of depression obviously will have a bearing on the number of cases that are identified, but there is no gold standard against which to judge such a decision. Regardless of the measure used to assess mood, distress in the physically ill appears to be a continuously distributed variable, suggesting that depression is not a disease but rather the tail end of a continuum, like hypertension (61). The value of classification of patients into depressive diagnoses lies in whether this distinction operationalizes the decision of whether to treat with antidepressants, or to treat at all. Thus, diagnostic distinctions require validation by an intervention trial. Since very few of these have been done for medically ill depressed patients, the practical value of making any depressive diagnosis in this population has so far not been established (61). Nevertheless, the selection of criteria still depends on the purpose of the diagnosis. If maximizing specificity is crucial, as, for example, in research where homogeneity of the clinical population is important, then an exclusive approach is best. If maximizing sensitivity is important, as, for example, in screening large medical populations where one does not want to miss a treatable condition, then the inclusive approach is best (62). For the experienced clinician evaluating a patient referred by medical colleagues, an etiological approach may be equally or more useful.

V. TREATMENT

The few studies in the literature that address treatment of depression in medically ill patients suggest that much of the excess medical morbidity and mortality caused by the depression can be reduced with effective therapy. Psychiatric consultation has been found to reduce the hospital length of stay among depressed medical patients to lengths comparable to those of nondepressed patients (35). A study of 200 depressed patients seen in a primary-care clinic found a 75% remission rate in the group randomized to receive collaborative care by a team that included a psychiatrist, compared to a 40% remission rate in the control group (63). In a 3-year follow-up study of 519 hospitalized depressed patients, those treated with electroconvulsive therapy had a significantly lower total mortality than those treated with inadequate courses of antidepressants, and there was a trend for patients treated with adequate trials of antidepressants also to have lower mortality (42). In particular, the death rate from MI was lower in the combined adequate treatment group than in the inadequate treatment group, despite the greater age of the adequately treated patients. The decrease in mortality was especially striking in the elderly patients; of those over the age of 60, the 1-year mortality of the inadequate treatment group was five times that of the group that received adequate treatment (42). One report expressed some nihilism about the treatment of depression in hospitalized medically ill patients (64); in a planned trial of nortriptyline, only seven of 40 eligible patients could be enrolled, and medical illnesses prevented more than 80% of eligible patients from participating in or completing the clinical trial. However, newer antidepressants with fewer side effects may prove more useful. Other investigators have suggested that interventions designed to improve functional independence, through rehabilitative approaches or the teaching of problem-solving techniques, may improve depressive symptoms whether or not they treat medical illness or pain (33,65).

VI. SUMMARY

In summary, comorbid depression in patients with medical illness is more common than would be expected by chance alone. The highest rates are found in patients with cardiovascular disease and cancer, but the strongest association is with the degree of psychological and functional disability and burden due to the medical illness. In this sense, depression in the medically ill elderly may be viewed as reactive, but patients with predisposing psychiatric and biological vulnerability also are at greater risk. Depression contributes to increased medical morbidity and mortality, and medical illness can affect the presentation, course, and outcome of depressive illness. This bidirectional relationship suggests that a model of "generalized vulnerability" may best explain the complex interactions of affective and medical disorders in the elderly, with functional disability, anxiety, and pain as mediating factors. The presence of common features, especially somatic symptoms, may interfere with the diagnosis of depression in medically ill elderly, and even with the identification of medical illness in depressed elderly. The determination of whether a specific symptom, or a depressive syndrome, is due to a comorbid medical condition can be difficult. Different methods for counting symptoms have therefore been proposed, each with advantages and disadvantages. In general, an exclusive approach works best for research purposes, an inclusive approach with an emphasis on somatic symptoms works best for population screening, and an etiological approach is most appropriate for the skill psychiatric clinician evaluating a medical patient. Treatment should focus on therapy of the underlying medical condition, but also must directly address functional impairment, pain, and anxiety. Much additional research is needed on the appropriate pharmacological treatment of depression in elderly patients who are frail and medically ill.

REFERENCES

1. Lacro JP, Jeste DV. Physical comorbidity and polypharmacy in older psychiatric patients. Biol Psychiatry 1994; 36:146–152.
2. Gierz M, Jeste DV. Physical comorbidity in elderly Veterans Affairs patients with schizophrenia and depression. Am J Geriatr Psychiatry 1993; 1:165–170.
3. Coulehan JL, Schulberg HC, Block MR, Janosky JE, Arena VC. Medical comorbidity of major depressive disorder in a primary medical practice. Arch Intern Med 1990; 150:2363–2367.
4. Unutzer J, Patrick DL, Simon G, Grembowski D, Walker E, Rutter C, Katon W. Depressive symptoms and the cost of health services in HMO patients aged 65 years and older: a 4-year prospective study. JAMA 1997; 277:1618–1623.
5. Kukull WA, Koepsell TD, Inui TS, Borson S, Okimoto J, Raskind MA, Gale JL. Depression and physical illness among elderly general medical clinic patients. J Affect Disord 1986; 10:153–162.
6. Borson S, Barnes RA, Kukull WA, Okimoto JT, Veith RC, Inui TS, Carter W, Raskind MA. Symptomatic depression in elderly medical outpatients. I. Prevalence, demography, and health service utilization. J Am Geriatr Soc 1986; 34:341–347.
7. Rapp SR, Vrana S. Substituting nonsomatic for somatic symptoms in the diagnosis of depression in elderly male medical patients. Am J Psychiatry 1989; 146:1197–1200.
8. Koenig HG, Meador KG, Shelp F, Goli V, Cohen HJ, Blazer DG. Major depressive disorder in hospitalized medically ill patients: an examination of young and elderly male veterans. J Am Geriatr Soc 1991; 39:881–890.
9. Koenig HG, O'Connor CM, Guarisco SA, Zabel KM, Ford SM. Depressive disorder in older medical inpatients on general medicine and cardiology services at a university teaching hospital. Am J Geriatr Psychiatry 1993; 1:197–210.
10. Kitchell MA, Barnes RF, Veith RC, Okimoto JT, Raskind MA. Screening for depression in hospitalized geriatric medical patients. J Am Geriatr Soc 1982; 30:174–177.
11. Carney RM, Rich MW, Tevelde A, Saini J, Clark K, Jaffe AS. Major depressive disorder in coronary artery disease. Am J Cardiol 1987; 60:1273–1275.
12. Carney RM, Freedland KE, Rich MW, Smith LJ, Jaffe AS. Ventricular tachycardia and psychiatric depression in patients with coronary artery disease. Am J Med 1993; 95:23–28.
13. Carney RM, Rich MW, Freedland KE, Saini J, TeVelde A, Simeone C, Clark K. Major depressive disorder predicts cardiac events in patients with coronary artery disease. Psychosom Med 1988; 50:627–633.
14. Ladwig KH, Roll G, Breithardt G, Budde T, Borggrefe M. Post-infarction depression and incomplete recovery 6 months after acute myocardial infarction. Lancet 1994; 343:20–23.
15. Schleifer SJ, Macari-Hinson MM, Coyle DA, Slater WR, Kahn M, Gorlin R,

Zucker HD. The nature and course of depression following myocardial infarction. Arch Intern Med 1989; 149:1785–1789.
16. Frasure-Smith N, Lesperance F, Talajic M. Depression following myocardial infarction: impact on 6-month survival. JAMA 1993; 270:1819–1825.
17. Aromaa A, Raitasalo R, Reunanen A, Impivaara O, Heliovaara M, Knekt P, Lehtinen V, Joukamaa M, Maatela J. Depression and cardiovascular diseases. Acta Psychiatr Scand 1994; 377(Suppl):77–82.
18. Massie MJ, Holland JC. Depression and the cancer patient. J Clin Psychiatry 1990; 51:12–17.
19. Koenig HG, Meador KG, Cohen HJ, Blazer DG. Depression in elderly hospitalized patients with medical illness. Arch Intern Med 1988; 148:1929–1936.
20. Moldin SO, Scheftner WA, Rice JP, Nelson E, Knesevich MA, Akiskal H. Association between major depressive disorder and physical illness. Psychol Med 1993; 23:755–761.
21. Kumar A, Miller D, Ewbank D, Yousem D, Newberg A, Samuels S, Cowell P, Gottlieb G. Quantitative anatomic measures and comorbid medical illness in late-life major depression. Am J Geriatr Psychiatry 1997; 5:15–25.
22. Derogatis LR, Morrow GR, Fetting J, Penman D, Piasetsky S, Schmale AM, Henrichs M, Carnicke CLM. The prevalence of psychiatric disorders among cancer patients. JAMA 1983; 249:751–757.
23. Crum RM, Cooper-Patrick L, Ford DE. Depressive symptoms among general medical patients: prevalence and one-year outcome. Psychosom Med 1994; 56:109–117.
24. Dalack GW, Roose SP. Perspectives on the relationship between cardiovascular disease and affective disorder. J Clin Psychiatry 1990; 51 [7, suppl]:4–9.
25. Pomerantz AS, de Nesnera A, West AN. Resolution of depressive symptoms in medical inpatients after discharge. Int J Psychiatry Med 1992; 22:281–289.
26. Moffic HS, Paykel ES. Depression in medical in-patients. Br J Psychiatry 1975; 126:346–353.
27. Winokur G, Black DW, Nasrallah A. Depressions secondary to other psychiatric disorders and medical illnesses. Am J Psychiatry 1988; 145:233–237.
28. Cassem EH. Depression and anxiety secondary to medical illness. Psychiatr Clin North Am 1990; 13:597–612.
29. Mossey JM, Knott K, Craik R. The effects of persistent depressive symptoms on hip fracture recovery. J Gerontol 1990; 45:M163–168.
30. Wells KB, Stewart A, Hays RD, Burnam MA, Rogers W, Daniels M, Berry S, Greenfield S, Ware J. The functioning and well-being of depressed patients: results from the Medical Outcomes Study. JAMA 1989; 262:914–919.
31. Lyness JM, Caine ED, Conwell Y, King DA, Cox C. Depressive symptoms, medical illness, and functional status in depressed psychiatric inpatients. Am J Psychiatry 1993; 150:910–915.
32. Parmelee PA, Katz IR, Lawton MP. The relation of pain to depression among institutionalized aged. J Gerontol 1991; 46:15–21.
33. Williamson GM, Schulz R. Pain, activity restriction, and symptoms of depression among community-residing elderly adults. J Gerontol 1992:P367–372.

34. Saravay SM, Steinberg MD, Weinschel B, Pollack S, Alovis N. Psychological comorbidity and length of stay in the general hospital. Am J Psychiatry 1991; 148: 324–329.
35. Ackerman AD, Lyons JS, Hammer JS, Larson DB. The impact of coexisting depression and timing of psychiatric consultation on medical patients' length of stay. Hosp Commun Psychiatry 1988; 39:173–176.
36. Fulop G, Strain JJ, Vita J, Lyons JS, Hammer JS. Impact of psychiatric comorbidity on length of hospital stay of medical/surgical patients: a preliminary report. Am J Psychiatry 1987; 144:878–882.
37. Saravay SM, Pollack S, Steinberg MD, Weinschel B, Habert M. Four-year follow-up of the influence of psychological comorbidity on medical rehospitalization. Am J Psychiatry 1996; 153:397–403.
38. Malzberg B. Mortality among patients with involution melancholia. Am J Psychiatry 1937; 93:1231–1238.
39. Bruce ML, Leaf PJ. Psychiatric disorders and 15-month mortality in a community sample of older adults. Am J Public Health 1989; 79:727–730.
40. Rabins PV, Harvis K, Koven S. High fatality rates of late-life depression associated with cardiovascular disease. J Affect Disord 1985; 9:165–167.
41. Koenig HG, Shelp F, Goli V, Cohen HJ, Blazer DG. Survival and health care utilization in elderly medical inpatients with major depression. J Am Geriatr Soc 1989; 37:599–606.
42. Avery D, Winokur G. Mortality in depressed patients treated with electroconvulsive therapy and antidepressants. Arch Gen Psychiatry 1976; 33:1029–1037.
43. Keitner GI, Ryan CE, Miller IW, Kohn R, Epstein NB. 12-month outcome of patients with major depression and comorbid psychiatric or medical illness (compound depression). Am J Psychiatry 1991; 148:345–350.
44. Wells KB, Rogers W, Burnam MA, Camp P. Course of depression in patients with hypertension, myocardial infarction, or insulin-dependent diabetes. Am J Psychiatry 1993; 150:632–638.
45. Moos RH, Mertens JR. Patterns of diagnoses, comorbidities, and treatment in late-middle-aged and older affective disorder patients: comparison of mental health and medical sectors. J Am Geriatr Soc 1996; 44:682–688.
46. Murphy JM, Monson RR, Olivier DC, Zahner GEP, Sobol AM, Leighton AH. Relations over time between psychiatric and somatic disorders: the Stirling County study. Am J Epidemiol 1992; 136:95–105.
47. Jenkins CD. Recent evidence supporting psychologic and social risk factors for coronary disease. N Engl J Med 1976; 294:987–994.
48. Wells KB, Golding JM, Burnam MA. Chronic medical conditions in a sample of the general population with anxiety, affective and substance use disorders. Am J Psychiatry 1989; 146:1440–1446.
49. Lyness J, Cox C, Curry J, Conwell Y, King D, Caine E. Older age and the underreporting of depressive symptoms. J Am Geriatr Soc 1995; 43:216–221.
50. Koenig HG, Cohen HJ, Blazer DG, Kirshnan KRR, Sibert TE. Profile of depressive symptoms in younger and older medical inpatients with major depression. J Am Geriatr Soc 1993; 41:1169–1176.

51. Caine ED, Lyness JM, King DA. Reconsidering depression in the elderly. Am J Geriatr Psychiatry 1993; 1:4–20.
52. Forsell Y, Jorm AF, Winblad B. Association of age, sex, cognitive dysfunction, and disability with major depressive symptoms in an elderly sample. Am J Psychiatry 1994; 151:1600–1604.
53. Weiner MF, Edland SD, Luszczynska H. Prevalence and incidence of major depression in Alzheimer's disease. Am J Psychiatry 1994; 151:1006–1009.
54. Rodin G, Voshart K. Depression in the medically ill: an overview. Am J Psychiatry 1986; 143:696–705.
55. Kinzie JD, Lewinsohn P, Maricle R, Teri L. The relationship of depression to medical illness in an older community population. Compr Psychiatry 1986; 27:241–246.
56. Endicott, J Measurement of depression in patients with cancer. Cancer 1984; 53: 2243–2248.
57. Linden M, Borchelt M, Barnow S, Geiselmann B. The impact of somatic morbidity on the Hamilton Depression Rating Scale in the very old. Acta Psychiatr Scand 1995; 92:150–154.
58. Cavanaugh S, Clark D, Gibbons R. Diagnosing depression in the hospitalized medically ill. Psychosomatics 1983; 24:809–815.
59. Koenig HG, Pappas P, Holsinger T, Bachar JR. Assessing diagnostic approaches to depression in medically ill older adults: how reliably can mental health professionals make judgments about the cause of symptoms? J Am Geriatr Soc 1995; 43: 472–478.
60. Chochinov HM, Wilson KG, Enns M, Lander S. Prevalence of depression in the terminally ill: effects of diagnostic criteria and symptom threshold judgments. Am J Psychiatry 1994; 151:537–540.
61. House A. Mood disorders in the physically ill—problems of definition and measurement. J Psychosom Res 1988; 32: 345–353.
62. Cohen-Cole SA, Stoudemire A. Major depression and physical illness: special considerations in diagnosis and biologic treatment. Psychiatr Clin North Am 1987; 10: 1–17.
63. Katon W, Von Korff M, Lin E, Simon G, Walker E, Bush T, Ludman E. Collaborative management to achieve depression treatment guidelines. J Clin Psychiatry 1997; 58 Suppl 1:20–23.
64. Koenig HG, Goli V, Shelp F, Kudler HS, Cohen HJ, Meador KG, Blazer DG. Antidepressant use in elderly medical inpatients: lessons from an attempted clinical trial. J Gen Intern Med 1989; 4:498–505.
65. Alexopoulos GS, Vrontou C, Kakuma T, Meyers BS, Young RC, Klausner E, Clarkin J. Disability in geriatric depression. Am J Psychiatry 1996; 153:877–885.

6

Comorbidity with Depression in Children and Adolescents

ELIZABETH JANE COSTELLO, ADRIAN ANGOLD, and MARK E. SWEENEY
Duke University Medical Center
Durham, North Carolina

I. INTRODUCTION

In this chapter we first examine what comorbidity with depression means for the development of child and adolescent psychopathology, and then review the available data on the prevalence of comorbidity and its development across childhood and adolescence. We concentrate on studies using representative, community-based samples, because information about comorbidity and risk factors from clinic-based samples is likely to be biased by the factors that give some children greater access to clinic settings than others. For example, children with a family history of one or other of the conditions may be more likely than children with no family pathology to be brought for treatment. This means that clinic-based samples cannot safely be used to study rates of comorbidity, or genetic or other risk factors associated with comorbidity. In this chapter, we use "comorbidity with depression" to refer to other psychiatric disorders seen in children with depression, "depressive comorbidity" to refer to depression seen in children with other disorders, "children" to include adolescents, and "parent" to include anyone who cares for a child.

II. BACKGROUND

Almost 30 years ago, the Isle of Wight and Inner City studies of Rutter and his colleagues found that there was a high degree of overlap between emotional and behavioral disorders (1,2). Historically, the now defunct concept of "masked depression" represented an early attempt to address the issue of comorbidity with depression. During the 1970s, as the issue of the frequent presence of depressive symptomatology in children with other disorders began to be more fully addressed, it was suggested that the presence of a wide range of symptoms represented *formes frustes* depressions. This notion was dispensed with when several groups (see e.g., 3,4) pointed out that when adult diagnostic criteria were applied to data from detailed systematic evaluations of psychopathology, the depressions were not "masked" but patently manifest. These authors emphasized the need to look for depression in children and adolescents whatever their presenting complaints.

III. RECENT EPIDEMIOLOGICAL STUDIES OF COMORBIDITY WITH DEPRESSION

In a previous publication (5) we reviewed the epidemiological literature from the 1970s and 1980s. The present review carries the story forward to 1996. Over the past 15 years a dozen or so community-based studies have published data that permit us to examine the size and correlates of comorbidity with depression in children and adolescents of various ages and nationalities. We present a summary of the findings from these studies, and then consider some methodological and substantive explanations for them.

A. Samples and Procedures

Samples are all the community studies that permit analyses of comorbidity rates to be made, and also meet the following criteria: (1) The sample was reasonably representative of the general population of children in the area from which it was drawn. (2) A standardized psychiatric interview was used to gather data. (3) The child was interviewed, and data were also collected from other informants, using either a standardized interview or questionnaires. (4) Decision rules for making diagnoses were specified, and the symptom specifications conformed in general to the *Diagnostic and Statistical Manual* (DSM-III, DSM-III-R, or DSM-IV) criteria for that disorder. (5) A diagnosis of depression could be made, either by specific subtypes (major depressive episode, dysthymia, bipolar disorder, etc.) or with subtypes combined. (6) At least one of the following other diagnoses could also be made: attention deficit hyperactivity disorder, conduct and/or oppositional defiant disorder, anxiety disorder, substance abuse/dependence. There are too few studies providing rates of comorbidity with any other diagnoses for a detailed review to be possible at this stage. If several subtypes of anxiety diagnosis were made in the study, they were combined into one category. (7) It was possible to calculate a prevalence ratio or odds ratio, if these were not provided in the original publication. The reason for using an interview with the child as the core of the diagnostic data is the nearly all epidemiological studies that have addressed the issue have found that depressive disorders are reported by children much more often than by their parents (6).

B. Results

Before examining the results in detail, it is important to note that studies used different assessment instruments, different numbers of informants, different rules for aggregating information from informants, different time frames for calculating prevalence rates, different definitions of depression (some included dysthymia and bipolar depression, some confined themselves to major depressive episode), and different criteria for the comorbid conditions. As Table 1 shows, they included different age ranges, and extended from 1983 to 1996, using any of three versions of the DSM. In the face of so much variability, the impressive thing is the extent of agreement on the amount of depressive comorbidity in children and adolescents.

Despite all these differences in design, instrumentation, age, and ethnicity of subjects, comorbidity in youth with depression was consistently well above the level expected by chance. In every case, the rate of every comorbid disorder was at least twice as high as depressed as in nondepressed children. Tables 2–5 provide the details for conduct disorder and/or oppositional defiant disorder (Table 2), anxiety disorders (Table 3), attention deficit/hyperactivity disorders (ADHD) (Table 4), and substance abuse or dependence (Table 5). In each table, studies are divided by diagnostic system used (DSM-III, DSM-III-R, DSM-IV), and within those categories, in order of the earliest date at which data were collected. Thus, the first five studies used DSM-III, beginning with the Ontario study in 1983; the second group, beginning with the New York State study in 1983, used DSM-III-R; and the third group, confined to the North Carolina studies, used DSM-IV. Each table shows, for each community study for which relevant data are available, the number of cases and prevalence of depressive disorders (percentages weighted to adjust for design characteristics of the study, if appropriate); the number of cases and prevalence of the comorbid condition; the number of comorbid cases; the proportion of children with depression who have the comorbid condition; the proportion of children with the comorbid condition who have depression; the prevalence ratio, i.e., the ratio of cases of the comorbid condition in children with depression to cases in children without depression; and, if it could be calculated from the data provided, the odds ratio, or ratio of the likelihood of the comorbid condition in the presence of depression to its likelihood in the absence of depression. For example, in Table 2 row 2,

Table 1 Studies Used in Review of Depressive Comorbidity

Study site	Number of children (screened) assessed	Age at interview (years)	Informants and method of diagnostic data collection	Comments
Using DSM-III				
1. Ontario, Canada, 1983 (25)	3294	6–17	Child 11–17: questionnaire Parent: questionnaire Teacher 6–11: questionnaire Questionnaires based on CBCL (26)	
2. Dunedin, New Zealand 1983–1984 (27)	934	11	Child: interview Parent: questionnaire Teacher: questionnaire DISC 1.3 (28) for child, Rutter A and B scales (29) for parent and teacher	
3. Pittsburgh, PA, 1984–1985 (30)	(789) 300	7–11	Child: interview Parent: interview DISC 1.3 (28)	
4. Puerto Rico, 1985–1986 (31)	(777) 386	4–16	Child: interview Parent: interview DISC 1.3 (28) plus psychiatrist	
Using DSM-III-R				
5. New York State, 1983 (32)	776	9–18	Child: interview Parent: interview DISC 1.3 (33)	

6. New York State, 1985 (32)	776	11–20	Child: interview Parent: interview DISC 1.3 (33)	
7. Dunedin, 1987–1988 (34)	943	15	Child: interview Parent: questionnaire Teacher: questionnaire	
8. Oregon 1987–1988 (15,17)	1508	14–17	Child: interview	
9. Pittsburgh, PA 1989–1991 (30)	278	12–18	Child: interview Parent: interview DISC 2.1 (33)	
10. United States, 1990–1992 (35)	479	15–17	Child: interview UM-CIDI (36,37)	Subjects aged 15–17 from the National Comorbidity Survey
11. Christchurch, New Zealand, 1992 (38)		15		
Using DSM-IV				
12. North Carolina, 1992–1996 (19)	(4,500) 1073	9–16	Child: interview Parent: interview CAPA (39)	Data from 4 annual interviews with each family, 1992–1996
13. North Carolina, American Indians, 1992–1996 (19)	346	9–16	Child: interview Parent: interview CAPA (39)	Data from 4 annual interviews with each family, 1992–1996

Table 2 Studies of Comorbidity of Depression and Conduct/Oppositional Defiant Disorder

	Prevalence of disorders				Comorbidity					
	Depression		Conduct/ oppositional disorder		Conduct/ oppositional disorders in depression		Depression in conduct/ oppositional disorders			
Study	*N*	%	*N*	%	*N*	%	(%)	Prevalence ratio	Odds ratio	95% Cl
Using DMS-III										
Dunedin 1983–84	14	1.8	72	9.2	11	78.6	15.2	42.7	NA	NA
Pittsburgh 1984–85	8	2.0	33	7.4	3	31.2	8.5	6.0	6 .6	2.4–17.8
Puerto Rico 1985–86	31	8.0	33	10.5	15	55.8	45.4	18.4	NA	NA
Using DMS-III-R/IV										
New York State 1983	26	3.4	55	7.1	6	23.7	10.9	4.3	NA	NA
New York State 1985	22	2.8	45	5.8	5	22.7	11.1	5.2	NA	NA
Dunedin 1987–88	40	4.2	85	9.0	13	32.5	15.3	5.5	NA	NA
Oregon 1987–88	342	20.4	94	7.3	36	12.4	34.4	18	2.2	1.5–3.2
Pittsburgh 1989–91	15	3.1	49	12.1	11	67.7	20.4	5.8	16.0	8.6–29.7
United States 1990–92	72	15.1	75	14.4	22	32.0	33.7	2.8	3.7	2.3–6.0
Christchurch 1992	47	6.6	NA	10.8	NA	NA	NA	NA	3.4	NA
North Carolina 1992–96	196	4.1	260	4.1	62	20.9	23.2	7.1	8.7	5.6–13.5
North Carolina 1992–96	26	2.1	63	5.1	5	19.2	7.9	4.0	4.7	1.7–12.9

NA = not available.

Table 3 Studies of Comorbidity of Depression and Anxiety Disorder

	Prevalence of disorders				Comorbidity					
	Depression		Anxiety disorder		Anxiety disorders in depression		Depression in anxiety disorders			
Study	*N*	%	*N*	%	*N*	%	(%)	Prevalence ratio	Odds ratio	95% CI
Using DMS–III										
Ontario 1983	86	5.5	261	16.7	50	58.1	19.2	9.7	NA	NA
Dunedin 1983–84	14	1.8	59	7.5	10	71.5	16.2	36.9	NA	NA
Pittsburgh 1984–85	8	2.0	58	11.4	3	37.5	6.6	4.9	6.9	2.7–17.4
Puerto Rico 1985–86	31	8.0	26	6.6	13	38.9	50.0	16.0	NA	NA
Using DSM-III-R/IV										
New York State 1983	26	3.4	152	19.6	11	42.3	7.2	3.2	NA	NA
New York State 1985	22	2.8	81	10.4	9	40.9	11.1	6.6	NA	NA
Dunedin 1987–88	40	4.2	101	10.7	12	30.0	11.9	3.9	NA	NA
Oregon 1987–88	342	20.4	124	8.8	67	21.0	48.7	3.7	4.4	3.1–6.3
Pittsburgh 1989–91	15	4.2	49	14.4	6	42.4	12.3	6.5	4.8	2.4–9.6
United States 1990–92	72	15.1	129	24.7	37	54.3	33.2	2.8	4.9	3.1–7.7
Christchurch 1992	47	6.6	104	12.8	NA	NA	NA	NA	4.6	NA
North Carolina 1992–96	196	4.1	155	2.9	52	18.5	25.7	8.1	9.8	6.1–15.5
North Carolina 1992–96	26	2.1	32	2.6	5	19.2	15.6	8.6	10.4	3.6–29.6

NA = not available.

Table 4 Studies of Comorbidity of Depression and Attention Deficit/Hyperactivity Disorder

Study	Prevalence of disorders				Comorbidity					
	Depression		ADHD in depression		ADHD in depression		Depression in ADHD	Prevalence	Odds	
	N	%	*N*	%	*N*	%	(%)	ratio	ratio	95% Cl
Using DSM-III										
Dunedin 1983–84	14	1.8	53	6.7	8	57.1	15.1	210.0	NA	NA
Pittsburgh 1984–85	8	2.0	11	2.2	1	12.5	9.1	11.0	5.4	1.1–25.6
Puerto Rico 1985–86	31	8.0	35	10.4	13	44.5	37.1	10.4	NA	NA
Using DSM-III-R/IV										
New York State 1983	26	3.4	93	12.0	12	46.2	12.9	7.1	NA	NA
New York State 1985	22	2.8	59	7.6	5	22.7	8.5	3.8	NA	NA
Dunedin 1987–88	40	4.2	20	2.1	0	0	0	—	—	—
Pittsburgh 1989–91	15	4.2	42	12.2	5	25.2	8.7	2.2	2. 6	1.1–5.8
North Carolina 1992–96	196	4.1	114	1.3	23	7.1	22.5	6.8	7.3	3.6–14.6
North Carolina 1992–96	26	2.1	15	1.2	3	11.5	20.0	11.5	13.0	3.4–49.1

NA = not available.

Table 5 Studies of Comorbidity of Depression and Substance Abuse/Dependence

Study	Prevalence of disorders				Comorbidity					
	Depression		Substance abuse/ dependence		Substance abuse/ dependence in depression		Depression in substance abuse/ dependence	Prevalence	Odds	
	N	%	*N*	%	*N*	%	(%)	ratio	ratio	95% Cl
Using DSM-III-R/IV										
Oregon 1987–88	342	20.4	148	8.3	78	20.1	49.3	3.8	4.5	3.2–6.4
Pittsburgh 1989–91	15	4.2	17	5.4	3	21.2	16.5	4.5	5.5	2.4–12.7
United States 1990–92	72	15.1	55	11.1	20	23.2	31.7	2.6	3.1	1.8–5.2
Christchurch 1992	47	6.6	53	7.7	NA	NA	NA	NA	4.4	NA
North Carolina 1992–96	196	4.1	53	0.9	9	5.2	23.9	7.4	7.8	3.5–17.5
North Carolina 1992–96	26	2.1	29	2.4	4	15.4	13.8	7.4	8.6	2.8–26.8

NA = not available.

an odds ratio of 6.6 means that the comorbid condition is 6.6 times as likely in depressed as in nondepressed children, and there is a 95% probability that the correct value lies between the confidence limits 2.4 and 17.8. The odds ratio is significantly different from chance if the 95% confidence interval does not contain 1.0.

Looking first at the prevalence of depressive disorders, the two studies with the highest prevalence were the National Comorbidity Survey (no. 10) and the Oregon study (no. 8). In both of these studies, the data for examining comorbidity were only available for lifetime prevalence estimates, which could be expected to be higher than, for example, the 3-month estimates from the CAPA (no. 13 and 14), or the 6-month estimates from the DISC 1.3 (no. 2–4). Apart from these two, the other studies present population-based prevalence estimates ranging from 1.8% to 8.0%. After making allowance for different prevalence intervals, the lower estimates tend to be in the younger samples.

Table 2 shows comorbidity with *conduct and/or oppositional disorders*. This ranged from 12.4% in the Oregon study (no. 8) to 78.6% in the Dunedin sample of 11-year-olds (no. 2). Most estimates fell into the 20–30% range. In most studies, comorbidity with depression was higher than rates of depression in children with conduct disorder, and the range of rates of depressive comorbidity was lower (7.9–45.4%) than the range of comorbidity with depression. The likelihood of conduct/oppositional disorder was 2–42 times higher in the presence of depression than in its absence, with most estimates in the threefold to sevenfold range.

The lowest reported rate of depressive comorbidity with *anxiety disorders* (Table 3) was 18.5% (no. 12), and the highest 71.5% (no. 2). In all but three studies, anxiety in depression was higher than the rate of depression in anxious children, which ranged from 6.6% (no. 3) to 50.0% (no. 4). Prevalence ratios ranges from 2.8 to 36.9, with the majority in the threefold to eightfold range.

The prevalence of *ADHD* in depressed children (Table 4) ranged from 7.1% (no. 11) to 57.1% (no. 2). Estimates were scattered widely across this range. Once again, depression in children with ADHD was lower than ADHD in depressed children, except for the two DSM-IV studies. Prevalence ratios were widely scattered, ranging from 2 to 12.

Information about comorbidity with *substance-related disorders* was available only for six studies, more recent ones with older subjects. Comorbidity with depression ranged from 5.2% (no. 12) to 23.2% (no. 10), with three of the five available estimates in the 20–23% range. Depression in adolescents with substance-related disorders was higher, ranging from 13.8% (no. 13) to 49.3% (no. 8). Substance-related disorders were 2.6–7.4 times more common in depressed than in nondepressed adolescents.

C. Conclusions About Comorbidity from Epidemiological Studies

Certain general themes emerge from this overview of community-based studies of comorbidity with depression. First, as the studies addressing this topic have accumulated over the past 15 years, estimates have begun to stabilize, despite some outliers. A majority of studies present estimates of comorbidity with anxiety, conduct/oppositional disorders, and ADHD within the 20–40% range. Comorbidity with substance-related disorders may be slightly lower, but there are fewer studies at present. This is supported by Levy and Deykin (7), using the adult Diagnostic Interview Schedule, who found 22% depressive comorbidity with substance abuse in a college-age sample, with a prevalence ratio of 2.7.

Second, the rates of comorbidity tend to be lower in DSM-III-R and DSM-IV studies than in DSM-III studies. At the same time, the former tend to have older subjects, so it is not clear whether we are looking at an age effect or a nosological effect. In the next section we attempt to disaggregate the possible reasons for this trend.

IV. POSSIBLE REASONS FOR THE OBSERVED PATTERNS OF COMORBIDITY

A. Methodological Interpretations

Before we draw conclusions about the extent of the problem of comorbidity with depression, it is essential to ensure that the comorbidity is real. There are many ways in which the methods of data collection could produce a spurious impression of comorbidity. Among them are the following:

1. There is no etiological or pathogenetic connection between depression and other disorders, but the detection of any one disorder makes the detection of another more likely.

This could occur in a clinical context because an alert clinician searches harder for the comorbid condition, or in community studies using unstructured methods for diagnosing psychiatric disorder. The studies described here all used procedures designed to avoid this risk: standardized protocols, interviewers blind to the reports of other informants, and computerized diagnostic procedures. It is highly unlikely that this explanation accounts for much of the observed comorbidity.

A variant on this explanation is that comorbidity might be more likely in populations with low rates of depression and high rates of the other disorder. However, the odds ratios shown in Tables 2–5 are not sensitive to the baseline prevalence rates, only to the extent to which they co-occur. The tables demonstrate that there is nothing about the base rates of individual disorders to explain the observed variations in comorbidity.

2. There is no etiological or pathogenetic connection between depression, anxiety, and disruptive behavior disorders, but the individual conditions share some symptoms in common, so the presence of one disorder reduces the number of symptoms required for the second disorder to reach the threshold for diagnosis:

For instance, irritability is allowed to be the basic mood state for the DSM-III-R diagnosis of depression. Irritability may be manifested as temper tantrums, arguments, touchiness, anger and resentment, or fighting, all of which are included as defining criteria for DSM-III-R oppositional defiant disorder or conduct disorder. In effect, the presence of one disorder constitutes a partial fulfillment of the criteria for the second disorder, and thus, in purely operational terms, partially implies the presence of the second disorder.

If such an effect were the sole cause of an association between two diagnoses, then the apparent "comorbidity" would be present only in those manifesting the shared symptoms, and not in those whose disorders did not involve such symptoms. Tables 2–5 show that comorbidity with depression is as common in disorders with no shared symptoms (e.g., substance abuse) as in those where symptoms may be shared, such as oppositional disorder. Thus, while shared symptoms may explain some comoribidity, they cannot be the whole story.

A subtype of this explanation is that comorbidity is particularly high in earlier studies because they used DSM-III, and lower in later studies because DSM-III-R and DSM-IV removed some methodological causes of comorbidity. Tables 2–5 show that the highest rates of comorbidity are found in the first Dunedin study and the DSM-III Puerto Rico study, both of which used DSM-III. There is no such consistency in the lowest rates, although several are to be found in the DSM-IV North Carolina studies. It is not immediately obvious why DSM-III should have generated such high rates of depressive comorbidity. A comparison of the DSM-III and DSM-IV criteria for a range of disorders shows no clear reasons for greater comorbidity in DSM-III studies at the level of the symptoms. One difference is that DSM-IV requires functional impairment for most diagnoses, whereas DSM-III required symptomatic distress but not necessarily functional impairment. However, the requirement of impairment seems more likely to increase than to decrease comorbidity.

3. There is no etiological or pathogenic connection between depression, anxiety, and disruptive behavior disorders, but the presence of one disorder makes a child, parent, or teacher more likely to report the presence of a second disorder than would have been the case if the first disorder had not been present.

The possible effects on clinician assessment described above under (1) could also apply to subject, teacher, or parent reports. For instance, a parent who observes that her child seems unhappy might talk to her about her feelings, and include questions about fears and worries that she would never have asked had not the depressive symptoms provided a clue to the fact that something was worrying the child. Thus even if fears and worries were really no more common in depressed children that nondepressed children, the parents of the former could report more anxiety problems because they had explored this area in ways that the parents of nondepressed children did not.

If this were the case, then one should see higher levels of comorbidity in studies using both parent and child reports than in stųdies using the child alone as informant (e.g., nos. 7 and 9). Odds ratios for the association with conduct/oppositional disorder and substance abuse/dependence in these two studies were indeed at the lower end of the range, but odds ratios for the association with anxiety were similar to those found in other studies. Thus, the hypothesis has some support from the data, but it does not extend to anxiety, an area where one might expect a strong effect if the "informant sensitivity" explanation were true.

4. There is no etiological or pathogenic connection between depression, anxiety, and disruptive behavior disorders, but the use of multiple informants describing the same phenomena in different terms leads to the spurious appearance of multiple disorders.

All of the epidemiological studies and most of the clinical studies of comorbidity have employed some means of combining information from different sources (parents, teachers, children) at either the symptom level or the diagnostic level. In most cases this has meant using a decision rule; for example, if either the parent or the child reports the presence of a symptom, then it is regarded as being present. This approach raises the problem that different individuals may interpret symptoms in different ways. Suppose, for instance, that a child tells her mother, and also tells the interviewer, that she is worried about going to school and cries every morning. It is possible that the parent may interpret this as a sign of the child's being depressed, and might report depressed mood, while the child's description leads her interviewer to record the presence of anxiety. Using the rule that positive ratings from any informant count toward a diagnosis, the same phenomenon would be counted twice under different headings, contributing to two diagnoses, and thereby creating spurious comorbidity.

The argument that comorbidity is a spurious effect of using multiple informants can be checked, first, by comparing rates in studies using one informant with those using multiple informants, as in (3) above, where we found limited support for the idea. Second, one can examine rates of comorbidity within a single study, using single versus multiple informants.

As an example, Table 6 shows the odds ratios for depressive comorbidity using a single informant (parent, child) versus two informants in the Great

Table 6 Depressive Comorbidity Based on Parent, Child, and Combined Data: The Great Smoky Mountains Study

	Comorbidity with anxiety disorders		Comorbidity with conduct/ oppositional disorder		Comorbidity with substance abuse/ dependence	
	Odds ratio	95% Cl	Odds ratio	95% Cl	Odds ratio	95% Cl
Child only	3.1	1.3–7.6	8.4	4.5–15.6	12.9	7.4–22.6
Parent only	13.4	7.9–23.0	22.3	15.3–32.6	1.8	0.4–7.4
Combined	8.1	6.1–15.5	8.7	5.6–13.5	7.8	3.5–17.5

Smoky Mountain Study; these data do not support hypothesis (4). In most cases comorbidity is higher with a single informant than when two informants are used. This argues against the multiple informants hypothesis.

These data also speak to hypothesis (3): When the parent is the informant, comorbidity is higher for anxiety and conduct/oppositional disorders than when child or multiple informants are considered, but the opposite is true for substance abuse/dependence (in this study ADHD diagnoses were based on parent information alone). Once again, the evidence is equivocal.

B. Conclusions About Methodological Explanations

Recent studies provide some limited support for the idea of "increased informant sensitivity," but little for other methodological interpretations.

C. Substantive Interpretations

If methodological explanations are ruled out or controlled through careful design of the research and its analysis, the observed rates of comorbidity can be seen as having some basis in children's symptoms. However, several possible substantive explanations need to be considered. In another paper (8) we set out five possible substantive reasons for comorbidity. Briefly, we postulate (1) that all child psychiatric disorders arise from the same underlying pathogenic process; (2) that depression and anxiety arise from the same pathogenic process, but the process is different for disruptive behavior disorders; (3) that some disorders, e.g., conduct disorder, are nonspecific accompaniments to an underlying pathogenic mechanism that gives rise to depression/anxiety; (4) that depression causes disruptive behavior disorders, or vice versa; (5) that a third factor modulates the relationship between depression and other disorders. In essence, all of these explanations have to do with the respective timing of the various disorders:

some antecedent factor causes depression and another condition, or depression causes or is caused by another condition. Until recently, there has been little prospective longitudinal research, and no longitudinal epidemiological research, with which to test the various versions of this theme. The clinical studies of Kovacs (9–14) and the community-based studies of Lewinsohn and others (15–22) will fill this gap, but the relevant papers are not yet published. There are also limits to the usefulness of observational studies for testing causal mechanisms; we need to use the data from cross-sectional studies to generate hypotheses to be tested in longitudinal and/or experimental studies. For example, a tentative conclusion to be drawn from Tables 2–5 is that comorbidity is more common in younger than in older children. However, the age of subjects in the DSM-III-R and DSM-IV studies is on the whole higher than that of subjects in the DSM-III studies, so that age is somewhat confounded with taxonomy. The effects of age on comorbidity can, however, be examined in the North Carolina studies, which have a sufficiently large sample of children aged 9–16 by the end of the fourth data collection wave, for whom DSM-IV diagnoses are available. Comorbidity with anxiety fell from 26.8% in the 9–12-year-olds to 13.5% in the 13–16-year-olds ($p = .03$), and comorbidity with conduct/oppositional disorders fell from 23.6% in the younger group to 19.3% in the older group (not significant). Comorbidity with ADHD also fell dramatically with age, but rates of ADHD were too low in the older group for estimates to be at all stable; the converse was true for substance abuse, which was extremely rare in the younger children. Thus, the North Carolina data provide some support for lower levels of comorbidity with depression in adolescence than in childhood.

If comorbidity with depression were indeed to be higher in younger children, why should this be? A methodological problem is the unreliability of psychiatric diagnoses, especially of anxiety and depression, in children below the age of about 9 (23,24). It is possible that younger children who say "yes" to one symptom are more likely to endorse another one, whereas older children are less likely to do this. Another hypothesis is that depression itself is uncommon before age 13, and that the cases that do occur, being so abnormal, might be expected to be particularly complex. An associated possibility is that the home and school environment for depressed prepubertal children may be particularly unsupportive and conducive to the development of associated disorders. These ideas need much more research.

D. Summary and Conclusions

This chapter has concentrated on the epidemiological literature on comorbidity, because community-based studies permit us to examine comorbidity without worrying about the possible distortions created by referral biases. However, we have shown elsewhere that comorbidity in community samples may be no lower than that seen in clinic settings (5). In general, a child or adolescent with a depressive disorder has a one-in-five to one-in-three chance of having another psychiatric disorder, and that disorder is as likely to be a disruptive behavior disorder as it is to be an internalizing disorder. While there is some evidence that parents of children with depression may be sensitized to their child's problems and more likely to report other symptoms than parents who are not aware of their child's depression, on the whole the other methodological explanations that we considered here did not explain the amount of comorbidity observed across this wide range of studies. Important longitudinal studies are now in progress, but we are still a long way from having a clear picture of the course and outcome of depression in comorbid children, and even further from understanding why depressed children are so vulnerable to other disorders, or what to do about it.

Thus, the bad news is that, having cleared the field for exploring substantive reasons for comorbidity with depression, we find ourselves stuck. The published data do not permit us to draw conclusions about possible causal mechanisms. A new generation of theory-driven studies is needed. The good news is that the basic work has been done; we now have a range of reasonably reliable psychiatric assessment instruments for children and adolescents, together with a core of studies that provide information on likely prevalence rates and effect sizes, so it is possible to calculate how big the next generation of hypothesis-testing studies will have to be. The next decade should be an exciting one.

REFERENCES

1. Rutter M, Tizard J, Whitmore K. Education, Health, and Behaviour. London: Longman, 1970.
2. Rutter M, Graham P, Chadwick OFD, Yule W. Adolescent turmoil: Fact or fiction? J Child Psychol Psychiatry 1976; 17:35–56.
3. Kovacs M, Beck AT. Cognitive-affective process in depression. In: Izard CE. Emotions in Personality and Psychopathology. New York: Plenum Press, 1979:415–442.
4. Pearce J. Depressive disorder in childhood. J Child Psychol Psychiatry 1977; 18: 79–82.
5. Angold A, Costello EJ. Depressive comorbidity in children and adolescents: empirical, theoretical, and methodological issues. Am J Psychiatry 1993; 150:1779–1791.
6. Brandenburg NA, Friedman RM, Silver SE. The epidemiology of childhood psychiatric disorders. J Am Acad Child Adolesc Psychiatry 1990; 29:76–83.
7. Levy JC, Deykin EY. Suicidality, depression, and substance abuse in adolescence. Am J Psychiatry 1989; 146, 11:1462–1467.
8. Angold A, Costello EJ. Comorbidity. J Child Psychol Psychiatry (in press).
9. Kovacs M, Feinberg TL, Crouse-Novak MA, Paulauskas SL, Finkelstein R. De-

pressive disorders in childhood. I. A longitudinal prospective study of characteristics and recovery. Arch Gen Psychiatry 1984; 41:229–237.
10. Kovacs M, Feinberg TL, Crouse-Novak MA, Paulauskas SL, Pollock M, Finklestein R. Depressive disorders in childhood. II. A longitudinal study of the risk for a subsequent major depression. Arch Gen Psychiatry 1984; 41:643–649.
11. Kovacs M, Paulauskas S, Gatsonis C, Richards C. Depressive disorders in childhood. III. A longitudinal study of comorbidity with and risk for conduct disorders. J Affect Disord 1988; 15:205–217.
12. Kovacs M, Gatsonis C, Paulauskas SL, Richards C. Depressive disorders in childhood. IV. A longitudinal study of comorbidity with and risk for anxiety disorders. Arch Gen Psychiatry 1989; 46:776–782.
13. Kovacs M, Akiskal HS, Gatsonis C, Parrone PL. Childhood-onset dysthymic disorder: clinical features and prospective naturalistic outcome. Arch Gen Psychiatry 1994; 51:365–374.
14. Kovacs M, Goldston D. Cognitive and social cognitive development of depressed children and adolescents. J Am Acad Child Adolesc Psychiatry 1991; 30(3):388–392.
15. Lewinsohn PM, Hops H, Roberts RE, Seeley JR, Andrews JA. Adolescent psychopathology. I. Prevalence and incidence of depression and other DSM-III-R disorders in high school students. J Abnorm Psychol 1993; 102:133–144.
16. Lewinsohn PM, Roberts RE, Seeley JR, Rohde P, Gotlib IH, Hops H. Adolescent psychopathology. II. Psychosocial risk factors for depression. J Abnorm Psychol 1994; 103:302–315.
17. Lewinsohn PM, Rohde P, Seeley JR. Adolescent psychopathology. III. The clinical consequences of comorbidity. J Am Acad Child Adolesc Psychiatry 1995; 34:541–519.
18. Lewinsohn PM, Gotlib IH, Seeley JR. Adolescent psychopathology. IV. Specificity of psychosocial risk factors for depression and substance abuse in older adolescents. J Am Acad Child Adolesc Psychiatry 1995; 34:1221–1229.
19. Costello EJ, Angold A, Burns BJ, Stangl DK, Tweed DL, Erkanli A, Worthman CM. The Great Smoky Mountains Study of Youth: goals, designs, methods, and the prevalence of DSM-III-R disorders. Arch Gen Psychiatry 1996; 53:1129–1136.
20. Feehan M, McGee R, Williams SM, Nada-Raja S. Models of adolescent psychopathology: childhood risk and the transition to adulthood. J Am Acad Child Adolesc Psychiatry 1995; 34:670–679.
21. Giaconia RM, Reinherz HZ, Silverman AB, Pakiz B, Frost AK, Cohen E. Ages of onset of psychiatric disorders in a community population of older adolescents. J Am Acad Child Adolesc Psychiatry 1994; 33:706–717.
22. Cohen P, Cohen J, Brook J. An epidemiological study of disorders in late childhood and adolescence. 2. Persistence of disorders. J Child Psychol Psychiatry 1993; 34: 869–877.
23. Edelbrock C, Costello AJ, Dulcan MK, Kalas R, Conover NC. Age differences in the reliability of the psychiatric interview of the child. Child Dev 1985; 56: 265–275.
24. Schwab-Stone M, Fallon T, Briggs M, Crowther B. Reliability of diagnostic report-

ing for children aged 6–11 years: a test-retest study of the Diagnostic Interview Schedule for Children-Revised. Am J Psychiatry 1994; 151:1048–1054.

25. Offord DR, Boyle MH, Szatmari P, Rae-Grant NI, Links PS, Cadman DT, Byles JA, Crawford JW, Munroe-Blum H, Byrne C, Thomas H, Woodward CA. Ontario child health study. II. Six-month prevalence of disorder and rates of service utilization. Arch Gen Psychiatry 1987; 44:832–836.
26. Achenbach TM, Edelbrock C. Manual for the Child Behavior Checklist and Child Behavior Profile. Burlington: University of Vermont, 1983.
27. Anderson JC, Williams S, McGee R, Silva PA. DSM-III disorders in preadolescent children: prevalence in a large sample from the general population. Arch Gen Psychiatry 1987; 44:69–77.
28. Costello AJ, Edelbrock CS, Dulcan MK, Kalas R, Klaric SH. Development and Testing of the NIMH Diagnostic Interview Schedule for Children in a Clinic Population: Final Report (contract no. RFP-DB-81-0027). Rockville, MD: Center for Epidemiologic Studies–NIMH, 1984.
29. Rutter M. A children's behaviour questionnaire for completion by teachers: preliminary findings. J Child Psychol Psychiatry 1967; 8:1–11.
30. Costello EJ, Costello AJ, Edelbrock C, Burns BJ, Dulcan MK, Brent D, Janiszewski S. Psychiatric disorders in pediatric primary care: prevalence and risk factors. Arch Gen Psychiatry 1988; 45:1107–1116.
31. Bird HR, Canino G, Rubio-Stipec M, Gould MS, Ribera J, Sesman M, Woodbury M, Huertas-Goldman S, Pagan A, Sanchez-Lacay A, Moscoso M. Estimates of the prevalence of childhood maladjustment in a community survey in Puerto Rico: the use of combined measures. Arch Gen Psychiatry 1988; 45:1120–1126.
32. Velez CN, Johnson J, Cohen P. A longitudinal analysis of selected risk factors of childhood psychopathology. J Am Acad Child Adolesc Psychiatry 1989; 28:861–864.
33. Shaffer D, Fisher PW, Schwab-Stone M, Piacentini J, Wicks J. The Diagnostic Interview Schedule for Children (DISC 2.1). Rockville, MD: National Institute of Mental Health, 1989.
34. McGee R, Feehan M, Williams S, Partridge F, Silva PA, Kelly J. DSM-III disorders in a large sample of adolescents. J Am Acad Child Adolesc Psychiatry 1990; 29:611–619.
35. Kessler RC, McGonagle KA, Zhao S, Nelson CB, Hughes M, Eshleman S, Wittchen HU, Kendler KS. Lifetime and 12-month prevalence of DSM-III-R psychiatric disorders in the United States: results from the National Comorbidity Study. Arch Gen Psychiatry 1994; 51:8–19.
36. Kessler RC. The National Comorbidity Survey of the United States. Int Rev Psychiatry 1994; 6:365–376.
37. Kessler RC. Building on the ECA: the National Comorbidity Survey and the Children's ECA. Int J Meth Psychiatr Meth 1994; 4:81–94.
38. Fergusson DM, Horwood LJ, Lynskey MT. Prevalence and comorbidity of DSM-III-R diagnoses in a birth cohort of 15 year olds. J Am Acad Child Adolesc Psychiatry 1993: 32:1127–1134.
39. Angold A, Cox A, Prendergast M, Rutter M, Simonoff E. The Child and Adolescent Psychiatric Assessment (CAPA): Version 3.0. Durham, NC: Duke University Medical Center, 1992.

7

Bipolar Disorder and Substance Abuse

SUSAN C. SONNE and KATHLEEN T. BRADY
Medical University of South Carolina
Charleston, South Carolina

I. INTRODUCTION

Recent data from the National Comorbidity Survey (Kessler et al., 1994) indicate that affective illness and substance abuse are among the most common psychiatric disorders in the United States today. Data from the National Institute of Mental Health Epidemiologic Catchment Area (ECA) study (Regier et al., 1990) found that bipolar disorder was the Axis I disorder associated with the highest risk for co-occurrence with alcohol or drug abuse. Over half of the individuals with bipolar I disorder met criteria for a substance use disorder sometime in their lives. In the substance abuse treatment-seeking population, estimates of the prevalence of bipolar disorder range from 15 to 30%, with particularly high rates in the cocaine-abusing population (Weiss et al., 1988a; Brady and Lydiard, 1992).

Although bipolar disorder and substance abuse co-occur frequently, the relationship between these disorders is not well understood. Meyer (1986) described several theories regarding the co-occurrence of substance abuse and psychopathology, including the notion that psychopathology may be a risk factor for developing substance use disorder, psychopathology may modify the course of the substance use disorder, or psychiatric symptoms may emerge during the course of chronic intoxication and withdrawal from substances. It appears that this relationship is not simply cause and effect, but is complex and multidirectional.

In spite of the alarming prevalence rates, there is little published data on specific psychotherapeutic or pharmacotherapeutic treatments for bipolar disorder in the presence of a substance use disorder. Preliminary data indicate that substance abuse may be a predictor of poor prognosis and poor medication response to lithium, but this has never been studied systematically.

II. PREVALENCE

The prevalence of comorbid bipolar disorder and substance abuse can be examined in several ways. One approach is to look at the prevalence of comorbidity in non-treatment-seeking community samples. Another approach is to study the frequency of comorbidity in treatment-seeking populations, evaluating either the frequency of bipolar disorder among those presenting for substance abuse treatment or, conversely, the frequency of substance use disorders in those presenting for treatment of affective symptoms. Regardless of the approach used, many studies indicate that these disorders co-occur more commonly than would be expected by chance alone.

The ECA study (Regier et al., 1990) revealed that 60.7% of patients with bipolar I disorder had a lifetime diagnosis of a substance use disorder with 46.2% having an alcohol diagnosis and 40.7% having a drug abuse or dependence diagnosis. Forty-eight percent of individuals with bipolar II disorder had a substance use disorder, with 39.2% having an alcohol use disorder and 21% having a drug abuse or dependence diagnosis. As can be seen in Table 1, alcohol and drug dependence were twice as likely to be found in bipolar patients compared to unipolar depressed patients. Again, bipolar disorder was associated with the highest risk of any Axis I disorder for coexistence with a drug or alcohol use disorder.

Data from the substance abuse treatment-seeking population show similarly high estimates for the co-occurrence of bipolar disorder and substance use disorders. While the prevalence of bipolar disorder in the U.S. population is slightly more than 1%, prevalence estimates in the substance abuse treatment-seeking population range from approximately 2% (Hesselbrock et al., 1985; Ross et al., 1988) to 15–30% (Nunes et al., 1989; Mirin et al., 1991), depending on the population studied and the diagnostic schema used. In examining drug-dependent individuals, Mirin and co-workers (1991) compiled data on 350 hospitalized, drug-dependent patients over a 10-year period. They found that 4.0% had bipolar disorder and 5.7% had cyclothymic disorders. Both the occurrence of bipolar disorder and cyclothymia were significantly more frequent among stimulant abusers (17.5%) than among opiate (5.4%) or sedative hypnotic (6.8%) abusers. Nunes et al. (1989) found that in a group of 30 treatment-seeking cocaine abusers, 30% met lifetime criteria for an affective disorder in the bipolar spectrum. Weiss and co-workers have published several studies on the psycho-

Table 1 Comorbid Affective Disorders and Substance Abuse ECA Data

	Any substance abuse or dependence		Alcohol dependence		Alcohol abuse		Drug dependence		Drug abuse	
	%	OR	%	OR	%	OR	%	OR	%	OR
Any affective disorder	32.0	2.6	4.9	2.2	6.9	1.3	11.3	4.4	8.1	4.1
Any bipolar disorder	56.1	6.6	27.6	4.6	16.1	3.3	21.8	8.3	11.7	5.2
Bipolar I	60.7	7.9	31.5	5.5	14.7	3.0	27.6	11.1	13.1	5.9
Bipolar II	48.1	4.7	20.8	3.1	18.4	3.9	11.7	3.7	9.3	3.9
Unipolar major depression	27.2	1.9	11.6	1.6	5.0	0.9	10.7	3.7	7.3	3.3

Odds ratio (OR) = the ratio of the odds of having the substance use disorder in a subject with mood disorder, compared to the odds in a subject without mood disorder.
Source: Adapted from Regier et al., 1990.

pathology of cocaine abusers. In a study of 30 cocaine abusers, 23% were found to have a mood disorder in the bipolar spectrum (Weiss et al., 1986), and in a larger study of 149 patients, cocaine abusers had a significantly higher rate of cyclothymia than abusers of other drugs (Weiss et al., 1988b). Gawin and Kleber (1986) also found that a significant percentage (20%) of cocaine abusers had affective disorders in the bipolar spectrum. Although the percentages vary somewhat depending on diagnostic criteria and methodology used, all studies suggest that a substantial number of cocaine abusers have bipolar spectrum disorders. Interestingly, several reports of cocaine use among cyclothymic and bipolar patients indicate that patients use cocaine to intensify and lengthen euphoric mood states rather than to self-medicate depressive episodes (Weiss et al., 1988b; Mirin et al., 1991).

In focusing on individuals seeking treatment for alcoholism, Hesselbrock and co-workers (1985) studied hospitalized alcoholics and found mania in 2% of this population. Lydiard and co-workers found that 4% of 49 alcoholic patients they interviewed met the criteria for bipolar disorder set forth by DSM-III-R (Brady and Lydiard, 1992). Ross and colleagues (1988) found that 1.9% of 501 patients seeking treatment for alcohol and drug use disorders had a lifetime diagnosis of mania. Table 2 summarizes data on the prevalence of bipolar disorder in individuals seeking treatment for substance abuse.

In summary, these data indicate that the percentage of bipolar disorder is higher in the drug-abusing population, particularly among those abusing co-

Table 2 Bipolar Spectrum Disorders in Individuals Seeking Treatment for Substance Abuse

Study	*N*	Mood disorder	%	Primary substance
Gawin and Kleber (1986)	30	Cyclothymia	17.0	Cocaine abuse
Weiss et al. (1988a)	149	Bipolar/cyclothymia	16.1	Cocaine abuse
Nunes et al. (1989)	30	Bipolar/cyclothymia/hyperthymia	30.0	Cocaine abuse
Mirin et al. (1991)	350	Bipolar/cyclothymia	9.7	Nonalcohol drug problems
Rounsaville et al. (1991)	298	Hyperthymia/cyclothymia/mania/hypomania	31.0	Cocaine abuse
Hesselbrock et al. (1985)	321	Mania	2.0	Alcoholism
Ross et al. (1988)	501	Mania	1.9	Drug and alcohol problems
Lydiard et al. (1987)	50	Bipolar disorder	4.0	Alcoholism

Source: Adapted from Brady and Lydiard, 1992.

caine, than in the alcoholic population. It is also clear that expanding the diagnostic schema to include bipolar spectrum disorders leads to higher prevalence estimates. In this regard, it is noteworthy that none of the studies that have assessed mood disorder in the alcoholic population have included patients with bipolar spectrum disorders (e.g., cyclothymia). Expanding the diagnostic schema to include bipolar spectrum disorders would most likely lead to higher prevalence estimates.

Studies designed to evaluate the prevalence of substance use disorders in individuals seeking treatment for bipolar disorder have also shown high rates of comorbidity (see Table 3). Reich and co-workers (1974) retrospectively surveyed records of 65 patients being treated for bipolar disorder and found that 31% of these patients had a history of excessive drinking. Patients reported that excessive alcohol use occurred predominantly during the manic phase of the illness. El-Guebaly (1975) reported a 21% prevalence of drug or alcohol abuse among 110 bipolar disorder patients surveyed. Estroff and colleagues (1985) found that of 36 patients who met DSM-III-R criteria for bipolar disorder, 58% of those presenting with mania and 50% with mixed or atypical features had histories of a substance use disorder. Keller and co-workers (1986) found that of 155 patients presenting with bipolar disorder, 5% of the pure manics, 8% of the pure depressives, and 13% of those with mixed or rapid-cycling disorder met criteria for a current alcohol use disorder.

Table 3 Substance Use Disorders in Individuals Seeking Treatment for Bipolar Spectrum Disorders

Study	*N*	Primary substance	%	Mood disorder
Reich et al. (1974)	65	Alcoholism	31.0	Bipolar disorder
El-Guebaly (1975)	110	Alcohol and drug abuse	21.0	Bipolar disorder
Miller et al. (1989)	60	Alcohol and drug abuse	25.0	Bipolar disorder
Salloum et al. (1996)	274	Unspecified	12.0	Bipolar disorder, manic phase
Brady et al. (1991)	20	Alcohol and drug abuse	30.0	Bipolar disorder
Winokur et al. (1995)	231	Alcoholism	30.3	Bipolar disorder, schizoaffective mania

III. DIAGNOSTIC ISSUES

Diagnosing bipolar disorder in the face of substance abuse can be difficult because drugs of abuse, particularly with chronic use, can mimic nearly any psychiatric disorder. Affective instability, in particular, is often associated with intoxication and withdrawal states. Both stimulant and alcohol intoxication can produce a syndrome indistinguishable from mania or hypomania, characterized by euphoria, increased energy, decreased appetite, grandiosity, and sometimes paranoia. For most substances of abuse, however, withdrawal states do not mimic mania. Manic symptoms that persist for a number of days after last substance use are not likely to be substance-induced. Long-acting stimulants (methamphetamine) and hallucinogens may be an exception to this rule as manic symptoms resulting from intoxication with these substances may last for several days. The differential diagnosis of depression is somewhat more difficult. Depression is a core feature of withdrawal from a number of substances of abuse, and studies have demonstrated that symptoms of withdrawal-related depression may persist for 2–4 weeks (Brown and Schuckit, 1988). Because of this phenomenon, it is likely that observation during lengthier periods of abstinence is important for the diagnosis of depression as compared to mania.

Bipolar spectrum disorders, such as cyclothymia, are even more difficult to reliably diagnose because of the shorter duration and more subtle nature of the psychiatric symptoms. However, as previously discussed, a number of studies using careful diagnostic techniques have noted the high prevalence of bipolar spectrum disorder among substance users. Because of diagnostic difficulties, it may be that this important diagnostic group is often overlooked. If mood dysregulation can contribute to substance abuse, recognition and treatment of these conditions may be important.

As a general guideline, it seems most reasonable to diagnose bipolar disorder if the symptoms clearly occur before the onset of the substance use disorder or if they persist during periods of abstinence from substances of abuse. The adequate period of abstinence for diagnostic purposes is not clearly defined at this point. Family history and severity of symptoms should also factor into diagnostic considerations.

Another issue in the validity of psychiatric diagnoses among substance abusers concerns the use of structured or semistructured interviews to maximize reliability and validity. In a recent publication, Kranzler and colleagues (1996) evaluated the concurrent, discriminant, and predictive validity of the Structured Clinical Interview for DSM-III-R (SCID) in substance users. They found only moderate validity in the diagnoses of affective disorders. Recently, two modified versions of the SCID have been developed (Hasin et al., 1996), which obtain data systematically on the chronological relationship between the onset of substance abuse and the onset of psychiatric symptoms. Further evaluation of the use of these instruments will be important in assessing diagnostic reliability and validity.

IV. CLINICAL COURSE OF COMORBID BIPOLAR DISORDER AND SUBSTANCE ABUSE

Despite the prevalence of substance use disorders in patients with bipolar disorder, few studies have specifically focused on the characteristics and presentation of this important group of bipolar patients. There is currently very little information on the treatment of patients with bipolar disorder complicated by substance abuse. Reich and co-workers (1974) found that excessive use of alcohol distinguished manic patients with a history of hospitalizations from those without one. Brady and colleagues (1991) reported that bipolar patients with a coexisting substance use disorder had twice as many lifetime hospitalizations as those bipolar patients without a substance use disorder.

There is some evidence to suggest that substance use disorders affect the presentation of bipolar disorder. Keller and colleagues (1986) found that a higher percentage of patients with mixed or rapid cycling bipolar disorder had concurrent alcoholism (13%). Such patients were also more likely to have a slower time to recovery than patients presenting with pure depression or pure mania. Sonne and colleagues (1994) compared a group of individuals with bipolar disorder and a coexisting substance use disorder to a group with bipolar disorder and no substance use disorder. They found that substance users had an earlier onset of mood disorder, were more likely to be male, had other comorbid Axis I disorders, and were significantly more likely to have dysphoric mania at the time of interview. Other investigators have reported similar results. Salloum and co-workers (1996) evaluated 274 manic subjects over a 5-year period. They found that 12% had a comorbid substance use disorder, with more males in the comorbid group compared to the non-substance users (67% vs. 45%, respectively). Also, the substance users were more likely to have a previous history of both manic and depressive episodes, compared to the non-substance users, who were more likely to have a previous history of manic episodes only. Blanco-Perez and colleagues (1996) also compared characteristics of substance-abusing and non-substance-abusing bipolar patients ($n = 136$ and 178, respectively). They found substance abuse to be associated with male gender, child trauma, earlier onset of bipolar disorder, higher number of hospitalizations, lower social support, and higher frequency of attempted suicide. These data suggest that bipolar patients with comorbid substance use disorders may have a more severe course of affective illness than bipolar patients who do not have a substance use disorder.

In a 5-year follow-up study, Winokur and co-workers (1995) evaluated a group of bipolar patients with and without alcoholism. In the alcoholic patients, bipolar illness and alcoholism were categorized as being either primary or secondary (primary being defined as that which came first). The patients with primary alcoholism had significantly fewer episodes of affective illness at follow-up, which may suggest that the patients with primary alcoholism had a less severe form of bipolar illness. Similarly, Feinman and Dunner (1996) conducted a retrospective chart review in which they studied three groups of bipolar individuals: those with bipolar disorder who had no lifetime history of alcohol or drug abuse, those who developed a substance use disorder after the onset of bipolar disorder, and those whose bipolar disorder began after the onset of a substance use disorder. They found that those who developed a substance use disorder after the onset of bipolar disorder had an earlier age of onset for bipolar disorder compared to the other group. They also found that those with a lifetime history of a substance use disorder had significantly more suicide attempts than those individuals who did not have a lifetime substance use diagnosis. Thus, there is growing evidence that the presence of a concomitant substance use disorder affects the course of bipolar disorder, and the order of onset of the two disorders may have prognostic implications.

However, when evaluating the effects of affective illness on substance use, some data indicate that patients with bipolar disorder and alcoholism do better in treatment than patients with other affective syndromes. O'Sullivan and colleagues (1988) found that alcoholics with bipolar disorder functioned better during a 2-year follow-up period than did primary alcoholics or alcoholics with unipolar depression. Similarly, Hasin and colleagues (1989) found that patients with bipolar II disorder were likely to have earlier remission of alcoholism than patients with schizoaffective disorder or bipolar I disorder. It is noteworthy that in these studies the treatment outcome measured was remission of alcoholism rather than affective stability, which may explain the discrepancy in the results of these studies.

In conclusion, it appears that substance use disorders may adversely affect the course and prognosis of affective disorders, leading to more frequent hospitalizations and more treatment-resistant symptoms. On the other hand, some data indicate that with good resolution of affective symptoms, individuals with bipolar disorder can have remission of their substance use disorder. This may be dependent on whether the bipolar illness is primary or secondary. It has been postulated that the presence of the affective syndrome, particularly mania, may precipitate or exacerbate substance abuse (Hasin et al., 1985). Alternatively, substance abuse and withdrawal are likely to worsen affective symptoms, thereby forming a vicious cycle of substance abuse and affective instability.

V. THEORETICAL IMPLICATIONS

An interesting theoretical perspective in this area comes from the literature on neuronal sensitization, or "kindling." It has been postulated that bipolar disorder is a phenomenon of neuronal sensitization because the course of the illness is often characterized by acceleration with successively shortened periods of remission between episodes of illness (Post et al., 1984). Cocaine and alcohol are the most common agents of abuse in patients with bipolar disorder (Brady and Lydiard, 1992). Acute cocaine intoxication and alcohol withdrawal both appear to produce neuronal sensitization (Brown et al., 1986; Post and Weiss, 1988). Because use of both of these substances is associated with neuronal sensitization, and it has been postulated that the course of bipolar disorder is also affected by neuronal sensitization, it is possible that this common mechanism is responsible for the morbidity and poor prognosis associated with substance abuse in bipolar patients. Carbamazepine and valproate are two antikindling anticonvulsant agents that have efficacy in the treatment of acute manic states. If neuronal sensitization, or "kindling," is one consequence of substance abuse and is important in the pathophysiology of bipolar disorder, an antikindling agent may be particularly efficacious in patients with comorbid bipolar disorder and a substance use disorder. There is also evidence to support the use of the antikindling agent carbamazepine in the treatment of alcohol withdrawal (Malcolm et al., 1989), which may make the antikindling agents even more useful for treating substance-abusing bipolar patients.

VI. PHARMACOTHERAPY

A. Lithium

Lithium has been used as the standard treatment of bipolar disorder for several decades. Unfortunately, lithium is effective in only 60–80% of classic bipolar patients (Calabrese et al., 1993). The response rate for lithium has been estimated to be as low as 50% when all bipolar subtypes have been considered. As many as 72–82% of patients with the rapid-cycling variant of bipolar disorder exhibit a poor response to lithium (Calabrese and Delucchi, 1989).

Substance abuse has been listed as a predictor of poor response to lithium in several studies (Tohen et al., 1990; O'Connell et al., 1991; Bowden, 1995). In a 4-year follow-up study of 24 bipolar patients after their first manic episode (Tohen et al., 1990), alcoholism was found to be a statistically significant predictor of a shorter time in remission from affective symptomatology. Another long-term lithium study (O'Connell et al., 1991) found the incidence of substance abuse to be substantially higher in the patients with a poor outcome (36%) compared to patients with a good outcome (7%). Gawin and Kleber (1984) conducted an open-label trial of lithium carbonate in cocaine abusers with cyclothymia and found it to be useful. However, Nunes and co-workers (1990) failed to replicate these findings in an open trial with 10 cocaine abusers with bipolar spectrum disorder.

Several studies suggest that manic patients exhibiting significant depressive symptoms (mixed manic episodes) respond less well to lithium than patients in the nonmixed state. Prien et al. (1988) found that over a 2-year period, lithium and lithium plus imipramine were highly effective as preventive treatments for a pure manic subgroup, but largely ineffective for a subgroup with mixed mania. Secunda et al. (1987) found that nine of 10 pure manic patients responded well to lithium compared to only two of seven patients with mixed mania. Keller et al. (1986) also found that patients with mixed mania were less responsive to lithium than were other bipolar patients. Preliminary data from a review by McElroy and associates (1992) suggest that bipolar patients with rapid-cycling or dysphoric or mixed mania may be particularly likely to respond to valproate as compared to lithium therapy.

B. Anticonvulsant Therapy

Ballenger and Post (1978) conducted the first double-blind, placebo-controlled trial demonstrating efficacy of the anticonvulsant carbamazepine as an antimanic agent. Subsequently, this finding has been replicated numerous times, and it is now recognized that both carbamazepine and valproate play a major role in the management of lithium-resistant patients. In a review by Post (1990) it was reported that 19 double-blind studies on the treatment of acute mania with carbamazepine demonstrated an average response rate of 70%. The study designs included comparison of carbamazepine with neuroleptics, lithium, and placebo.

Recently the anticonvulsant divalproex sodium (Depakote; valproate) was FDA approved for the acute treatment of manic episodes associated with bipolar disorder (Abbott Laboratories, 1995). Part of the evidence supporting the approval of valproate for the treatment of mania comes from a large multicenter trial (Bowden et al., 1994) that showed valproate to be more effective than placebo and as effective as lithium, with response rates of 48%, 25%, and 49% for valproate, placebo, and lithium, respectively, in a group of bipolar patients without a substance use disorder.

Freeman and co-workers (1992) conducted a 3-week, randomized, double-blind comparison of lithium ($n = 13$) and valproate ($n = 14$) in the treatment of acute mania. Both lithium and valproate were effective in decreasing manic symptoms. Although lithium was slightly more effective overall, valproate was more effective in decreasing the symptoms of mixed mania. Schaff and colleagues (1993) found 47 of 63 (75%) patients with bipolar spectrum disorders, who were previously considered treatment resistant to either lithium, carbamazepine, or a combination of the two, responded positively to the addition of valproate to their treatment regimens. Jacobsen (1993) found that 26 of 33 patients with rapid-cycling mood who were diagnosed with either cyclothymia or bipolar II disorder had marked or moderate cessation of mood cycling with low doses of valproate (125–500 mg). The anticycling responses consisted of suppression of both hypomanic and depressive episodes.

Numerous studies have concluded that patients with mixed and/or rapid cycling bipolar disorder are more likely to respond to anticonvulsant medications than to lithium (Freeman et al., 1992; Calabrese et al., 1992). As stated previously, bipolar patients with concomitant substance use disorders appear to have more mixed and/or rapid-cycling bipolar disorder than patients with bipolar disorder who do not abuse substances. Therefore, substance-abusing bipolar patients may respond better to anticonvulsant medications (e.g., valproate) than to lithium therapy. In fact, in an open-label pilot study, Brady and colleagues (1995) found valproate to be safe and effective in nine mixed-manic bipolar patients with concurrent substance dependence, who previously had either not tolerated or not responded to lithium.

Both valproate and alcohol consumption are known to cause transient elevations in liver transaminases and, in rare cases, fatal liver failure. Therefore, the safe use of valproate in the alcoholic population has recently been in question because of the potential for hepatotoxicity in patients who are already at risk for this complication. However, there is recent preliminary evidence from our site that liver transaminases do not dramatically increase in alcoholic patients who are receiving valproate even if they are actively drinking (unpublished data). Additionally, chronic alcohol use may cause decreased white blood cell and decreased platelet counts, which may also complicate the use of valproate in the alcoholic population. These preliminary data have not shown any clinically significant decreases in platelet counts of alcoholic individuals who were receiving valproate for as long as 2 years (unpublished data). Table 4 shows laboratory data for 20 alcoholics before and after valproate treatment. As can be seen, there

Table 4 Average Test Results Before and During Treatment with Depakote

	Normal range	Baseline	<2 months	2–8 months	>8 months	Test statistic
AST (IU/L)	10–42	31.4 ($n = 19$)	35.1 ($n = 19$)	37.1 ($n = 16$)	24.8 ($n = 5$)	NS
ALP (IU/L)	40–120	81.8 ($n = 20$)	85.8 ($n = 19$)	76.3 ($n = 16$)	58.2 ($n = 4$)	NS
T. Bili (mg/dl)	0.1–1.3	0.9 ($n = 19$)	0.9 ($n = 18$)	0.9 ($n = 16$)	0.8 ($n = 4$)	NS
LD (IU/L)	90–180	162.0 ($n = 19$)	162.2 ($n = 19$)	169.7 ($n = 15$)	146.5 ($n = 4$)	NS
GGT (U/L)	8–64	80.3 ($n = 16$)	68.2 ($n = 17$)	67.3 ($n = 12$)	70.7 ($n = 3$)	NS
ALT (IU/L)	10–60	43.9 ($n = 14$)	37.9 ($n = 15$)	40.5 ($n = 13$)	21.3 ($n = 3$)	NS
WBC (K/mm^3)	4.8–10.8	8.4 ($n = 16$)	7.3 ($n = 10$)	7.1 ($n = 12$)	—	NS
PLT (K/mm^3)[a]	140–440	280.0 ($n = 18$)	248.4 ($n = 9$)	226.7 ($n = 10$)	—	$p < .05$

[a]Paired Student's t-test for baseline versus 2–8 months = 10.06, $p < 0.001$; for ANOVA $F = 25.35$, $p = 0.001$.

are no significant elevations in liver transaminase and no clinically significant changes in platelets or white blood cell counts.

Currently valproate is the only anticonvulsant medication that is FDA approved for the treatment of bipolar disorder. However, a number of studies support the use of carbamazepine in the treatment of bipolar disorder, specifically in the treatment of mixed mania and rapid cycling. There are also a number of studies that have found carbamazepine effective in the treatment of bipolar disorder when lithium therapy has failed (Okuma et al., 1989).

C. Other Agents

When acute mania is being treated, the other traditional agents (e.g., neuroleptics, benzodiazepines) are also useful in the substance-abusing population. However, when substance-abusing bipolar individuals are being managed with benzodiazepines on an outpatient basis, it may be prudent to use agents that have a longer onset of action (e.g., clonazepam, oxazepam) since those agents appear to have less abuse potential.

VII. PSYCHOTHERAPEUTIC TREATMENTS

Psychotherapeutic interventions are useful in the treatment of both bipolar affective disorder and substance use disorders and are a critical element in the treatment of the substance-abusing bipolar patient. It is fairly well accepted that the use of medications for mood stability is an essential component of the treatment of bipolar patients. Although most experts agree that psychotherapy can be an important adjunct to pharmacotherapeutic interventions in bipolar patients, there is less consensus concerning the most appropriate psychotherapeutic treatment.

However, mood stabilization alone will rarely be an effective treatment for a substance use disorder. Adjunctive therapy and psychosocial rehabilitation are necessary.

A wide range of psychotherapeutic interventions have been used in the treatment of bipolar disorder. These include psychodynamic, interpersonal, cognitive, behavioral, and family therapy (APA Practice Guidelines, 1994). Judgments concerning the effectiveness of these treatments are primarily based on clinical consensus rather than controlled clinical trial, however; formal studies of several of these treatments are currently being conducted.

Psychotherapeutic and psychosocial interventions are mainstays in the treatment of the substance use disorders. Several recent studies have demonstrated success with cognitive behavioral therapy interventions (Carroll et al., 1994) as well as with behaviorally oriented contingency management programs (Higgins et al., 1994). Many of the principles of cognitive behavioral therapy are common to the treatment of affective disorder as well as substance use disorders. Emphasis on developing therapies to specifically treat individuals with comorbid psychiatric and substance use disorders by combining techniques used to treat both disorders will be a fruitful area for further work. In the meantime, substance use disorders should be aggressively treated in bipolar patients as soon as they are psychiatrically stable enough to participate in and benefit from treatment. It is also important to recognize that all individuals with bipolar disorder are at risk for developing a substance use disorder and should therefore be informed about the risks of substance abuse and counseled in the early warning signs of substance abuse. In particular, patients should be warned about the dangers of self-medication with substances of abuse.

VIII. CONCLUSION

Substance abuse/dependence is very common among patients with bipolar disorder. It has been estimated that over 50% of bipolar patients have a concomitant substance use disorder. There is currently very little published data on the treatment of bipolar disorder complicated by substance abuse. There is evidence that substance abuse affects the course and presentation of bipolar disorder and is associated with increased hospitalizations and more mixed manic states. While studies have suggested that these patients are more likely to be lithium nonresponders, this area requires further investigation. If both bipolar disorder and substance use are associated with neuronal sensitization (kindling), it is possible that antikindling anticonvulsant agents may be more useful to treat these concomitant disorders than more conventional lithium therapy. Psychotherapeutic interventions specific to this population need to be further investigated.

REFERENCES

Abbott Laboratories. Divalproex Sodium (Depakote) product information. North Chicago: May 1995.

American Psychiatric Association Practice Guidelines. Practice guidelines for the treatment of patients with bipolar disorder. Am J Psychiatry 1994; 151(Suppl):1–36.

Ballenger JC, Post RM. Therapeutic effects of carbamazepine in affective illness: a preliminary report. Commun Psychopharmacol 1978; 2:159–179.

Blanco-Perez CR, Blanco C, Grimaldi JAR, Rueda CA, Mayo JA, O'Connell RA. Substance abuse and bipolar disorder. Proceedings of the American Psychiatric Association, New York, May 1996, NR 90, p. 90.

Bowden CL. Predictors of response to divalproex and lithium. J Clin Psychiatry 1995; 56(Suppl 3):25–30.

Bowden CL, Brugger AM, Swann AC, Calabrese JR, Janicak PG, Petty F, Dilsaver SC, Davis JM, Rush AJ, Small JG, Garza-Trevino ES, Risch SC, Goodnick PJ, Morris DD. Efficacy of Divalproex vs lithium and placebo in the treatment of mania. JAMA 1994; 271:918–924.

Brady KT, Lydiard RB. Bipolar affective disorder and substance abuse. J Clin Psychopharmacol 1992; 12(Suppl):17s–22s.

Brady KT, Casto S, Lydiard RB, Malcolm R, Arana GW. Substance abuse in an inpatient psychiatric sample. Am J Drug Alcohol Abuse 1991; 17:389–397.

Brady KT, Sonne SC, Anton R, Ballenger JC. Valproate in the treatment of acute bipolar affective episodes complicated by substance abuse: a pilot study. J Clin Psychiatry 1995; 56:118–121.

Brown ME, Anton RF, Malcolm R, Ballenger JC. Alcoholic detoxification and withdrawal seizures: clinical support for a kindling hypothesis. Biol Psychiatry 1986; 43:107–113.

Brown SE, Schuckit M. Changes in depression among abstinent alcoholics. J Stud Alcohol 1988; 49:412–417.

Calabrese JR, Delucchi GA. Phenomenology of rapid cycling manic depression and its treatment with valproate. J Clin Psychiatry 1989; 50(Suppl):30–34.

Calabrese JR, Markovitz PJ, Kimmel SE, Wagner SC. Spectrum of efficacy of valproate in 78 rapid-cycling bipolar patients. J Clin Psychopharmacol 1992; 12(Suppl): 53s–56s.

Calabrese JR, Rapport DJ, Kimmel SE, Reece B, Woyshville MJ. Rapid cycling bipolar disorder and its treatment with valproate. Can J Psychiatry 1993; 38(Suppl):s57–s61.

Carroll KM, Rounsaville BJ, Gordon LT. Psychotherapy and pharmacotherapy for ambulatory cocaine abusers. Arch Gen Psychiatry 1994; 51:177–187.

El-Guebaly N. Manic-depressive psychosis and drug abuse. Can J Psychiatry 1975; 20: 595–598.

Estroff TW, Dackis CA, Gold MS, et al. Drug abuse and bipolar disorders. Int J Psychiatry Med 1985–86; 15:37–40.

Feinman JA, Dunner DL. The effect of alcohol and substance abuse on the course of bipolar affective disorder. J Affect Disord 1996; 37:43–49.

Freeman TW, Clothier JL, Pazzaglia R, Lesem MD, Swann AC. A double-blind comparison of valproate and lithium in the treatment of acute mania. Am J Psychiatry 1992; 149:108–111.

Gawin FH, Kleber HD. Cocaine abuse treatment: open pilot trial with desipramine and lithium carbonate. Arch Gen Psychiatry 1984; 41:903–909.

Gawin FH, Kleber HD. Abstinence symptomatology and psyciatric diagnosis in cociane abusers: clinical observations. Arch Gen Psychiatry 1986; 43:107–113.

Hasin D, Endicott J, Lewis C. Alcohol and drug abuse in patients with affective syndromes. Compr Psychiatry 1985; 26:283–295.

Hasin DS, Endicott J, Keller MB. RDC alcoholism in patients with major affective syndromes: two-year course. Am J Psychiatry 1989; 146:318–323.

Hasin DS, Trautman KD, Miele GM, et al. Psychiatric Research Interview for Substance and Mental Disorders (PRISM): reliability in substance abusers. Am J Psychiatry 1996; 9:1195–1201.

Hesselbrock MN, Meyer RE, Keener JJ. Psychopathology in hospitalized alcoholics. Arch Gen Psychiatry 1985; 42:1050–1055.

Higgins ST, Budney AJ, Bickel WK, Foerg FE, Donham R, Budger GJ. Incentives improve outcome in outpatient behavioral treatment of cocaine dependence. Arch Gen Psychiatry 1994; 51:568–576.

Jacobsen FM. Low-dose valproate: a new treatment for cyclothymia, mild rapid cycling disorders, and premenstrual syndrome. J Clin Psychiatry 1993; 54:229–234.

Keller MB, Lavori PW, Coryell W, Andreasen NC, Endicott J, Clayton PJ, Klerman GL, Hirschfeld RM. Differential outcome of pure manic, mixed/cycling, and pure depressive episodes in patients with bipolar illness. JAMA 1986; 255:3138–3142.

Kessler RC, McGonagle KA, Zhao S, Nelson CB, Hughes M, Eshleman S, Wittchen HU, Kendler KS. Lifetime and 12-month prevalence of DSM-III-R psychiatric disorders in the United States: results from the National Comorbidity Survey. Arch Gen Psychiatry 1994; 51:8–19.

Kranzler HR, Kadden RM, Babor TF, Tennen H, Rounsaville BJ. Validity of SCID in substance abuse patients. Addiction 1996; 91:859–868.

Lydiard RB, Howell EF, Ballenger JC, Malcolm R. Prevalence of anxiety and mood disorders in hospitalized alcoholics. Presented at the Annual Meeting of the American College of Neuropsychopharmacology, San Juan, Puerto Rico, December 1987.

Malcolm R, Ballenger JC, Sturgis ET, Anton R. Double-blind controlled trial comparing carbamazepine to oxazepam treatment of alcohol withdrawal. Am J Psychiatry 1989; 146:617–621.

McElroy SL, Keck PE, Pope HG, Hudson JI, Faedda GL, Swann AC. Clinical and research implications of the diagnosis of dysphoric or mixed mania or hypomania. Am J Psychiatry 1992; 149:1633–1644.

Meyer RE. How to understand the relationship between psychopathology and addictive disorders: another example of the chicken and the egg. In: Meyer RE, ed. Psychopathology and Addictive Disorders. New York, Guilford Press, 1986:3–16.

Miller FT, Busch F, Tanenbaum JH. Drug abuse in schizophrenia and bipolar disorder. Am J Drug Alcohol Abuse 1989; 15:291–295.

Mirin SM, Weiss RD, Griffin ML, Michael JL. Psychopathology in drug abusers and their families. Compr Psychiatry 1991; 32:36–51.

Nunes EV, Quitkin FM, Klein DF. Psychiatric diagnosis in cocaine abuse. Psychiatry Res 1989; 25:105–114.

Nunes EV, McGrath PJ, Wager S, Quitkin FM. Lithium treatment for cocaine abusers with bipolar spectrum disorders. Am J Psychiatry 1990; 147:655–657.

O'Connell RA, Mayo JA, Flatow L, Cuthbertson B, O'Brien BE. Outcome of bipolar disorder on long-term treatment with lithium. Br J Psychiatry 1991; 159:123–129.

O'Sullivan K, Rynne C, Miller J, O'Sullivan MS, Fitzpatrick V, Hux M, Cooney J, Clare A. A follow-up study on alcoholics with and without co-existing affective disorder. Br J Psychiatry 1988; 152:813–819.

Okuma T, Yamashita I, Takahashi R, Itoh H, Kurihara M, Otsukis, Watanabe S, Sarai K, Hazama H, Inanaga K. Clinical efficacy of carbamazepine in affective, schizoaffective, and schizophrenic disorders. Pharmacopsychiatry 1989; 22:47–53.

Post RM. Non-lithium treatment for bipolar disorder. J Clin Psychiatry 1990; 51(Suppl): 9–16.

Post RM, Weiss SRB. Psychomotor stimulant vs. local anesthetic effects of cocaine: role of behavioral sensitization and kindling. In: Clout D, Asghar K, Brown R, eds. Mechanism of Cocaine Abuse and Toxicity, Rockville NIDA, research monograph 88. 1988:217–238.

Post RM, Rubinow DR, Ballenger JC. Conditioning, sensitization, and kindling: implications for the course of affective illness. In: Post RM, Ballenger JC, eds. Neurobiology of Mood Disorders. Baltimore: Williams & Wilkins, 1984:432–466.

Prien RF, Himmelhock JM, Kupfer DJ. Treatment of mixed mania. J Affect Disord 1988; 15:9–15.

Regier CA, Farmer ME, Rae DS, Locke BZ, Keith SJ, Judd LL, Goodwin FK. Comorbidity of mental disorders with alcohol and other drug abuse results from the epidemiologic catchment area (ECA) study. JAMA 1990; 264:2511–2518.

Reich LH, Davies RK, Himmelhoch JM. Excessive alcohol use in manic-depressive illness. Am J Psychiatry 1974; 131:83–86.

Ross HE, Glaser FB, Germanson T. The prevalence of psychiatric disorders in patients with alcohol and other drug problems. Arch Gen Psychiatry 1988; 45:1023–1031.

Rounsaville BJ, Anton SF, Carroll K, Budde D, Prusoff BA, Gawin F. Psychiatric diagnoses of treatment seeking cocaine abusers. Arch Gen Psychiatry 1991; 48:43–51.

Salloum IM, Mezzich JE, Kerisci L, Janoski T, Cornelius JR, Daley D, Jorge MR. Implication of substance abuse versus non-substance abuse in bipolar disorder. Proceedings of the 1996 American Psychiatric Association, New York, May 1996, NR348, p. 161.

Schaff MR, Fawcett J, Zajecka JM. Divalproex sodium in the treatment of refractory affective disorders. J Clin Psychiatry 1993; 54:380–384.

Secunda SK, Swann A, Katz MM, Koslow SH, Croughan J, Chang S. Diagnosis and treatment of mixed mania. Am J Psychiatry 1987; 144:96–98.

Sonne SC, Brady KT, Morton WA. Substance abuse and bipolar affective disorder. J Nerv Ment Dis 1994; 182:349–352.

Tohen M, Waternaux CM, Tsuang MT, Hunt AT. Four year follow-up of twenty-four first-episode manic patients. J Affect Disord 1990; 19:76–86.

Weiss RD, Mirin SM, Michael JL, et al. Psychopathology in chronic cocaine abusers. Am J Drug Alcohol Abuse 1986; 12:17–29.

Weiss RD, Mirin SM, Griffin ML, Michael JL. Psychopathology in cocaine abusers: changing trends. J Nerv Ment Dis 1988a; 176:719–725.

Weiss RD, Mirin SM, Griffin ML, Michael JL. A comparison of alcoholic and nonalcoholic drug abusers. J Stud Alcohol 1988b; 49:510–515.

Winokur G, Coryell W, Akiskal HS, Maser JD, Keller MB, Endicott J, Mueller T. Alcoholism in manic-depressive (bipolar) illness: familial illness, course of illness, and the primary-secondary distinction. Am J Psychiatry 1995; 152:365–372.

8

The Co-occurrence of Bipolar Disorder with Medical Illness

KENJI W. SAX and STEPHEN M. STRAKOWSKI
University of Cincinnati
Cincinnati, Ohio

I. INTRODUCTION

The term 'comorbidity' was originally used to define conditions that are etiologically distinct, but co-occur in a single patient (1). Without knowing the underlying etiology of psychiatric illnesses, studies of comorbidity in psychiatry are limited, since it is difficult to determine whether a medical condition is the cause of, or simply co-occurs with, a given psychiatric disorder. Alternatively, studies of comorbid medical and psychiatric conditions may clarify the etiology of both. For example, if a medical condition can be shown to represent a risk factor for a psychiatric disorder, understanding the pathophysiology of the medical condition may lead to understanding the etiology of the psychiatric illness. Second, studies of comorbidity help to delineate treatment algorithms in patients with these complex co-occurring disorders. Clarifying the relationships among psychiatric illnesses and co-occurring medical conditions may aid in determining which disorder requires more immediate treatment or whether both syndromes should be treated concurrently. Third, with the increased attention during the past few years to controlling medical costs, there are often fewer resources to treat these complicated patients who have more than one syndrome. Understanding how co-occurring syndromes interact and respond to treatment may alter the manner in which health care is delivered and reimbursed.

Despite the importance of understanding interactions between medical and psychiatric illnesses, the actual number of systematic studies examining syndrome co-occurrence is relatively small. Early studies of comorbidity focused on the co-occurrence of depressive disorders with medical conditions (2) and led to the concept of secondary depression (3). In contrast to the studies in unipolar depression, there are relatively few systematic studies examining medical comorbidity in bipolar disorder, with the majority of data coming from case studies. Unfortunately, due to variability in the methods of data collection, these case studies are severely limited when trying to generalize findings across studies (see Refs. 4,5 for review).

In this chapter, we review articles pertaining to the co-occurrence of medical and psychiatric disorders, and extend our previous publications (4) by adding new references and expanding our discussion of medical comorbidity with bipolar disorder. Relevant articles that were published in English by December 31, 1995 were identified using Paperchase. References from these articles were also examined for inclusion in this review. Papers are presented only if data were provided separately for co-occurrence of mania or bipolar disorder with other medical syndromes. While the majority of the literature is related to medical illnesses that produce secondary mania, a number of articles show a relationship between bipolar disorder, which includes primary mania, and certain medical syndromes. Hence, this review is divided into two sections: (1) medical disorders associated with secondary mania, and (2) medical comorbidity in bipolar disorder.

II. MANIA SECONDARY TO MEDICAL ILLNESSES

Secondary mania, i.e., mania resulting from a concurrent medical condition, was considered to be relatively uncommon and therefore received little attention before the seminal review by Krauthammer and Klerman in 1978 (6). They identified 21 cases that met their criteria for secondary mania, which were classified into five general categories corresponding to the medical condition associated with the symptoms: (1) drugs, including steroids, central nervous system (CNS) stimulants, and toxins; (2) metabolic disturbances; (3) infections; (4) neoplasms; and (5) epilepsy. To differentiate secondary from primary mania and from delirium, cases were excluded if there was a clear previous history of mania or other affective illness, or a disoriented or confusional state associated with the manic symptoms. In reviewing the general characteristics of these cases, Krauthammer and Klerman found a median age of onset of 41 years, which was considerably older than the median age of onset of bipolar illness, approximately 25 years. Although family history data were limited in their sample, of the 10 subjects with information on family history, nine reported a negative family history of affective illness. This was in sharp contrast to their data on bipolar illness, which showed a positive family history in over 85% of patients. By differentiating cases of secondary mania from those associated with bipolar disorder (i.e., primary mania), they suggested that mania is a heterogeneous syndrome with multiple etiologies and, therefore, not exclusively a presentation of manic-depressive illness (i.e., bipolar disorder), even though patients with secondary mania appeared very similar phenomenologically to patients with primary mania.

Cummings (7) later extended the list of medical conditions associated with secondary mania by adding a number of disorders that were not identified by Krauthammer and Klerman (6), including disorders associated with the extrapyramidal system, multiple sclerosis, and thyroid dysregulation. Based on the focal lesions and degenerative neurological disorders producing secondary mania, Cummings tentatively suggested the pathophysiological mechanisms producing mania involved midline neural structures including the thalamus, hypothalamus, and basal ganglia, as well as nuclei with connections to the limbic system. He also observed that focal lesions producing secondary mania were predominantly right-hemispheric, and, drawing from studies of primary mania (i.e., mania associated with bipolar disorder), implicated both norepinephrine and serotonin in the development of secondary mania. Thus, Cummings extended the assertion by Krauthammer and Klerman (6) that mania is a syndrome with multiple etiologies, and hypothesized that it involves dysfunction in right-hemispheric midline structures with monoaminergic projections.

Another article that appeared a year earlier presented a similar review, but included neurosyphilis and herpes simplex encephalitis in the list of medical conditions causing secondary mania (8). Combined with more recent reviews of the literature provided by Strakowski et al. (4) and Heilä et al. (5), Table 1 presents the array of organic conditions that have been reported to be associated with secondary mania.

While many medical illnesses have been linked to secondary mania, studies of traumatic brain injury have been useful in terms of localizing brain areas associated with the manic syndrome. The relationship between mania and brain injury has been examined in both patient case series and controlled studies, although instances of the latter are relatively few (9–14). Manic symptoms are less common than depressive symptoms as a sequela of brain injury, although there are numerous reports of irritable mood, assaultive behavior, racing thoughts, poor sleep, and, less frequently, euphoric mood. In the only prospective, longitudinal study of secondary mania in individuals following closed-head injury, Jorge et al. (15) found that over the 12 months following hospitalization, 9% of patients with closed-head injury subsequently developed symptoms severe enough to meet DSM-III-R (16) criteria for mania. Neuroanatomical findings in these patients indicated an association between bilateral temporal basal polar lesions and the presence of manic symptoms. Other studies have reported a preponderance of damage to structures functionally connected to limbic struc-

Table 1 Medical Illnesses Associated with Secondary Mania (see Ref. 4–8 for review)

Head trauma	
Epidural hematoma	Concussion
Traumatic brain injury	
Neurological abnormalities	
Glioma	Arteriovenous malformation
Meningioma	Normal-pressure hydrocephalus
Metastases	Idiopathic basal ganglia calcification
Stroke	Tuberous sclerosis
Neurological damage following heart surgery	Cerebral sarcoidosis
	Wolfram syndrome
Familial cerebellar atrophy	Subcortical gray matter heterotopia
Subarachnoid hemorrhage	
Other CNS disorders	
CNS systemic lupus erythematosus	Epilepsy
Dialysis dementia	Huntington's disease
Electrical trauma	Klein-Levin syndrome
Idiopathic dystonia	Klinefelter's syndrome
Infectious diseases	
Cytomegalovirus	AIDS
Herpes simplex	Q fever
St. Louis type A encephalitis	Influenza
Japanese B encephalitis	Enteric fever
Neurosyphilis	Cholera, tetanus, and typhoid immunization
HIV	Lyme borreliosis
Metabolic disorders	
Cushing's disease	Polycythemia
Hemodialysis	Intravenous calcium replacement
Hyperthyroidism	Vitamin B_{12} deficiency
Uremia	Wilson's disease

tures including the basotemporal or orbitofrontal cortex, caudate nuclei, and thalamus. However, damage to metencephalic structures including pontine infarction (17) and cerebellar atrophy (18) have also been linked to secondary mania, possibly through their connections to diencephalic structures such as the hypothalamus. Moreover, secondary mania is a more common sequela of brain injuries involving right-sided subcortical structures than other brain regions (11). One notable exception to this pattern is from a case study which reported left-sided arteriovenous malformation involving limbic structures in a 33-year-old woman with recurrent unipolar mania who was left-handed (19), suggesting that it may be injury to the nondominant hemisphere rather than the right hemisphere specifically that is associated with mania. In addition to structural damage, the development of posttraumatic seizure disorder may also play a role in secondary mania following brain injury, particularly foci located in temporal or temporoparietal areas (9). Specifically, the presence of epileptogenic activity appears to be associated with irritable mood and assaultive behavior. In summary, although a number of different cortical and subcortical areas have been implicated in the development of secondary mania, particularly in the right hemisphere, there is evidence to suggest involvement of limbic structures in the pathophysiology of mania.

The degree to which patients who develop secondary mania after brain trauma have higher rates of affective illness in their families is unclear. There is limited information based on relatively few subjects that indicates no such association is present (15), whereas other findings point toward a relationship between injury to right-hemispheric structures with limbic connections, a positive family history of affective illness, and secondary mania (14). In one other positive study, no family history of bipolar illness was present; however, approximately one-third of the subjects had one or more relatives with a history of depression (9).

Documented approaches to treating mania secondary to brain injury are primarily from observations made from small case series, since controlled studies examining the therapeutic efficacy of mood-stabilizing agents are lacking. However, the armamentarium used to treat primary mania (i.e., bipolar disorder) appears to be effective in treating secondary mania due to brain injury, and includes lithium, carbamazepine, and valproic acid (20).

In addition to brain trauma, individual cases of CNS abnormalities, including neoplasms, malformations, and neurodegenerative disorders producing secondary mania, have been reported. They include brain-stem tumor (21), arteriovenous malformation (22), acoustic neurinoma (23), cerebral sarcoidosis (24,25), familial cerebellar cortical atrophy (18), gray matter heterotopia (26), intracranial chondroma of the frontoparietal region (27), idiopathic basal ganglia calcification (28), normal pressure hydrocephalus (29), Wolfram syndrome (30), tuberous sclerosis (31), and cerebral infarct (32). Eight of these patients reported localization of the abnormalities unilaterally: six in the right-hemisphere (21–23,27,31,32) and two in the left-hemisphere (26,28). Although the latter cases are inconsistent with the general observation of right-hemispheric dysfunction in secondary mania, both patients were left-handed. As previously indicated, mania may be associated with injury to the nondominant hemisphere rather than to the right hemisphere per se. Consistent with this pattern, five of the six patients with right-hemispheric abnormalities were right handed.

Determining the neuroanatomical structures involved in the expression of mania secondary to medical illnesses may be of heuristic value when examining the etiology of primary mania (i.e., bipolar disorder). More specifically, the anatomical structures implicated in the development of secondary mania may be the same regions involved in the development of primary mania. Neuroendocrinological and morphological research in bipolar disorder supports this contention, implicating midline subcortical structures such as the hypothalamus in the development of mania (33). For example, morphometric studies have reported third-ventricular enlargement in bipolar patients relative to controls, which may reflect hypothalamic abnormalities since these nuclei are laterally adjacent to the third ventricle (34,35). In addition, the suprachiasmatic nucleus of the hypothalamus is involved in circadian rhythm regulation, which is abnormal in bipolar disorder (36,37). Data from neuropsychological studies fairly consistently corroborate these findings, including the prominence of right-sided deficits (33). Abnormalities in midsagittal areas have also been found to correlate with impaired neuropsychological functioning (38), suggesting that the phenomenologically similar presentation of primary and secondary mania may be due to a common pathophysiological mechanism, even though the underlying causes of each are different. Therefore, studies of medical comorbidity provide, albeit indirectly and relatively unsystematically, potential clues to the origins of bipolar disorder.

In addition to reports of secondary mania in individuals with brain trauma and structural abnormalities, there have been numerous case reports of secondary mania occurring with other medical and neurological conditions including metabolic disorders and infectious diseases (see Table 1). Indeed, in a retrospective chart review of 755 patients evaluated by a psychiatric consult/liaison service (39), 13 (87%) of the 15 diagnoses of mania found were attributed to a medical condition, with the most common being the use of corticosteroids (54%) and HIV-related complications (23%). Additionally, there has been one case of secondary mania attributed to hyperbaric chamber pressure in an individual participating in a deep-diving experiment (40).

As previously stated, generalizing across a large number of individual case reports makes establishing meaningful associations tenuous at best. In addition, data from uncontrolled trials of various medications including lithium, antipsychotics, and benzodiazepines to treat secondary mania provide little toward the development of treatment strategies. In some cases these medications are administered prior to or concurrent with treatment of the underlying medical condition. Unless there is a clear pathophysiological link between the medical illness and manic symptomatology, assumptions about the presence of secondary, as opposed to primary, mania are weak. If, on the other hand, manic symptoms remitted following treatment exclusively for the medical syndrome, it would provide a rationale for assuming their direct association with the medical syndrome (i.e., secondary mania). One fairly clear example of the latter case involved an individual with meningeal cryptococcosis presenting with mania (41). Initially treated as a case of bipolar disorder, this individual was placed on chlorpromazine and lithium, which reduced the affective lability and motoric excitement, but produced emotional withdrawal, disorientation, and a deterioration in motoric functioning. Upon reevaluation, the underlying medical condition was identified, all psychotropic medications were discontinued, and antibiotic therapy was introduced. The patient soon returned to the previous baseline that consisted of a relatively high level of functioning. Unfortunately, not all cases are as clear. Walter-Ryan and Fahs (42) presented the case of what was initially thought to be a manic episode secondary to hyperthyroidism (i.e., thyroid storm). However, several months after discontinuing psychotropic medication, the individual again suffered a manic episode and was treated successfully with the same medication. This time, results of thyroid studies indicated normal functioning. Whether the initial manic episode resulted from hyperthyroidism or was primary mania coinciding with the medical condition is unknown. However, this case highlights the difficulty in determining causality even when the evidence for associations between manic symptoms and the underlying medical condition seem compelling.

Another limitation of generalizing from individual case studies involves the relative absence of structured diagnostic instruments and longitudinal assessments used to systematically evaluate whether symptoms are due to mania or the result of delirium (4). Finally, not all articles provide neurobiological information that might implicate specific brain regions in the development of manic symptomatology. Taken in concert, these factors limit a clear understanding of the relationship between mania and many medical conditions (43). More systematic studies are needed that incorporate standardized assessment tools, modern neuroimaging techniques, comprehensive biochemical evaluation, and controlled treatment protocols (4). Also, consistent reporting of handedness may be useful when interpreting abnormalities in brain structure, if they are present. Finally, family history data aid in determining whether the manic episode is secondary to a medical condition or whether it may represent a first episode of bipolar mania, as high rates of familial affective illness characterize patients with bipolar disorder. Implementing more systematic and comprehensive approaches to data collection will foster clinicians' ability to understand and treat cases of mania coexisting with medical syndromes.

III. MEDICAL COMORBIDITY IN BIPOLAR DISORDER

In contrast to medical conditions that produce secondary mania, there are a number of medical conditions that co-occur with bipolar disorder more commonly than expected. In these cases, the underlying etiologies of "functional" mania and medical conditions are distinct and therefore represent separate disorders. These studies have helped to identify medical illnesses that are more common in bipolar patients than in the general population and have provided a better understanding of the effects of comorbidity on outcome. One question that is as yet unanswered is: What factors are associated with bipolar disorder that increase the risk of developing a medical syndrome, or vice versa?

Black et al. (44–46) retrospectively examined medical comorbidity in patients with bipolar mania or schizoaffective disorder, manic type. They used the term "complicated" mania to describe mania coexisting with a concurrent major medical condition, which included cases of mania secondary to a medical illness and cases of comorbid medical disorders and primary mania (i.e., bipolar disorder). Since in many cases it was difficult to determine whether the manic syndrome preceded or followed the co-occurring illness, Black and colleagues chose to differentiate between complicated (i.e., occurring with a medical illness) and uncomplicated (i.e., without a medical illness) mania, rather than between primary and secondary mania. Results from their retrospective review of psychiatric records showed that 21% of patients had been diagnosed with a coexisting medical condition. When compared to matched controls with similar psychiatric diagnoses but no concurrent medical diagnoses, the complicated manics were older, had an older age of illness onset, and showed a poorer course of illness. Despite the likely inclusion of patients with secondary mania, these findings indicate that medical comorbidity may be an important indicator of poor outcome.

Similarly, Strakowski et al. (47,48) examined medical comorbidity in a prospective study of patients with a first episode of mania diagnosed using the Structured Clinical Interview for DSM-III-R (SCID-P) (49). Unlike the studies of Black et al. (44–46), patients with secondary mania were excluded. Strakowski et al. found that 18% of the 60 patients had a comorbid medical diagnosis, with the most common illnesses being temporal lobe epilepsy (4%) and pneumonia (3%). Medical comorbidity was associated with an older age; however, unlike previous observations (44–46), these patients had shorter hospitalizations, decreased use of antipsychotic medication, and less severe symptomatology at discharge.

In addition to these phenomenological studies of comorbidity, there have been a few studies of specific relationships between medical illnesses and bipolar disorder, specifically multiple sclerosis, Tourette's disorder, and migraine. Bipolar disorder appears to be more common in multiple sclerosis than in the general population. For example, in their epidemiological study of a county population, Schiffer et al. (50) found that bipolar disorder and multiple sclerosis occurred together almost twice as frequently as expected by chance. High rates of co-occurrence were also observed by Joffe et al. (51), who studied 100 patients from a multiple sclerosis clinic and found that 13% met criteria for bipolar disorder, which is in sharp contrast to rates in the general population of 1% (33). It is unclear whether manic symptoms in patients with multiple sclerosis are due to brain injury or represent an increased risk of developing bipolar disorder. Using family history data, Joffe and colleagues (51) found that first-degree relatives of these patients did not demonstrate higher rates of affective illness than the general population, suggesting mania was secondary to the multiple sclerosis disease process. If this is the case, further research is warranted to identify the specific brain regions affected and to determine whether findings are consistent with those reported earlier of right-sided subcortical lesions. Results from a more recent study suggest that in some patients with co-occurring mania and multiple sclerosis, manic symptoms may precede the onset of other symptoms associated with multiple sclerosis (52). This retrospective chart review examined 2720 consecutive admissions to psychiatric units and found 10 patients who were diagnosed with multiple sclerosis in addition to a psychiatric syndrome. Seven had psychiatric hospitalizations prior to their diagnosis of multiple sclerosis, although in several of the cases, the severity of manic symptoms may have obscured other signs and symptoms of multiple sclerosis. Clarifying relationships between multiple sclerosis and bipolar disorder may lead to improved understanding of the pathophysiology of both disease processes.

In addition to multiple sclerosis, there have been reports of associations between bipolar and Tourette's disorders. In a recent epidemiological study (53), minimal risk ratios were calculated to determine genetic risk indicators for comorbid Tourette's and bipolar disorders. The estimated risk of developing bipolar disorder in individuals with Tourette's was more than four times higher than expected by chance. In addition, males were at a greater risk for comorbidity than females. Separate etiological processes leading to dysfunctions in common neural pathways, perhaps located in the basal ganglia, were hypothesized to underlie the increased likelihood of bipolar disorder co-occurring with Tourette's disorder.

Although the majority of studies examining migraine and psychiatric comorbidity have focused on depressive and anxiety-spectrum disorders, associations between bipolar disorder and migraine have been observed. For example, Merikangas et al. (54) found that in patients with migraine, the likelihood of a past diagnosis of hypomania or mania was three times the rate in individuals without migraine. Examining the association from the opposite perspective, Younes et al. (55) studied male children with bipolar disorder and found a history of migraine headaches was significantly more common in patients (29%) than in normal controls (0%). Similar to research on Tourette's disorder, it is unclear whether bipolar disorder and migraine share a common pathophysiological pathway (56). However, based on a recent review by Keck et al. (57), it does appear that migraine may be more strongly associated with major depression and anxiety disorders than bipolar disorder. Nonetheless, with recent advances in functional imaging techniques, it may be useful to examine cortical activation in individuals with comorbid migraine and bipolar disorder to determine whether interactions between comorbid disorders produce quantitative differences in brain functioning as compared to bipolar disorder alone.

As previously mentioned, some studies of comorbidity have shown an association between poorer outcome in bipolar disorder and the presence of a co-occurring medical illness. Based on a limited case series, Strakowski et al. (58) found this association in patients with obstructive sleep apnea. This finding does not suggest that obstructive sleep apnea is more common in bipolar disorder than expected by chance. However, it does suggest that obstructive sleep apnea may affect treatment response in such a way that the illness is prolonged. In addition, the authors speculated that weight gain due to lithium therapy may have contributed to either the development or increase in the severity of sleep apnea.

Rather than examining prevalence rates of specific medical conditions in patients with bipolar disorder, several studies have compared their rates of comorbidity with those in other psychiatric populations. In a recent report from the NIMH Collaborative Study on the Psychobiology of Depression (59), only 3% of patients with bipolar disorder or schizoaffective mania had been physically ill at the time of intake, which was significantly lower than the rate found in patients with unipolar depression. Moreover, patients with bipolar disorder had a smaller number of medical conditions requiring treatment and fewer lifetime medical hospitalizations. This is in sharp contrast to another study that found 50% of patients with bipolar disorder had a concurrent medical condition, compared with 43% of patients with schizophrenia (60). There are also data indicating relatively high rates of missed medical diagnoses in women with bipolar disorder, which suggests that medical illness may be more common than previously reported (61). A major limitation of these findings is the lack of information regarding the prevalence of medical illnesses in the population from which the patients were drawn.

In summary, there is a lack of systematic, controlled, prospective, longitudinal studies examining relationships between mania and comorbid medical diagnoses. The result has been a lack of clear understanding of both the physiological processes and the efficacy of various forms of treatment. In case studies, it is necessary to include all potentially useful information, such as handedness, family history of affective illness, and a thorough evaluation of personal psychiatric history. Additionally, using standardized, structured assessment tools enhances the validity of diagnoses. Ultimately, understanding interactions between medical illnesses and bipolar disorder may provide the impetus to develop more effective treatment strategies for co-occurring conditions.

IV. DISCUSSION

As Krauthammer and Klerman (6) originally observed, the study of affective disorders, and indeed, psychiatric disorders in general, involves the "continual search for more homogeneous clinical entities." Their effort to differentiate secondary mania, which has a known etiology, from primary or "functional" mania, where the cause is not known, was sustained in subsequent studies. These findings support the proposal that mania is a heterogeneous syndrome with a number of different causes, perhaps affecting common neurophysiological pathways. Completely understanding these interactions and their effects on treatment is an enormous undertaking, and one that can only be accomplished with more systematic methods of data acquisition.

Studies examining secondary mania in individuals with a major medical illness have focused on identifying pathophysiological pathways linking the two. However, in some cases there was not a clear differentiation between primary and secondary mania (41,42). Under ideal circumstances, treating the medical condition and determining whether it results in a reduction in manic symptoms would provide potentially important evidence toward differentiating primary from secondary mania. However, the obvious importance of appropriately managing the acute manic episode takes precedence in clinical settings. As previously stated, many of the studies presented were limited by their retrospective designs, preponderance of individual case studies, lack of comparison groups, and uncontrolled medication trials. Nonetheless, results from these studies have provided an indication of specific brain regions associated with secondary mania, which might prove useful in studies examining the pathophysiology of bipolar disorder. For example, the implication of midline subcortical structures (e.g., thalamus, hypothalamus) underlying the expression of secondary mania along with an association with right-hemispheric dysfunction may provide a basis for studies of the neurophysiological etiology of bipolar disorder. Future studies incorporating functional neuroimaging techniques may provide potentially valuable information on the neural processes associated with secondary mania and, ultimately, bipolar disorder (35).

In contrast to studies of mania secondary to a medical illness, studies of comorbid medical syndromes and bipolar disorder are significantly less common. Although the existing studies indicate that prevalence rates of certain syndromes are significantly higher in bipolar disorder than expected by chance, the lack of prevalence rates from the general population used in comparison limits these findings. With this in mind, the data suggest that multiple sclerosis, Tourette's disorder, and migraine may be more common in bipolar disorder than in the general population. However, it is unclear whether these syndromes share a common pathophysiological process, or whether the presence of one disorder increases the risk of developing another (e.g., a vulnerability indicator). Further information is needed to address this question, including careful examination of the chronology of onset of each syndrome to determine their temporal relationship. In addition, neuroimaging studies may help to clarify the neurobiological basis for comorbidity. Prospective, longitudinal studies of large numbers of patients with bipolar disorder that include thorough medical evaluations and comparison groups are necessary to better understand the way in which these comorbid syndromes develop and interact (4). These kinds of studies may lead to improved understanding of syndrome comorbidity, which, in turn, may contribute to the development of appropriate treatment algorithms, and perhaps ultimately, a clearer understanding of the neurophysiology of bipolar disorder.

REFERENCES

1. Feinstein A. The pre-therapeutic classification of comorbidity in chronic disease. J Chronic Dis 1970; 23:455–468.
2. Robins E, Guze SB. Classification of affective disorders: the primary-secondary, the endogenous-reactive and the neurotic-psychotic. In: Williams TA, Katz MM, Shield JA, eds. Recent Advances in the Psychobiology of the Depressive Illnesses: DHEW Publication No. 70-9053. Washington, DC: US Government Printing Office, 1972.
3. Winokur G. The concept of secondary depression and its relationship to comorbidity. Psychiatr Clin North Am 1990; 13:567–583.
4. Strakowski SM, McElroy SL, Keck PE Jr, West SA. The co-occurrence of mania with medical and other psychiatric disorders. Int J Psychiatry Med 1994; 24:305–328.
5. Heilä H, Turpeinen P, Erkinjuntti T. Case study: mania associated with multiple sclerosis. J Am Acad Child Adolesc Psychiatry 1995; 34:1591–1595.
6. Krauthammer C, Klerman GL. Secondary mania: manic syndromes associated with antecedent physical illness or drugs. Arch Gen Psychiatry 1978; 30:74–79.
7. Cummings JL. Organic psychoses: delusional disorders and secondary mania. Psychiatr Clin North Am 1986; 9:293–311.
8. Stasiek C, Zetin M. Organic manic disorders. Psychosomatics 1985; 26:394–402.
9. Shukla S, Cook BL, Mukherjee S, Godwin C, Miller MG. Mania following head trauma. Am J Psychiatry 1987; 144:93–96.
10. Robinson RG, Boston JD, Starkstein SE, Price TR. Comparison of mania and depression after brain injury: causal factors. Am J Psychiatry 1988; 145:172–178.
11. Starkstein SE, Boston JD, Robinson RG. Mechanisms of mania after brain injury: twelve case reports and review of the literature. J Nerv Ment Dis 1988; 176:87–100.
12. Starkstein SE, Robinson RG, Honig MA, Parikh RM, Joselyn J, Price TR. Mood changes after right-hemisphere lesions. Br J Psychiatry 1989; 155:79–85.
13. Starkstein SE, Mayberg HS, Berthier ML, Fedoroff P, Price TR, Dannals RF, Wagner HN, Leiguarda R, Robinson RG. Mania after brain injury: neuroradiological and metabolic findings. Arch Neurol 1990; 27:652–659.
14. Starkstein SE, Pealson GD, Boston J, Robinson RG. Mania after brain injury: a controlled study of causative factors. Ann Neurol 1987; 44:1069–1073.
15. Jorge RE, Robinson RG, Starkstein SE, Arndt SV, Forrester AW, Geisler FH. Secondary mania following traumatic brain injury. Am J Psychiatry 1993; 150:916–921.
16. American Psychiatric Association. DSM-III-R: Diagnostic and Statistical Manual of Mental Disorders Revised. 3rd ed. Washington, DC: The Association, 1987.

17. Drake ME Jr, Pakalnis A, Phillips B. Secondary mania after ventral pontine infarction. J Neuropsychiatry 1990; 2:322–325.
18. Yadalam KG, Jain AK, Simpson GM. Mania in two sisters with similar cerebellar disturbance. Am J Psychiatry 1985; 142:1067–1069.
19. Berthier ML, Starkstein SE, Robinson RG, Leiguarda R. Limbic lesions in a patient with recurrent mania. J Neuropsychiatry 1990; 2:235–236.
20. Wise MG, Taylor SE. Anxiety and mood disorders in medically ill patients. J Clin Psychiatry 1990; 51:27–32.
21. Greenberg DB, Brown GL. Mania resulting from brain stem tumor. J Nerv Ment Dis 1985; 173:434–436.
22. Gross RA, Herridge P. A manic-like illness associated with right frontal arteriovenous malformation. J Clin Psychiatry 1988; 49:119–120.
23. Mark M, Modai I, Aizenberg D, Heilbronn Y, Elizur A. Bipolar disorder associated with an acoustic neurinoma. Hosp Commun Psychiatry 1991; 42:1258–1260.
24. Walbridge DG. Rapid-cycling disorder in association with cerebral sarcoidosis. Br J Psychiatry 1990; 157:611–613.
25. McLoughlin D, McKeon P. Bipolar disorder and cerebral sarcoidosis. Br J Psychiatry 1991; 158:410–413.
26. Bourgeois JA, Nisenbaum J, Drexler KG, Dobbins KM, Hall MJ. A case of subcortical grey matter heterotopia presenting as bipolar disorder. Compr Psychiatry 1992; 33:401–410.
27. Salazar-Calderon Perriggo VH, Oommen KJ, Sobonya RE. Silent solitary right parietal chondroma resulting in secondary mania. Clin Neuropathology 1993; 12:325–329.
28. Trautner RJ, Cummings JL, Read SL, Benson DF. Idiopathic basal ganglia calcification and organic mood disorder. Am J Psychiatry 1988; 145:350–353.
29. Kwentus JA, Hart RP. Normal pressure hydrocephalus presenting as mania. J Nerv Ment Dis 1987; 175:500–502.
30. Nanko S, Yokoyama H, Hoshino Y, Kumashiro H, Mikuni M. Organic mood syndrome in two siblings with Wolfram syndrome. Br J Psychiatry 1992; 161:282.
31. Khanna R, Borde M. Mania in a five-year-old child with tuberous sclerosis. Br J Psychiatry 1989; 155:117–119.
32. Fawcett RG. Cerebral infarct presenting as mania. J Clin Psychiatry 1991; 52:352–353.
33. Goodwin FK, Jamison JR. Manic-Depressive Illness. New York: Oxford University Press, 1990:504–507.
34. Dewan MJ, Haldipur CV, Lane EE, Ishpahani A, Boucher MF, Major LF. Bipolar affective disorder. I. Comprehensive quantitative computed tomography. Acta Psychiatr Scand 1988; 77:670–676.
35. Strakowski SM, Wilson DR, Tohen M, Woods BT, Douglass AW, Stoll AL. Structural brain abnormalities in first-episode mania. Biol Psychiatry 1993; 33:602–609.
36. Wehr TA, Sack DA, Duncan WC, Mendelson WB, Rosenthal NE, Gillin JC, Goodwin FK. Sleep and circadian rhythms in affective patients isolated from external time cues. Psychiatry Res 1985; 15:327–339.
37. Kripke DF, Mullaney DJ, Atkinson M, Wolf S. Circadian rhythm disorders in manic-depressives. Biol Psychiatry 1978; 13:335–351.

38. Coffman JA, Bornstein RA, Olson SC, Schwarzkopf SB, Nasrallah HA. Cognitive impairment and cerebral structure by MRI in bipolar disorder. Biol Psychiatry 1990; 27:1188–1196.
39. Rundell JR, Wise MG. Causes of organic mood disorder. J Neuropsychiatry 1989; 1:398–399.
40. Stoudemire A, Miller J, Schmitt F, Logue P, Shelton D, Latson G, Bennett P. Development of an organic affective syndrome during a hyperbaric diving experiment. Am J Psychiatry 1984; 141:1251–1254.
41. Thienhaus OJ, Khosla N. Meningeal cryptococcosis misdiagnosed as a manic episode. Am J Psychiatry 1984; 141:1459–1460.
42. Walter-Ryan WG, Fahs JJ. The problem with parsimony: mania and hyperthyroidism. J Clin Psychiatry 1987; 48:289–290.
43. McAllister TW. Neuropsychiatric sequelae of head injuries. Psychiatr Clin North Am 1992; 15:395–413.
44. Black DW, Winokur G, Bell S, Nasrallah A, Hulbert J. Complicated mania: comorbidity and immediate outcome in the treatment of mania. Arch Gen Psychiatry 1988; 45:232–236.
45. Black DW, Winokur G, Hulbert J, Nasrallah A. Predictors of immediate response in the treatment of mania: the importance of comorbidity. Biol Psychiatry 1988; 24:191–198.
46. Black DW, Hulbert J, Nasrallah A. The effect of somatic treatment and comorbidity on immediate outcome in manic patients. Compr Psychiatry 1989; 30:74–79.
47. Strakowski SM, Tohen M, Stoll AL, Faedda GL, Goodwin DC. Comorbidity in mania at first hospitalization. Am J Psychiatry 1992; 149:554–556.
48. Strakowski SM, Tohen M, Stoll AL, Faedda GL, Mayer PV, Kolbrener ML, Goodwin DC. Comorbidity in psychosis at first hospitalization. Am J Psychiatry 1993; 150:752–757.
49. Spitzer RL, Williams JB, Gibbon M, First MG. Structured Clinical Interview for DSM-III-R patient edition (SCID-P). New York, NY: New York State Psychiatric Institute, Biometrics Research Department, 1990.
50. Schiffer RB, Wineman NM, Weitkamp LR. Association between bipolar affective disorder and multiple sclerosis. Am J Psychiatry 1986; 143:94–95.
51. Joffe RT, Lippert GP, Gray TA, Sawa G, Horvath Z. Personal and family history of affective illness in patients with multiple sclerosis. J Affect Disord 1987; 12: 63–65.
52. Pine DS, Douglas CJ, Charles E, Davies M, Kahn D. Patients with multiple sclerosis presenting to psychiatric hospitals. J Clin Psychiatry 1995; 56:297–306.
53. Kerbeshian J, Burd L, Klug MG. Comorbid Tourette's disorder and bipolar disorder: an etiologic perspective. Am J Psychiatry 1995; 152:1646–1651.
54. Merikangas KR, Angst J, Isler H. Migraine and psychopathology: results of the Zurich cohort study of young adults. Arch Gen Psychiatry 1990; 47:849–853.
55. Younes RP, DeLong R, Neiman G, Rosner B. Manic-depressive illness in children: treatment with lithium carbonate. J Child Neurol 1986; 1:364–368.
56. Hudson JI, Pope HG. Affective spectrum disorder: does antidepressant response identify a family of disorders with a common pathophysiology? Am J Psychiatry 1990; 147:552–564.

57. Keck PE Jr, Merikangas KR, McElroy SL, Strakowski SM. Diagnostic and treatment implications of psychiatric comorbidity with migraine. Ann Clin Psychiatry 1994; 6:165–171.
58. Strakowski SM, Hudson JI, Keck PE Jr, Wilson DR, Frankenburg FR, Alpert JE, Teschke GC, Tohen M. Four cases of obstructive sleep apnea associated with treatment-resistant mania. J Clin Psychiatry 1991; 52:156–158.
59. Winokur G, Coryell W, Endicott J, Akiskal H. Further distinctions between manic-depressive illness (bipolar disorder) and primary depressive disorder (unipolar depression). Am J Psychiatry 1993; 150:1176–1181.
60. Ghadirian AM, Engelsmann F. Somatic illness in manic-depressive and schizophrenic patients. J Psychosom Res 1985; 29:281–286.
61. D'Ercole A, Skodol AE, Struening E, Curtis J, Millman J. Diagnosis of physical illness in psychiatric patients using Axis III and a standardized medical history. Hosp Commun Psychiatry 1991; 42:395–400.

9

Bipolar Disorder and Comorbid Axis I Disorders

CARLOS A. ZARATE, JR.
University of Massachusetts Medical School
Worcester, Massachusetts

MAURICIO TOHEN
Lilly Research Laboratories
Indianapolis, Indiana
and McLean Hospital, Harvard Medical School
Boston, Massachusetts

I. INTRODUCTION

Outcome studies of mania have been conducted ever since the diagnosis has been recognized. Kraepelin recognized the importance of outcome data by differentiating the major psychoses into three types—dementia praecox, manic-depressive illness, and paranoia (1). Dementia praecox was referred by him as an illness with a deteriorating course, in contrast to manic-depressive illness, which was episodic with full recovery between episodes, and described to have a good prognosis (1). Throughout the years, many other outcome studies have been conducted; however, the findings have been inconsistent. Possible explanations for these discrepancies include: nonsystematic sampling; loss of patients to follow-up; differences in diagnostic criteria utilized; how outcome measures were collected and analyzed; and not taking into account the number of previous affective episodes (2–7). Similarly, recent data suggest that psychiatric and medical comorbidity may affect the course and treatment response in mania. In contrast to psychiatry, studies of comorbidity in medicine have been conducted for many decades (8). However, recently, an increase interest in studying comorbidity in bipolar disorder has begun (9): (1) to attempt to differentiate primary and secondary psychiatric illnesses; (2) to identify of the effects of comorbidity on response to treatment and on outcome; and (3) to evaluate the effects of comorbidity on patterns of hospital reimbursement (10,11). With the exception of substance abuse/dependence, psychiatric comorbidity in mania has been little studied. This chapter will review Axis I comorbid psychiatric (other than substance use) disorders, which are reviewed in Chapter 7.

II. DEFINITION OF COMORBIDITY

The term "comorbidity" derives from general medicine and indicates the presence of two or more disorders that may co-occur simultaneously (intraepisodically), or over a lifetime (longitudinally) (12). Comorbidity in mania (complicated mania) has been defined previously by Black and colleagues as the presence of nonaffective DSM-III-R Axis I psychiatric diagnoses or serious or potentially life-threatening medical illness, but not well-controlled conditions such as chronic hypertension (13–15). Psychiatric comorbidity has also been defined as the presence of an antecedent or concurrent psychiatric syndrome in addition to the principal diagnosis (13–16).

III. PSYCHIATRIC COMORBIDITY AND BIPOLAR DISORDER

Comorbidity in population-based studies is highly prevalent. Recent data from the National Comorbidity Survey (NCS) (17) indicate that 19% of the population in the United States have a psychiatric disorder at some time in their lives, and 27% have a substance use disorder. The concept of comorbidity in mania was first introduced by Krauthammer and Klerman, who reported 21 cases of mania associated with medical or pharmacological conditions; as a result, they proposed the concept of secondary mania (18). Following this initial report, Cummings and Black et al. reported on manic syndromes occurring in the context of antecedent or coexistent psychiatric disorders (13–15,19). In the McLean First-Episode Mania Project (11,16), the comorbidity in 60 manic and mixed-state bipolar patients was 42%. In the same project, women were found to be 2.7 times more likely to have a comorbid diagnosis than men. The University of Cincinnati Mania First-Episode Project (20–22) reported a much higher rate of psychiatric comorbidity than the previous study—66% (47/71) of bipolar patients—finding no differences in rates of psychiatric comorbidity between first- and multiple-episode manic patients—71% ($n = 24$) versus 62% ($n = 23$), respectively (22).

IV. THE CO-OCCURRENCE OF MANIA AND AXIS I PSYCHIATRIC DISORDERS

After substance abuse/dependence, probably the most prevalent Axis I psychiatric disorders estimated in an epidemiological survey are panic disorder and obsessive-compulsive disorder (OCD). Other Axis I comorbid psychiatric disorders reported to be comorbid with mania are bulimia nervosa, impulse control disorder, and attention deficit hyperactivity disorder.

A. Panic Disorder

The co-occurrence of panic disorder in patients with major depression has been described for many years (23); however, the relationship between mania and panic disorder has been little researched. The base prevalence rate of panic disorder in mania in the Epidemiologic Catchment Area (ECA) Study was 1.6% (24). Further analysis of three ECA sites concluded that rates of panic disorder in bipolar disorder was much higher than population estimates (25). Other studies have reported higher rates of panic disorder in mania ranging from 7% to 16% (11,16,20,21; Table 1). In bipolar patients with the rapid-cycling form of the illness, rates of panic disorder have been reported to be as high as 40% (26). However, McElroy and colleagues did not find differences in the rates of panic disorder in patients with mixed compared to pure mania (21). In a reanalysis of the ECA survey database, the lifetime prevalence of panic disorder among subjects with bipolar disorder was 21% compared to 10% among subjects with unipolar depression and 0.8% among comparison subjects (27). The odds ratio for meeting criteria for panic disorder was 19.0 among subjects with bipolar disorder compared with comparison subjects and 10.8 among subjects with uni-

Table 1 Prevalence Rates of Axis I Disorders[a] in Patients with Bipolar Affective Disorders

Study	Manic subjects (*n*)	Anxiety disorder (%)[b]	OCD (%)	Bulimia (%)	ICD (%)	ADD (%)
Black et al. (13,14,16)	438	—	—	2	—	—
Strakowski et al. (11,16)	60	7	8	7	—	—
Strakowski et al. (11,16)	39	15[b]	13	15	23	—
McElroy et al. (21,22)	71	16[c]	10	9	13	—
Kruger et al. (32)	61	—	—	13	13	—
West et al. (42)	14	—	—	—	—	57

OCD = obsessive-compulsive disorder; ICD = impulse control disorder; ADD = attention deficit disorder.

[a]Does not include substance use disorders.

[b]Percent refers to rate of comorbidity in all patients with mania.

[c]Percent includes patients with anxiety disorders (panic disorder, agoraphobia, simple phobia, and social phobias) in general.

Source: Adapted from Ref. 9.

polar depression compared to comparison subjects (27). The converse relationship of the comorbidity of bipolar spectrum disorder in patients with panic disorder appears to be high. One study explored the spectrum of intraepisodic and longitudinal comorbidity of 140 DSM-III-R panic disorder patients, 67% of whom concomitantly met the criteria for agoraphobia and who were consecutively admitted to an ambulatory service over a 2-year period (28). The authors found that comorbidity with bipolar disorders included 2% with mania, 5% with hypomania, 6.4% with cyclothymia, for a total of 14%; an additional 34% of panic disorder patients ultimately met the criteria for hyperthymic temperament (28).

Before a diagnosis of panic disorder is made in patients with bipolar disorder, other diagnoses should be ruled out; these include mixed states of bipolar disorder, hyperthyroidism, hypoxia, attention deficit disorder, alcohol/drug intoxication or withdrawal syndromes, other anxiety disorders (e.g., obsessive-compulsive disorder, posttraumatic stress disorder, social phobia), and agitated bipolar depression.

B. Obsessive-Compulsive Disorder

Some authors suggest that patients with OCD and major depression may share a common pathophysiology because of the similarities of treatment response to antidepressants (29). However, estimates of the co-occurrence of OCD with mania have been little examined. Initial case reports and treatment trials suggested that OCD may co-occur in patients with bipolar disorder (30,31). Recently, prospective and controlled studies have reported rates of OCD in bipolar patients ranging from 8% to 13% (11,16,20–22; Table 1). Boyd and colleagues, in a reanalysis of three ECA sites, observed OCD to be much more prevalent in bipolar disorder than in the general population (25). The McLean First-Episode Mania Project reported similar rates of comorbid OCD in first-episode mania to patients with new-onset DSM-III-R schizophrenia (11,16). Some authors found that DSM-III-R bipolar mixed patients are more likely to be associated with OCD than pure mania, 21% versus 4% (21). However, they found no differences in rates of OCD between first-episode and multiple-episode manic patients (22). A more recent study of a sample of 149 inpatients with DSM-III major affective disorder who had received a clinical structured diagnostic interview found that the frequency of OCD syndrome was not significantly different between subjects with major depression (35%, $n = 105$) and bipolar disorder (35%, $n = 37$) (32). Some studies of antidepressant clinical trials in OCD have rates of switches into mania as high as 20%, thus suggesting that a possible relationship with bipolar disorder exists (33,34). Another study, involving patients with body dysmorphic disorder, which has been reported to be part of the

OCD spectrum, reported that up to 22% of patients also met criteria for bipolar disorder (35). Another syndrome that has been reported to be part of the OCD spectrum is Tourette's disorder. Kerbeshian et al., utilizing an epidemiological approach, found that 15 of 205 patients with Tourette's disorder had comorbid bipolar disorder, a rate that was more than four times higher than the level expected by chance (36).

Before OCD is diagnosed in patients with bipolar disorder, other differential diagnosis should be ruled out, including eating disorders, paraphilias, gambling, alcohol dependence or abuse, major depression (e.g., with obsessive brooding), movement disorders secondary to neuroleptics (e.g., tardive Tourette's), and Tourette's disorder.

C. Bulimia Nervosa

The co-occurrence of bulimia nervosa and depression has been well described (37); however, the association between bulimia nervosa and mania lacks systematic evaluation. Few studies have observed high rates of bipolar disorder in patients with bulimia nervosa and their relatives (38), suggesting an association between these disorders. The rates of comorbid bulimia in bipolar disorder have been reported to range between 2 and 15%, as reported in Refs. 11, 13, 14, 16, and 21; Table 1). Kruger et al. studied 61 patients meeting DSM-III-R criteria for bipolar disorder and found that eight subjects (13%) met DSM-IV criteria for binge-eating disorder and 15 (25%) met criteria for a partial binge-eating syndrome. The rates reported in this study were found to be much higher than the rates found in community samples (39). Another study reported that bulimia nervosa was found more frequently in patients with mixed rather than pure mania (21).

Studies on the converse relationship of the comorbidity of bipolar spectrum disorder in patients with bulimia have been more sparse (40). Nevertheless, an increased rate of bipolar disorder, especially bipolar II disorder, has been found in several epidemiological studies of patients with bulimia nervosa (40).

D. Impulse Control Disorders

High rates of comorbid impulse control disorders (pathological gambling, kleptomania, pyromania, and trichotillomania) have been reported to occur in patients with affective illness (41). In bipolar disorder, rates of comorbid impulse control disorder have been reported to range from 13 to 23% (11,16,21,32; Table 1). One study reports that comorbid impulse control disorder predates the onset of bipolar disorder in the majority of the cases (20). Another study found no differences in the rates of impulse control disorder between patients with the mixed and pure forms of bipolar disorder (21).

E. Attention Deficit Hyperactivity Disorder

Another Axis I psychiatric disorder that has been reported to be comorbid with bipolar disorder is attention hyperactivity disorder. A recent study suggests that attention deficit hyperactivity disorder is highly prevalent in bipolar patients. In this study, eight (57%) of 14 adolescent bipolar patients who were hospitalized for treatment of acute mania or hypomania also met criteria for attention deficit hyperactivity disorder (42). Another study examined the co-occurrence of comorbid disorders in hospitalized bipolar adolescents ($n = 10$) compared with unipolar depressed adolescents ($n = 33$), and with adolescents with nonaffective psychiatric disorders ($n = 11$). The authors found that attention deficit hyperactivity disorder, as well as conduct disorder, psychosis, and any DSM-III-R psychoactive substance use disorder, were all significantly more common in the bipolar group than in the unipolar depressed group. In addition, comorbid anxiety disorder was present in 40–45% of the subjects in the unipolar and bipolar groups, but in none of the control group subjects (43).

IV. BIPOLAR DISORDER AND MULTIPLE COMORBIDITY

The presence of any psychiatric diagnosis seems to increase the odds of having other psychiatric disorders (44). In the ECA study, 54% of subjects who were mentally ill had two or more conditions. Similarly, the University of Cincinnati Mania First-Episode Project (22) reported high rates of multiple comorbidity (defined as more than one Axis I diagnosis other than bipolar disorder) of 45%. In contrast, the McLean First-Episode Mania Project (11,16,45), reported a much lower rate of 22%.

V. DIAGNOSTIC DIFFICULTIES IN PATIENTS WITH BIPOLAR DISORDER AND COMORBID AXIS I CONDITIONS

There is much inherent difficulty in diagnosing bipolar affective disorder in the face of comorbid psychiatric conditions because substantial overlap exists between the symptoms of bipolar disorder and those of other psychiatric disorders (46). This is particularly true of bipolar disorder and stimulant abuse. For example, stimulant intoxication can produce a syndrome indistinguishable from mania or hypomania, and substantial depressive symptoms can emerge during stimulant withdrawal. In addition, the phenomenological overlap between bipolar disorder and attention deficit hyperactivity disorder is extensive, which often makes it difficult to distinguish between these two syndromes (46). Core symptoms of both conditions include impaired attention, distractibility, racing thoughts, and hyperactivity. In general, it is recommended to diagnose a comorbid psychiatric disorder only if it occurs before the onset of bipolar disorder or it occurs during periods when affective symptoms are not prominent.

VI. GENERAL INDICATIONS FOR MEDICATIONS IN COMORBID OCD AND PANIC

The pharmacological treatment of patients with OCD and panic disorder commonly includes the use of antidepressants such as the selective serotonin-reuptake inhibitors. In general, these agents should be used more cautiously in the management of OCD and panic disorder in patients with bipolar disorder than in patients without bipolar disorder because of complications that may occur. Complications of antidepressant therapy in bipolar disorder include switching into hypomania or mania and cycle acceleration (26,34). Similarly, anxiolytics commonly used in the management of panic disorder will need to be used cautiously in patients with bipolar disorder because of the high lifetime prevalence (60%) of comorbid substance abuse found to be associated with this diagnosis. Figures 1 and 2 provide a general outline on how to manage comorbid OCD and panic disorder in patients with bipolar disorder.

If patients are currently manic or present with mixed manic-depressive features, then it is recommended to treat the bipolar disorder first before treating the OCD (sequential treatment). On the other hand, if patients are currently in the depressed phase of their bipolar illness, than it is recommended to treat both the bipolar disorder and OCD concurrently (integrated treatment). Other potential problems of managing comorbid OCD and panic disorder in bipolar disorder patients include the increased risk for drug-drug interactions, side effects, and noncompliance (because of multiple medications).

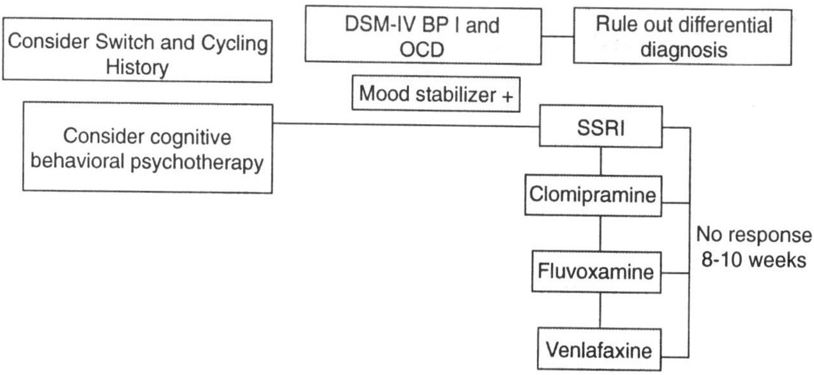

Figure 1 Pharmacotherapy of the co-occurrence of mania and OCD.

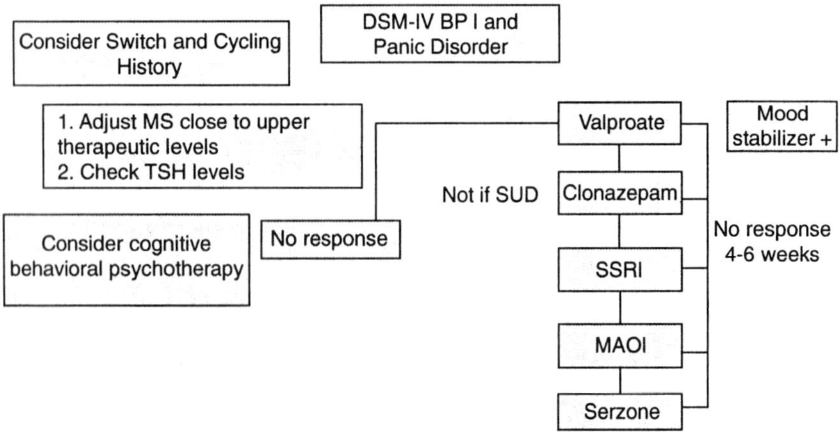

Figure 2 Pharmacotherapy of the co-occurrence of mania and panic disorder.

VII. CONCLUSION

To understand the association between bipolar disorder and comorbid disorders, it is important to know the temporal sequence of onset. To identify the onset sequence longitudinal studies must start at the onset of the illness. Risk factors must also be identified. Studies of psychiatric comorbidity in mania suggest that several disorders co-occur more frequently with bipolar disorder than is expected by base rate estimates. Future research will require prospective evaluation of bipolar patients and comparison groups that are followed longitudinally to determine how these co-occurring syndromes develop, interact over time, and affect outcome and response to treatment.

REFERENCES

1. Kraepelin E (1921): Manic-depressive Insanity and Paranoia. (translated R. M. Barclay). Edited by GM Robertson. Edinburgh: E & S Livingstone. Reprinted, New York: Arno Press, 1976.
2. Hastings DW. Follow-up results in psychiatric illness. Am J Psychiatry 1958; 114: 1057–1060.
3. Bratfos O, Haug JO. The course of manic-depressive psychosis. Acta Psychiatr Scand 1968; 44:89–112.
4. Shobe FO, Brion P. Long term prognosis in manic-depressive illness. Arch Gen Psychiatry 1971; 24:334–337.
5. Fleiss JL, Dunner DL, Stallone F, Fieve RR. The life table. A method for analyzing longitudinal studies. Arch Gen Psychiatry 1976; 33:107–112.

6. Keller MB, Lavori PW, Friedman B, Nielsen E, Endicott J, McDonald-Scott P, Andreasen NC. The longitudinal interval follow-up evaluation (LIFE): a comprehensive method for assessing outcome in prospective longitudinal studies. Arch Gen Psychiatry 1987; 44:540–548.
7. Zarate CA Jr, Tohen M. Outcome of mania in adults. In: Shulman K, Tohen M, Kutcher SP, eds. Mood Disorders Throughout the Life Span. New York: Wiley, 1996:281–297.
8. Feinstein A. The pre-therapeutic classification of comorbidity in chronic disease. J Chronic Diseases 1970; 23:455–468.
9. Strakowski SM, McElroy SL, Keck PW Jr, West SA. The co-occurrence of mania with medical and other psychiatric disorders. Int J Psychiatry Med 1994; 24:305–328.
10. Ridgely SM, Goldman HH, Willenbring M. Barriers to the care of persons with dual diagnoses: organizational and financing issues. Schizophr Bull 1990; 16:123–132.
11. Strakowski SM, Tohen M, Stoll AL, Faedda GL, Mayer ML, Kolbrener ML, Goodwin DC. Comorbidity in psychosis at first-hospitalization. Am J Psychiatry 1993; 150:752–757.
12. Maser JD, Cloninger CR, eds. Comorbidity of Mood and Anxiety Disorders. Washington, DC: American Psychiatric Press, 1990.
13. Black DW, Winokur G, Bell S, Nasrallah A, Hulbert J. Complicated mania: comorbidity and immediate outcome in the treatment of mania. Arch Gen Psychiatry 1988; 45:232–236.
14. Black DW, Winokur G, Hulbert J, Nasrallah A. Predictors of immediate response in the treatment of mania: the importance of comorbidity. Biol Psychiatry 1988; 24:191–198.
15. Black DW, Hulbert J, Nasrallah A. The effect of somatic treatment and comorbidity on immediate outcome in manic patients. Compr Psychiatry 1989; 30:74–79.
16. Strakowski SM, Tohen M, Stoll AL, Faedda GL, Goodwin DS. Comorbidity in mania at first-hospitalization. Am J Psychiatry 1992; 149:554–556.
17. Kessler RC, McGonagle KA, Zhao S, Nelson CB, Hughes M, Eshleman S, Wittchen HU, Kendler KS. Lifetime and 12-month prevalence of DSM-III-R psychiatric disorders in the United States: results from the National Comorbidity Survey. Arch Gen Psychiatry 1994; 51:8–19.
18. Krauthammer C, Klerman GL. Secondary mania: manic syndromes associated with antecedent physical illness or drugs. Arch Gen Psychiatry 1978; 35:1333–1339.
19. Cummings JL. Organic psychoses: delusional disorders and secondary mania. Psychiatr Clin North Am 1986; 9:293–311.
20. Strakowski SM, Keck PE Jr, McElroy SL, Lonczak HS, West SA. Chronology of comorbid and principal syndromes in first-episode psychosis. Compr Psychiatry 1995; 36:106–112.
21. McElroy SL, Strakowski SM, Keck PE Jr, Tugrul KL, West SA, Lonczak HS. Differences and similarities in mixed and pure mania. Compr Psychiatry 1995; 36:187–194.
22. Keck PE, McElroy SL, Strakowski SM, West SA, Hawkins JM, Huber TJ, New-

man RM, DePriest M. Outcome and comorbidity in first-compared with multiple-episode. 1995; 51:8–19.
23. DiNardo PA, Barlow DH. Syndrome and symptom co-occurrence in the anxiety disorders. In: Maser JD, Cloninger CR, eds. Comorbidity of Mood and Anxiety Disorders. Washington, DC: American Psychiatric Press, 1990:205–230.
24. Eaton WW, Dryman A, Weissman MM. Panic phobia. In: Robins LN, Regier DA, eds. Psychiatric Disorders in America: The Epidemiologic Catchment Area Study. New York: The Free Press, 1991:155–179.
25. Boyd JH, Burke JD, Gruenberg CE, Holzer CE III, Rae DS, George LK, Karno M, Stoltzman T, McEvoy L, Nestadt S. Exclusion criteria of DSM-III: a study of co-occurrence of hierarchy-free syndromes. Arch Gen Psychiatry 1984; 41:983–989.
26. Calabrese JR, Delucchi GA. Spectrum efficacy of valproate in 55 patients with rapid-cycling bipolar disorder. Am J Psychiatry 1990; 147:431–434.
27. Chen Y-W, Dilsaver SC. Comorbidity of panic disorder in bipolar illness: evidence from the Epidemiologic Catchment Area Survey. Am J Psychiatry 1995; 152:280–282.
28. Savino M, Perugi G, Simonini E, Soriani A, Cassano GB, Akiskal HS. Affective comorbidity in panic disorder: Is there a bipolar connection? J Affect Disord 1993; 28:155–163.
29. Hudson JI, Pope HG. Affective spectrum disorder: does antidepressant response identify a family of disorders with a common pathophysiology? Am J Psychiatry 1990; 147:552–564.
30. Baer L, Minichiello WE, Jenike MA. Behavioral treatment in two cases of obsessive-compulsive disorder with concomitant bipolar affective disorder. Am J Psychiatry 1985; 142:358–360.
31. Keck PE Jr, Lipinski JF, White K. An inverse relationship between mania and obsessive-compulsive disorder: a case report. J Clin Psychopharmacol 1986; 6:123–124.
32. Kruger S, Cooke RG, Hasey GM, Jorna T, Persad E. Comorbidity of obsessive compulsive disorder in bipolar disorder. J Affect Disord 1995; 34:117–120.
33. Insel TR, Murphy DL, Cohen RM, Alterman I, Kitts C, Linnoila M. Obsessive-compulsive disorder: a double-blind trial of clomipramine and clorgyline. Arch Gen Psychiatry 1983; 40:605–612.
34. Jefferson JW, Griest JH, Perse TL, Rosenfeld R. Fluvoxamine-associated mania/hypomania in patients with obsessive-compulsive disorder. J Clin Psychopharmacol 1991; 11:391.
35. McElroy SL, Phillips KA, Keck PE Jr, Hudson JI, Pope HG Jr. Body dysmorphic disorder: does it have a psychotic subtype? J Clin Psychiatry 1993; 54:389–395.
36. Kerbeshian J, Burd L, Klug MG. Comorbid tourette's disorder and bipolar disorder: an etiologic perspective. Am J Psychiatry 1995; 152:1646–1651.
37. Hudson JI, Pope HG Jr, Yurgelun-Todd D, Jonas JM, Frankenburg FR. A controlled study of lifetime prevalence of affective and other psychiatric disorders in bulimic outpatients. Am J Psychiatry 1987; 144:1283–1287.
38. Kassett JA, Gershon ME, Maxwell ME, Guroff JJ, Kazuba DM, Smith AL, Brandt HA, Jimerson DC. Psychiatric disorders in the first-degree relatives of probands with bulimia nervosa. Am J Psychiatry 1989; 146:1468–1471.

39. Kruger S, Shugar G, Cooke RG. Comorbidity of binge eating disorder and the partial binge eating syndrome with bipolar disorder. Int J Eating Disord 1996; 19: 45–52.
40. Mury M, Verdoux H, Bourgeois M. Comorbidite trouble bipolaire et trouble des conduites alimentaires. Aspects epidemiologigues et therapeutigues. Encephale 1995; 21:545–553.
41. McElroy SL, Hudson JI, Pope HG Jr, Aizley HG. The DSM-III-R impulse control disorders not elsewhere classified: clinical characteristics and relationship to other psychiatric disorders. Am J Psychiatry 1992; 149:318–327.
42. West SA, McElroy SL, Strakowski SM, Keck PE Jr, McConville J. Attention deficit hyperactivity disorder in adolescent mania. Am J Psychiatry 1995; 152:271–273.
43. Borchardt CM, Bernstein GA. Comorbid disorders in hospitalized bipolar adolescents compared with unipolar depressed adolescents. Child Psychiatry Hum Dev 1995; 26:11–18.
44. Regier DA, Farmer ME, Rae DS, Locke BZ, Keith SJ, Judd LL, Goodwin FK. Comorbidity of mental disorders with alcohol and other drug abuse: results from the Epidemiologic Catchment Area (ECA) Study. JAMA 1990; 264:2511–2518.
45. Tohen M, Zarate CA Jr, Zarate SB, Gebre-Medhin P, Pike S. The McLean/Harvard First-Episode Mania Project: pharmacologic treatment and outcome. Psychiatri Ann 1996; 26:S444–S448.
46. Blacker D, Tsuang MT. Contested boundaries of bipolar disorder and the limits of categorical diagnosis in psychiatry. Am J Psychiatry 1992; 149:1473–1483.

10

Bipolar Disorder and Comorbid Axis II Disorders

CARLOS A. ZARATE, JR.
University of Massachusetts Medical School
Worcester, Massachusetts

MAURICIO TOHEN
Lilly Research Laboratories
Indianapolis, Indiana
and McLean Hospital, Harvard Medical School
Boston, Massachusetts

I. INTRODUCTION

A number of studies have suggested that personality disorders are frequent in treatment settings and may complicate treatment and worsen the prognosis of Axis I conditions (1–3). Thus, it is important to estimate the influence of Axis II disorders on the outcome of bipolar disorder as major public health implications. This chapter will review comorbid Axis II personality disorders and bipolar disorder; it will not review the association between developmental disorders and bipolar disorder as the available information on this topic is scarce.

II. PERSONALITY DISORDERS IN THE GENERAL POPULATION

Previous research has suggested that the prevalence of personality disorders varies depending on the population under study and the methodology employed (4). The rates of personality disorder in the general population, with the possible exception of antisocial personality disorder, are relatively unknown. Estimates of prevalence rates range from 11% reported in a random sample of adults in Iowa City ($n = 235$) (5) based on self-completed Personality Diagnostic Questionnaire (6) to 18% (7) using the Structured Interview for DSM-III Personality

Disorders (8) in a sample ($n = 797$) of relatives of patients and controls (9). In a more recent study, a total of 810 adults from the population of eastern Baltimore were examined using a semistructured format that allowed DSM-III criteria (10). They found that the prevalence of personality disorders was 5.9% (11). The latter study suggests that personality disorders are relatively common in the community.

III. THE CO-OCCURRENCE OF MANIA AND AXIS II PSYCHIATRIC DISORDERS

Results from clinical and community studies indicate substantial comorbidity between personality disorders and Axis I conditions (5,7,12–14). Because of the dearth of information that exists on estimates of personality disorders in the general population, it is difficult to make any definite conclusions of whether or not personality disorders are more or less prevalent in bipolar disorder than in the general population.

Flick et al. studied the prevalence of personality disorders in 352 outpatients with anxiety and mood disorders. Subjects were diagnosed using the Structured Clinical Interview for DSM-III-R (15). They found that patients with bipolar disorder were more likely to have a diagnosis of a personality disorder than patients with major depression, panic disorder with agoraphobia, generalized anxiety disorder, and substance abuse (15). Mezzich et al. noted that only 3% of 205 bipolar disorder patients met criteria for a personality disorder, but there was no indication of the patients' clinical condition at the time of the personality assessment (16). Charney et al. (17) studied 30 bipolar disorder patients during the depressed phase and noted that seven (23%) met criteria for a personality disorder. Both Gaviria et al. (18) and Baxter et al. (19) examined the relationship between personality disorder and bipolar disorder and reported a rate of 11% of 88 and 4% of 26 patients, respectively. Boyd et al. (20) found that 4% of 46 patients with bipolar disorder had an antisocial personality. In a retrospective review, Black et al. (21) found that 55 (13%) of 438 individuals had a comorbid personality disorder along with their bipolar disorder. Of these, 13 had a diagnosis of antisocial personality disorder. One study using the Structured Interview for DSM-III Personality (SIDP) (22) found that 62% of 26 inpatients with bipolar disorder were assessed to have one or more personality disorders. Histrionic, borderline, passive-aggressive, and antisocial personality disorders were the most frequently diagnosed (23). Similarly, Turley et al. (24) examined the personality disorders of recent-onset DSM-III-R bipolar disorder patients using the revised Millon Clinical Multiaxial Inventory (MCMI-II) (25). They found, however, that after the bipolar symptoms had settled, 81% of 21 patients received at least one MCMI-II personality disorder diagnosis. In the same study, narcissistic and antisocial personality disorders were the most prevalent disorders in their sample, followed by histrionic and passive-aggressive disorders (24). The results of Pica et al. (23) contrast with Millon's MCMI-II validity data (25), which presented a personality disorder profile for 49 patients with DSM-III-R bipolar disorder in which histrionic and passive-aggressive personality patterns were the most prominent, followed by self-defeating and dependent patterns (16). Another study, by O'Connell et al. (26), demonstrated, in a systematic way, the relationship between bipolar disorder and personality disorders. In their study of 50 bipolar disorder patients with euthymic mood, O'Connell et al. used the Personality Disorders Questionnaire (27), a self-report inventory, and found that 58% of 29 patients met criteria for one or more personality disorders, with borderline (30%) and histrionic (20%) personality disorders the most prevalent. Recently, Peselow et al. (28) studied 66 outpatients who had a DSM-III-R bipolar disorder. All patients underwent the Structured Interview for DSM-III Personality Disorders during their hypomanic and euthymic phases of illness. In this study, 57% of the cohort met criteria for at least one personality disorder during the hypomanic phase, and 55% met criteria for at least one personality disorder after successful treatment.

Studies on the converse relationship of the comorbidity of bipolar disorder in patients with personality disorder have been more sparse. In an epidemiological study of 810 adults drawn from the community, Samuels and colleagues (11) found that bipolar disorder was more common in subjects with any personality disorder than subjects without a personality disorder (odds ratio = 3.5) [6 of 95 (6.3%) vs. 12 of 667 (1.8%); $p = 0.02$].

Comparisons of rates of personality disorders found to be comorbid in bipolar disorder are limited by a number of factors including differences in the population under study; differences in diagnostic criteria used; and how outcome measures were collected and analyzed.

Some authors have suggested that borderline personality represents an atypical but primary disturbance of affect (29,30); others suggest that borderline personality may be best viewed as occurring on a spectrum of bipolar disorders (31). Yet others view borderline personality as a distinct illness from affective or other personality disorders (32) in phenomenology (33) and response to treatment (34).

In summary, studies of the prevalence of specific personality in manic patients have found high rates of primarily DSM-III-R cluster B (antisocial, borderline, narcissistic, and histrionic) personality disorders (Table 1). The most consistently reported personality disorder to be comorbid with mania has been antisocial personality disorder followed by borderline, narcissistic, and histrionic personality disorders (13,21,23,26,35). The rates of cluster A (paranoid, schizoid, schizotypal) and cluster C personality disorders (avoidant, dependent, obsessive-compulsive, and passive-aggressive) have been reported inconsistently, ranging from 0 to 19% of bipolar patients (8,13,21,23,26,35,36; Table 1).

Table 1 Prevalence Rates of Personality Disorders in Patients with Bipolar Affective Disorders

Study	Manic subjects (*n*)	Any type of personality disorder (%)	Antisocial (%)	Borderline (%)	Narcissistic (%)	Histrionic (%)
Charney et al. (17)	30	23	—	—	—	—
Gaviria et al. (18)	88	11	—	12	—	—
Baxter et al. (19)	26	4	—	4	—	—
Boyd et al. (20)	46	4	—	—	—	—
Black et al. (21)	438	13	3	0	—	0
Koenigsberg et al. (13)	171	9	0	1	0	0
Wolf et al. (35)	31	23	23	—	—	—
Pica et al. (23)	26	62	15	12	4	27
O'Connell et al. (26)	50	58	16	30	14	20
Mezzich et al. (16)	205	3	—	—	—	—
Peselow et al. (28)	66	57	—	—	—	—

IV. DIAGNOSTIC DIFFICULTIES IN PATIENTS WITH BIPOLAR DISORDER AND COMORBID AXIS II CONDITIONS

One of the problems that affects the investigation of borderline personality disorder is that many patients have symptoms of multiple diagnoses. For example, there is a significant overlap in criteria among bipolar II, borderline personality disorder, and hysteroid dysphoria (37,38). Frequently, patients with long-standing recurrent behavioral disturbances, unstable interpersonal relationships, and periodic affective symptoms are often misdiagnosed as having a cluster B personality disorder when in fact they may have bipolar disorder. A major hazard that may occur with this approach is that the patient may be regarded as less deserving of medical care (39) or that psychopharmacological treatments may be withheld as patients with personality disorders are believed not to respond as well to pharmacotherapy as patients with affective disorders (40). Akiskal and Akiskal (41) suggest that there are several variants of bipolar disorder. They described a cyclothymic, hyperthymic, and irritable temperament in individuals who had cyclothymic mood disorders. Cyclothymic temperament has traits that are often confused with those of borderline personality disorder, and hyperthymic temperament has traits often confused with those of narcissistic or compulsive personality.

V. GENERAL INDICATIONS FOR MEDICATIONS IN COMORBID AXIS II PERSONALITY DISORDERS

The pharmacotherapy of the personality-disordered patient has been reviewed in detail elsewhere (42). The majority of treatment trials involve patients with borderline personality disorder. Few studies have been conducted in other Axis II disorders. To date, no medication has clearly and consistently emerged as efficacious for any Axis II disorder. In general, it is recommended that drug therapy be syndrome oriented (i.e., impulsive syndrome, depressive syndrome, etc.), regardless of the specific personality disorder. For example, antipsychotics may be used for transient psychosis or paranoia; antidepressants (e.g., selective serotonin-reuptake inhibitors, monoamine oxidase inhibitors) for concurrent panic attacks, phobias, compulsive symptoms as well as depressive syndromes; and mood stabilizers for cyclothymic or impulsive presentations.

VI. CONCLUSION

Future research will need to evaluate the relationship between personality disorders and affective disorders to examine its influence on the course of illness and response to treatment.

REFERENCES

1. Tyrer P, Casey P, Gall J. Relationship between neurosis and personality disorder. Br J Psychiatry 1983; 142:404–408.
2. Pfohl B, Stangl D, Zimmerman M. The implications of DSM-III personality disorders for patients with major depression. J Affect Disord 1984; 7:309–318.
3. Shea MT, Glass DR, Pilkonis PA, Watkins J, Docherty JP. Frequency and implications of personality disorders in a sample of depressed outpatients. J Personal Disord 1987; 1:27–42.
4. Widiger TA, Rogers JH. Prevalence and comorbidity of personality disorders. Psychiatric Ann 1989; 19:132–136.
5. Reich J, Yates W, Nduaguba M. Prevalence of DSM-III personality disorders in the community. Soc Psychiatry Psychiatr Epidemiol 1989; 24:12–16.
6. Hyler SE, Rieder RO, Williams JBW, Spitzer RL, Hendler J, Lyons M. Personality Diagnostic Questionnaire (PDQ). New York: New York State Psychiatric Institute, 1983.
7. Zimmerman M, Coryell W. DSM-III personality disorder diagnoses in a nonpatient sample: demographic correlates and comorbidity. Arch Gen Psychiatry 1989; 682–689.
8. Stangl D, Pfohl B, Zimmerman M, Bowers W, Corenthal C. A structured interview for the DSM-III personality disorders: a preliminary report. Arch Gen Psychiatry 1985; 42:591–596.
9. Maier W, Lichtermann D, Klinger T, Heun R, Hallmayer J. Prevalences of personality disorders (DSM-III-R) in the community. J Personal Disord 1992; 6:187–196.
10. Spitzer RI, Williams JBW. Structured Clinical Interview for DSM-III-R Personality Disorders (SCID-II). New York: New York State Psychiatric Institute, Biometrics Research, 1986.
11. Samuels JF, Nestadt G, Romanoski AJ, Folstein MF, McHugh PR. DSM-III personality disorders in the community. Am J Psychiatry 1994; 151:1055–1062.

12. Alnæs R, Torgersen S. The relationship between DSM-III symptom disorders (Axis I) and personality disorders (Axis II) in an outpatient population. Acta Psychiatr Scand 1988; 78:485–492.
13. Koenigsberg HW, Kaplan RD, Gilmore M, Cooper AM. The relationship between syndrome and personality disorder in DSM-III: experience with 2,463 patients. Am J Psychiatry 1985; 142:207–212.
14. Regier DA, Farmer ME, Rae DS, Locke BZ, Keith SJ, Judd LL, Goodwin FK. Comorbidity of mental disorders with alcohol and other drug abuse: results from the Epidemiologic Catchment Area Study. JAMA 1990; 264:2511–2518.
15. Flick SN, Roy-Byrne PP, Cowley DS, Shores MM, Dunner DL. DSM-III-R personality disorders in a mood and anxiety disorders clinic: prevalence, comorbidity, and clinical correlates. J Affect Disord 1993; 27:71–79.
16. Mezzich JE, Ahn CW, Fabrega H, Pilkonis PA. Patterns of psychiatric comorbidity in a large population presenting for care. In: Maser JD, Cloninger CR, eds. Comorbidity of Mood and Anxiety Disorders. Washington, DC: American Psychiatric Press, 1990.
17. Charney DS, Nelson JC, Quinlan DM. Personality traits and disorder in depression. Am J Psychiatry 1981; 138:1601–1604.
18. Gaviria M, Flaherty JH, Val E. A comparison of bipolar patients with and without borderline personality disorder. Psychiatr J Univ Ottawa 1982; 7:190–195.
19. Baxter LR, Phelps ME, Mazziotta JC, Schwartz JM, Gerner RH, Selin CE, Sumida RM. Cerebral metabolic rates for glucose in mood disorders: studies with positron emission tomography and fluorydeoxyglucose F 18. Arch Gen Psychiatry 1985; 42: 441–447.
20. Boyd JH, Burke JD, Gruenberg E, Holzer CE, Rae DS, George LK, Karno M, Stoltzman R, McEvoy L, Nestadt G. Exclusion criteria of DSM,-III: a study of co-occurrence of hierarchy free symptoms. Arch Gen Psychiatry 1984; 41:983–989.
21. Black DW, Winokur G, Bell S, Nasrallah A, Hulbert J. Complicated mania: comorbidity and immediate outcome in the treatment of mania. Arch Gen Psychiatry 1988; 45:232–236.
22. Pfhol B, Stangl D, Zimmerman M. Structured Interview for DSM-III Personality, 2nd ed. Iowa City: University of Iowa, Department of Psychiatry, 1983.
23. Pica S, Edwards J, Jackson HJ, Bell RC, Bates GW, Rudd RP. Personality disorders in recent-onset bipolar disorder. Compr Psychiatry 1990; 31:499–510.
24. Turley B, Bates GW, Edwards J, Jackson HJ. MCMI-II personality disorders in recent-onset bipolar disorders. J Clin Psychol 1992; 48:320–329.
25. Millon T. Manual for the MCMI-II. Minneapolis, MN: NCS, 1987.
26. O'Connell RA, Mayo JA, Sciutto MS. PDQ-R personality disorders in bipolar patients. J Affect Disord 1991; 23:217–221.
27. Hyler SE, Rieder RO. Personality Diagnostic Questionnaire—Revised (PDQ-R). New York: New York State Psychiatric Institute, 1987.
28. Peselow ED, Sanfilipo MP, Fieve RR. Relationship between hypomania and personality disorders before and after successful treatment. Am J Psychiatry 1995; 152:232–238.
29. Liebowitz MR, Klein DF. Interrelationship of hysteroid dysphoria and borderline personality disorder. Psychiatr Clin North Am 1981; 4:67–87.

30. Liebowitz MR. A medication approach. J Personal Disord 1987; 1:325–327.
31. Akiskal HS, Akiskal K. Cyclothymic, hyperthymic, and depressive temperaments as subaffective variants of mood disorder. In: Tasman A, Riba MB, eds. Review of Psychiatry. Washington, DC: American Psychiatric Press, 1992:43–62.
32. Barash A, Frances A, Hurt S, Clarkin J, Cohen S. Stability and distinctiveness of borderline personality disorder. Am J Psychiatry 1985; 142:1484–1486.
33. Gunderson JC, Phillips KA. A current view of the interface between borderline personality disorder and depression. Am J Psychiatry 1991; 148:967–975.
34. Soloff PH, George A, Nathan S, Schultz PM, Ulrich RF, Perel JM. Progress in pharmacotherapy of borderline personality disorders. Arch Gen Psychiatry 1986; 43:691–697.
35. Wolf AW, Schubert DSP, Patterson MB, Grande TP, Brocco KJ, Pendleton L. Associations among major psychiatric diagnoses. J Consult Clin Psychol 1988; 56: 292–294.
36. Hyler SE, Reider RO, Williams JBW. The personality diagnostic questionnaire: developments and personality results. J Personal Disord 1988; 2:229–237.
37. Akiskal HS, Khani MK, Scott-Strauss A. Cyclothymic temperamental disorders. Psychiatr Clin North Am 1979; 2:527–554.
38. Akiskal HS. Characterologic manifestations of affective disorders. Integr Psychiatry 1984; (May–June):83–88.
39. Lewis L, Appleby L. Personality disorder: the patients psychiatrists dislike. Br J Psychiatry 1988; 153:44–49.
40. Tyrer SP, Brittlebank AD. Misdiagnosis of bipolar affective disorder as personality disorder. Can J Psychiatry 1993; 38:587–589.
41. Akiskal HS, Akiskal K. Cyclothymic, hyperthymic, and depressive temperaments. In: Frances AJ, Hales RE, eds. Psychiatry Update: American Psychiatric Association Annual Review, vol 5. Washington, DC: American Psychiatric Press, 1986.
42. Triebwasser J, Sederer L. Borderline and antisocial personality disorders. In: Sederer L, Rothschild AJ, eds. Acute Care Psychiatry. Baltimore, MD: Williamson Wilkins, 1997.

11

Comorbidity and Bipolar Disorder in Old Age

KENNETH ISRAEL SHULMAN and ANU SINGH
Sunnybrook Health Science Center
University of Toronto
Toronto, Ontario, Canada

I. INTRODUCTION

The demographic pressures of a growing elderly population will necessitate a greater understanding of psychiatric illness in order to provide high-quality care in addition to effective and efficient utilization of limited health care resources. Advantages of studying an elderly cohort include the opportunity to describe the lifelong course of affective illness retrospectively. Familial patterns of inheritance may be elucidated given the prolonged exposure in first-degree relatives. Finally, there has been relatively little study of mania in geriatric patients with physical illness. It is precisely the high rate of medical illness in the elderly that invites the examination of comorbidity and its significance.

The relevance of comorbidity to clinical practice became widely apparent following the results of two large population studies in the United States. Respondents with comorbidity in the Epidemiologic Catchment Area (ECA) Study (1) displayed a higher utilization of services. Both the ECA (2) and the National Comorbidity Survey (NCS) (3) revealed similar high rates of comorbid lifetime disorders. As roughly one-sixth of the NCS respondents accounted for the majority of lifetime disorders and an even greater percentage of 12-month disorders, it appears that comorbidity is generally associated with a more serious course of illness. This applies a fortiori to an elderly population as funding for health services becomes tied to indicators of severity and outcome.

Limitations to the investigation of comorbid conditions and bipolar disorder arise from the conventional definition of comorbidity itself as conditions that are etiologically distinct may co-occur in a single patient (4). In the area of psychiatry, distinguishing disorders on the basis of known etiology becomes difficult, and the emphasis is often on phenomenology for diagnosis. Krauthammer and Klerman (5), in a review of 21 cases, introduced the term "secondary mania," suggesting that the manic syndrome is in fact a heterogeneous one of multiple etiologies. Black et al. (6), in a retrospective chart review, chose to move away from the term "secondary mania," preferring "complicated mania" to define manic syndromes occurring in the context of antecedent or coexistent nonaffective psychiatric disorders or concurrent serious medical disorders. They did not attempt to separate the cases felt to be secondary to a coexisting condition as this would imply causality.

Longitudinal studies of comorbidity and bipolar disorder become paramount to further our understanding of the possible relationships that may exist between mania and other medical and psychiatric disorders. When associations are observed, such studies could determine whether bipolar disorder and comorbid conditions represent risk factors for each other, similar manifestations of different etiological mechanisms, or variable presentations of a shared underlying pathophysiology. The availability of structural and functional brain imaging of manic patients may help clarify the neuropathophysiological basis of bipolar disorder and how it relates to commonly co-occurring conditions. A clearer understanding of these relationships will ultimately lead to further development of successful treatments, improved outcome, and, hopefully, prevention.

In this chapter we review the limited data available regarding comorbidity and bipolar disorder in old age. We also review relevant data from mixed-age studies of secondary mania where inferences may be drawn for an elderly population (7,8).

II. NEUROLOGICAL DISORDERS

Shulman and Post (9) first reported an association of heterogeneous cerebral organic disorders with mania in old age. This was confirmed in a subsequent retrospective cohort study that compared an elderly group of inpatients suffering from mania with an age- and sex-matched group of depressives (10). A preponderance of neurological disorders was found in the manic group (36% vs. 8% of depressives). Table 1 describes the features of the 18 patients and the nature of the neurological disorders. As seen from Table 1, one-third of the patients had clear evidence of cerebrovascular disease while almost one-quarter had alcohol-related disorders. Because of the retrospective nature of the study, it was difficult to establish an exact temporal relationship between the first episode of mania and the onset of the neurological disorder. However, in almost all cases,

Table 1 Demographic and Clinical Data for 18 Elderly Patients with Mania and Neurological Disorders at Index Hospitalization

Patient	Sex	Family history of affective disorder	Age at onset of affective disordcr (years)	Age at first manic episode (years)	Neurological disorder
1	M	Negative	82	82	Chronic alcoholism, peripheral neuropathy
2	F	Positive	20	20	Frontal lobotomy, bilateral encephalomalacia
3	F	Negative	50	50	Chronic alcoholism, dementia
4	F	Negative	67	67	Chronic alcoholism, seizures/delirium
5	M	Negative	69	70	Chronic alcoholism, blackouts/delirium
6	M	Negative	68	68	Cerebral contusions
7	F	Positive	41	46	Parkinson's disease
8	F	Negative	39	43	Right cerebral infarct
9	F	Negative	83	83	Multiple cerebral infarcts
10	F	Negative	43	58	Encephalopathy/neuroleptic malignant syndrome
11	M	Negative	58	58	Closed head injury
12	M	Negative	80	80	Recurrent cerebral contusions (boxing), lacunar infarct
13	F	Positive	71	71	Left cerebral hemorrhage 20 years before onset of affective disorder
14	F	Positive	39	39	Cerebral infarct
15	M	Positive	84	85	Dementia
16	M	Negative	76	76	Embolic cerebral infarct, mild dementia
17	F	Negative	19	19	Right capsular necrosis, cerebral vasculitis (rheumatoid)
18	F	Positive	68	68	Parkinson's disease

mania was the first affective episode or occurred in very close temporal proximity to the first depression. This compares to a mean latency of approximately 15 years between first depression and first mania for other elderly bipolars (9,10). This close temporal relationship certainly suggests a significant association.

A subgroup of elderly patients with first-episode mania were more likely to present with neurological abnormalities than were multiple-episode patients (71% vs 28%) (11). Table 2 describes the demographic characteristics, mortality, and comorbidity in 14 elderly patients with very-late-onset mania. The medical comorbidity also resulted in significant rates of subsequent hospitalization and death. During a follow-up period of 3–10 years, nine of the 14 patients required medical hospitalization and four were institutionalized in nursing homes. The presence of a neurological disorder was associated with death in five (83%) of the six patients who died during follow-up. Tohen et al. (11) noted that the clinical profile of very-late-onset mania was generally associated with neurological comorbidity and a high risk of death secondary to cerebrovascular disease. Authors of one other report of de novo mania in old age (12) were unable to demonstrate any obvious organic causes for their six first-episode cases. However, they were limited to computerized tomography in brain imaging.

Table 2 Demographic Characteristics, Mortality, and Comorbidity in 14 Elderly Patients with Late Onset of First-Episode Mania

Patient	Age (years)	Sex	Cause of death during follow-up	Neurological disorder
1	67	F		Seizures/delirium
2	68	F		
3	83	F		Multiple cerebral infarcts
4	71	F		Left cerebral hemorrhage
5	71	F	Septicemia	
6	77	F		
7	69	F		Infarct
8	80	F		Cerebral infarct
9	68	M	Cerebrovascular disease	Cerebral infarct
10	82	M	Cardiovascular disease	Gait disturbance, neuropathy
11	76	M	Cerebrovascular disease	Cerebral infarct
12	74	M	Pneumonia	Cerebral infarcts
13	80	M	Cerebrovascular disease	Recurrent cerebral contusions (boxing), Parkinson's disease
14	78	M		

A. Cerebrovascular Lesions

A number of case series and case-control studies involving cerebrovascular lesions in mania have been reported by Robinson et al. (13) and Starkstein et al. (14–17). A mixture of cortical as well as subcortical lesions was found mainly in the basal region of the right temporal lobe and the orbitofrontal regions of the cortex. Based on these data, right-hemisphere strokes predominated and in turn produced changes in central neurotransmitters (diaschisis) (13). The relationship of these lesions to the development of mania appears to be a function of their basotemporal connections to the limbic system, which modulates emotions.

The same group (18) further subdivided the manic group into "bipolar" (those with depression and mania) and "manic-only." Differences in lesion size and location were found. The bipolar group sustained right-sided subcortical lesions near the head of the caudate and thalamus associated with significant cognitive impairment, while the manic-only group had larger cortical lesions in the orbitofrontal and right basal temporal areas.

A series of case reports has also accumulated over the past decade also implicating right-sided cerebrovascular lesions. Jampala and Abrams (19) first described a preponderance of right cerebral infarctions associated with mania. Cummings and Mendez (20) and Kulisevsky et al. (21) both report cases of mania associated with cerebral infarcts in the right thalamic and subthalamic regions. In the case of Kulisevsky et al. (21) mania was accompanied by hemiballismus. Fawcett (22) described a case of mania in a 61-year-old man with a right frontal infarct. However, in this case, no neurological signs were found other than the manifestation of a manic syndrome.

Cerebrovascular complications of cardiac surgery have been reported in three cases of secondary mania. In the first of these case reports, Henriksen (23) found "diffuse brain damage" following cardiac surgery that resulted in decreased cerebral blood flow. More recently, Wilson and McLaughlin (24) reported a case of secondary mania after a mitral valvuloplasty, and Isles and Orrell (25) described a similar clinical presentation after open heart surgery. In the latter case, the 54-year-old male patient had sustained a right-sided cerebrovascular accident prior to the surgery but mania did not become manifest until the postoperative period.

B. Dementia and Mania

Originally, Spicer et al. (26) tried to explain the increase in incidence of mania late in life by suggesting that this was a manifestation of a dementing process. A number of subsequent studies failed to support an association between mania and the development of a dementing illness late in life (9,10,27,28). However, a number of studies have demonstrated significant cognitive impairment in a group of elderly manic patients (28,29). Broadhead and Jacoby (28) completed the Kendrick cognitive battery and found that 32% of the entire elderly manic group scored within the demented range on two subtests. Similarly, Stone (27), in a retrospective study, found that 14 of 92 patients who underwent cognitive testing showed persistent specific short-term memory loss. However, only three of the 14 patients with memory impairment went on to a clinical dementia in a 3-year follow-up.

Young and Klerman (30) reviewed mania in old age with a focus on age of onset; despite a trend for late-onset cases to show more cognitive impairment, they did not confirm a statistically significant difference between early- and late-onset elderly manic patients. Berrios and Bakshi (29) found significantly more cognitive impairment in a group of elderly manics compared to depressives. Manic patients also had higher Hachinski scores reflecting cerebrovascular disease. One can only conclude that the high prevalence of cognitive impairment in an elderly manic population without the development of a progressive dementia reflects the wide variety of pathologies found in reports of secondary mania but with a particular emphasis on cerebrovascular disease (29).

C. Other Neurological Conditions

Head trauma has been reported as comorbid with mania in patients with and without previous mood disorders (31–34). Jorge et al. (35) studied a series of 66 patients with closed head injury during the first year after the trauma. They found that 9% of their patients met criteria for mania during the follow-up period, but it was the presence of a temporal basal polar lesion that appeared to be the most significant variable associated with secondary mania even when the effect of other lesion locations was taken into account. This appears to be a higher frequency than that seen following stroke.

Some tumors have been associated with mania including “brain stem tumors” (36); an acoustic neurinoma (37); and a craniopharyngioma with extension into the third ventricle close to limbic structures (38).

Other isolated and anecdotal medical conditions in a mixed-age population are summarized by Strakowski et al. (8). They include a wide variety of medical and neurological conditions comorbid with mania including: central nervous system tumors, normal-pressure hydrocephalus, neurosyphilis, hyperthyroidism, and hemodialysis. Single cases of such exotic conditions as Lyme borreliosis, polycythemia, tuberous sclerosis, and Wolfram syndrome have been associated with mania. The unusual nature of these conditions no doubt increased their likelihood of publication.

Rundell and Wise (39) found 13 cases of “organic” manic syndrome out of 755 consultations and noted a preponderance of corticosteroid use in half of these patients (54%) and HIV-related complications in about one-quarter of this group (23%). Khouzam et al. (40) reported three new cases of secondary mania in elderly patients aged 64–85. The medical conditions associated with these three case reports included neurosyphilis, progression of melanoma, steroid treatment, sleep deprivation, and tricyclic treatment.

Manic syndromes occurred in 8% of AIDS patients attending an outpatient clinic (41). Those without risk factors for mood disorder such as family or prior history developed mania later in the course of HIV infection more often associated with comorbid dementia. With growing numbers of AIDS patients one can expect an increasing incidence of mania comorbid with an HIV-infected population.

Other anecdotal reports include a variety of endocrine conditions. B_{12} deficiency produces mania and a gait disturbance (42), and thyrotoxicosis (43) and hydrocortisone replacement for Addison's disease (44) have resulted in mania. Despite the clear limitations of anecdotal case reports and case series, a trend emerges for a wide variety of lesions and medical conditions to affect the brain structure associated with emotions, namely the basal ganglia, thalamus, and limbic aspects of the frontal and temporal lobes.

III. NEUROIMAGING

Following up the work of Robinson et al. (13), Fujikawa et al. (45) have examined the relationship of cerebrovascular disease and mania. Their methodology included the use of magnetic resonance imaging (MRI) to determine the incidence and location of silent cerebral infarctions (SCIs) in late- compared to early-onset mania. They also attempted to compare the incidence of SCIs in elderly manic patients compared to age- and sex-matched depressives. The definition of SCI was a high-intensity lesion greater than 5 mm in diameter and the minimum criterion for an SCI was the finding of four small cerebral infarcts or one large cerebral infarct. The results revealed that late-onset mania had a higher chance of being associated with a silent cerebral infarction (65% vs. 55% in late-onset depressives). This is consistent with the findings of Shulman et al. (10) where clinical data showed that the rate of neurological disorder (especially cerebrovascular disease) was higher than for age- and sex-matched elderly depressives.

Earlier another group showed that there was an age-related increase in the incidence of silent cerebral infarctions (46). From an incidence of 6% in the 40s to 50s, the incidence rose to greater than 20% in manic patients over the age of 60. Those patients with silent cerebral infarctions tend to have a relatively low family history of mood disorder consistent with the original speculations of Krauthammer and Klerman (5) when they first defined the notion of secondary mania. The same group of patients with SCIs also had a higher proportion of risk factors for cerebrovascular disease such as hypertension.

Recent work by Migliorelli et al. (47) utilized single-photon emission computerized tomography (SPECT) in a small, but controlled, study of primary mania. Manic patients were noted to have a general decrease in cerebral blood flow particularly in the basal portion of the right temporal lobe. Further, Migliorelli et al. (47) found a left/right asymmetry with a significant decrease in cerebral blood flow to the right basal temporal cortex, and like Robinson et al. (13), they suggest that lesions in the caudate and thalamus with connections to the frontal lobes are associated with secondary mania. In support of the work by Fujikawa et al. (45), they hypothesize that cerebral infarctions are more common in mania than in depression and play an etiological role in the manifestation of late-onset mania.

The occurrence of subcortical hyperintensities (SCHs) in elderly subjects with mania has been reported (48). These authors hypothesize that "signal hyperintensity" as found on the MRI is secondary to a focal loss of a brain tissue. The clinical significance of these hyperintensities is still under question but it is suggested that this could be due to normal aging but also a wide variety of cerebral pathologies. McDonald et al. (48) found a general increase in SCH in an elderly group of manic patients with a mean age at index of 68 years. These hyperintensities were not found in the periventricular region. Work with younger bipolar patients shows an interesting trend toward an increase in white matter hyperintensities in bipolar compared to depressive patients (49). Those individuals who revealed hyperintensities on MRI also had a significantly higher mean age than bipolar patients without hyperintensities. In this group of younger patients, the hyperintensities were largely located in the interior half of the frontal lobe and common risk factors associated with hyperintensities were hypertension, cardiovascular disease, and diabetes mellitus.

The neuroimaging data support a general finding of increased cerebrovascular pathology in patients suffering from mania. While a considerable amount of the data on neuroimaging in mania comes from mixed age groups, it is not unreasonable to extrapolate this finding to an elderly bipolar population where the comorbidity of clinical neurological diseases has already been demonstrated (10,11).

IV. COMORBIDITY AND OUTCOME

Limited data relating comorbidity to outcome have been reported in the literature. In a mixed age population, Black et al. (6) reported a case-control study of 438 manic patients meeting Research Diagnostic Criteria for either mania ($n = 396$) or schizoaffective disorder-manic type ($n = 42$) hospitalized at the University of Iowa Psychiatric Hospital during the 12-year period from 1970 to 1981 as identified by a chart review. Fifty-seven patients were considered to have a complicated form of mania as their index episode was preceded or accompanied by a nonaffective DSM-III psychiatric disorder or a serious or potentially life-threatening medical illness but not a well-controlled condition. Of the complicated manics, 18 had coexisting medical conditions, and 39 had at least one additional nonaffective psychiatric diagnosis. The mean age of the uncomplicated manic group was 38.5 years compared with a mean age of 50.8 years for the medically complicated group, and 33.8 years for the psychiatrically complicated group. The main comorbid diagnoses consisted of alcohol abuse/dependence, mixed substance abuse, antisocial personality, and medical disorders. Of the complicated group, 71.9% had only one additional medical or psychiatric disorder, 26.3% had two, and 1.8% had three.

The medical cluster of complicated manics were older, had an older age at onset, had more prior psychiatric hospitalizations, had more organic features, had no suicide attempts, had poor recovery rates, and high death rates. The psychiatric cluster were more likely to be male, divorced or separated, have fewer prior psychiatric hospitalizations, an early age at onset, prior suicide attempts, and poor recovery rates. There was no significant difference between the two clusters with respect to their poor recovery rates. Of the uncomplicated manics, 64.9% received adequate treatment compared to only 33.4% of the complicated manics. Of the manic patients receiving adequate treatment, the uncomplicated group had significantly higher recovery rates than the complicated group (74.3% vs. 42.1%). Significantly more uncomplicated than complicated manics (68.4% vs. 4.6%) had recovered at the time of discharge from hospital. Overall, only comorbidity was associated with poor outcome and this association was significant for women but not for men.

In a separate report, Black et al. (50) reported predictors of immediate response to the treatment of mania focusing on the issue of comorbidity. Overall, 80% of their manic patients had a good immediate outcome compared to 20% with poor outcome. Comorbidity as an independent variable revealed that those manic patients with a significant comorbid medical condition had a good outcome in less than 10% of cases while more than a quarter of those patients were reported to have a poor outcome. The three variables that predicted good outcome at discharge based on regression analysis were the absence of comorbidity, a duration of lithium treatment greater than 2 weeks, and an episode lasting less than a month.

Shulman et al. (10) considered a number of variables that influenced outcome in their group of elderly manic patients. Neurological disorders were significantly associated with subsequent psychiatric hospitalizations but surprisingly did not influence mortality rates. Overall the manic group had a significantly higher mortality rate compared to age- and sex-matched depressives. At the end of the 6-year follow-up period (range 3–10 years), half of the manic group were dead compared to only one-fifth of the depressives. Figure 1 illustrates the survival analysis comparing the two groups. While the overall prevalence of neurological disorders was significantly higher in the manic group, it may be that

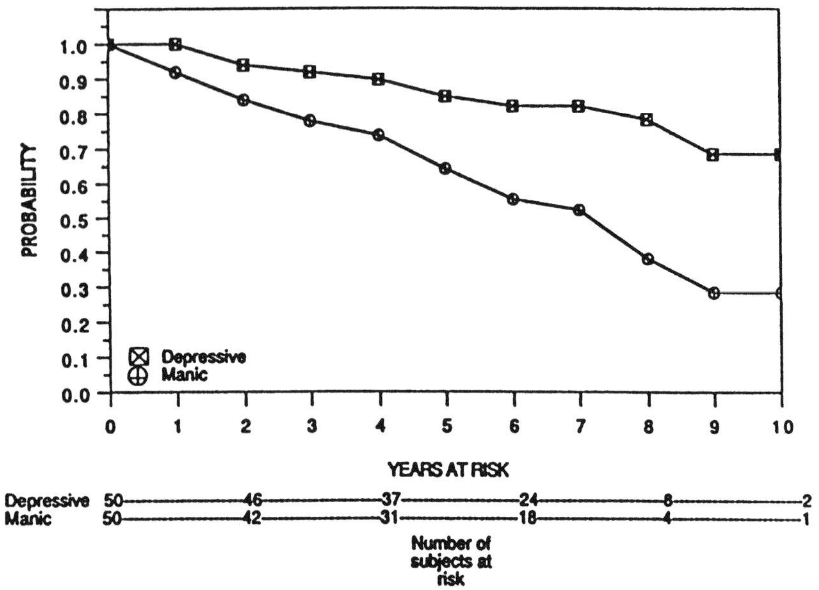

Figure 1 Cumulative probability of death for 50 elderly patients with mania and 50 elderly patients with unipolar depression at index hospital admission.

there was insufficient statistical power to show a difference when neurological disorders were isolated in terms of mortality rates.

V. SUMMARY

Comorbidity of medical and neurological disorders with bipolar disorder in old age offers unique opportunities to understand the underlying pathogenesis of the manic syndrome. The evidence accrued from systematic retrospective studies, cross-sectional analyses, case series, and numerous anecdotal case reports suggests a predominant role for cerebrovascular pathology. Other central nervous system disturbances such as head trauma, alcoholism, and a variety of pharmacological and endocrine challenges can produce the same final common pathway of a manic syndrome. Furthermore, a pattern emerges of heterogeneous right-sided lesions affecting the basal-temporal region with connections to the frontal and limbic system.

While helping to elucidate a possible pathogenesis for primary mania, comorbidity associated with mania in old age also carries a worse outcome. It appears to produce more cognitive impairment, higher rates of relapse, and higher mortality rates. Clinically, these findings are important in evaluating prognosis and emphasize the need to look carefully for neurological diseases when mania presents in late life especially as a first episode. Ultimately, the coarse neurological findings and heterogeneous medical comorbidity associated with mania in old age must be translated into neurotransmitter changes that can further define the underlying pathogenesis. Indeed, the elderly offer an important perspective that may shed light on bipolar disorders in all age groups.

REFERENCES

1. Heizer JE, Pryzbeck TK. The co-occurrence of alcoholism with other psychiatric disorders in the general population and its impact on treatment. J Stud Alcohol 1988; 49:219–224.
2. Regier DA, Narrow WE, Rae DS, Manderscheid RW, Locke BZ, Goodwin FK. The de facto US mental and addictive disorders service system. Epidemiologic Catchment Area prospective 1-year prevalence rates of disorders and services. Arch Gen Psychiatry 1993; 50:85–94.
3. Kessler RC, McGonagle KA, Zhao S, Nelson CB, Hughes M, Eshleman S, Wittchin H-U, Kendler KS. Lifetime and 12-month prevalence of DSM-III-R psychiatric disorders in the United States: results from the National Comorbidity Survey. Arch Gen Psychiatry 1994; 51:8–19.
4. Feinstein A. The pre-therapeutic classification of comorbidity in chronic disease. J Chronic Dis 1970; 23:455–468.
5. Krauthammer C, Klerman GL. Secondary mania: manic syndromes associated with antecedent physical illness or drugs. Arch Gen Psychiatry 1978; 30:74–79.
6. Black DW, Winokur G, Bells S, Nasrallah A, Hulbert J. Complicated mania: comorbidity and immediate outcome in the treatment of mania. Arch Gen Psychiatry 1988; 45:232–236.
7. Verdoux H, Bourgeois M. Manies secondaries a des pathologies organiques cerebrales. Anns Med-Psychol 1995; 153:161–168.
8. Strakowski SM, McElroy S, Keck P, West S. The co-occurrence of mania with medical and other psychiatric disorders. Int J Psychiatry Med 1994; 24:305–328.
9. Shulman K, Post F. Bipolar affective disorder in old age. Br J Psychiatry 1980; 136:26–32.
10. Shulman KI, Tohen M, Satlin A, Mallya G, Kalunian D. Mania compared with unipolar depression in old age. Am J Psychiatry 1992; 149:341–345.
11. Tohen M, Shulman KI, Satlin A. First-episode mania in late life. Am J Psychiatry 1994; 151(1):130–132.
12. Charron M, Fortin L, Paquette I. De novo mania among elderly people. Acta Psychiatr Scand 1991; 84:503–507.
13. Robinson RG, Starkstein SE, Price TR. Poststroke depression and lesion location. Stroke 1988; 19:125.
14. Starkstein SE, Pearlson GD, Boston J, Robinson RG. Mania after brain injury. A controlled study of causative factors. Ann Neurol 1987; 44:1067–1073.
15. Starkstein SE, Boston JD, Robinson RG. Mechanism of mania after brain injury:

Twelve case reports and review of the literature. J Nerv Ment Dis 1988; 176:87–100.
16. Starkstein SE, Robinson RG, Honig MA, Parikh RM, Joselyn J, Price TR. Mood changes after right-hemisphere lesions. Br J Psychiatry 1989; 155:79–85.
17. Starkstein SE, Mayberg HS, Berthier ML, Fedoroff P, Price TR, Robinson RG. Mania after brain injury: neuroradiological and metabolic findings. Ann Neurology 1990; 27:652–659.
18. Starkstein SE, Fedoroff P, Berthier ML, Robinson RG. Manic-depressive and pure manic states after brain lesions. Biol Psychiatry 1991; 29:149–158.
19. Jampala VS, Abrams R. Mania secondary to left and right hemisphere damage. Am J Psychiatry 1983; 140:1197–1199.
20. Cummings JL, Mendez MF. Secondary mania with focal cerebrovascular lesions. Am J Psychiatry 1984; 141:1084.
21. Kulisevsky J, Berthier ML, Pujol J. Hemiballismus and secondary mania following a right thalamic infarction. Neurology 1993; 43:1422–1424.
22. Fawcett RG. Cerebral infarct presenting as mania. J Clin Psychiatry 1991; 52(8): 352–353.
23. Henriksen L. Evidence suggestive of diffuse brain damage following cardiac operations. Lancet 1984; i:816–820.
24. Wilson D, McLaughlin T. Cerebrovascular disease and secondary mania. Gen Hosp Psychiatry 1990; 12:271–275.
25. Isles LJ, Orrell MW. Secondary mania after open-heart surgery. Br J Psychiatry 1991; 159:280–282.
26. Spicer CC, Hare EH, Slater E. Neurotic and psychotic forms of depressive illness: evidence from age-incidence in a national sample. Br J Psychiatry 1973; 123:535–541.
27. Stone K. Mania in the elderly. Br J Psychiatry 1989; 155:220–224.
28. Broadhead J, Jacoby R. Mania in old age: a first prospective study. Int J Geriatr Psychiatry 1990; 5:215–222.
29. Berrios GE, Bakshi N. Manic and depressive symptoms in the elderly: their relationships to treatment outcome, cognition and motor symptoms. Psychopharmacology 1991; 24:31–38.
30. Young RC, Klerman GL. Mania in late life: focus on age at onset. Am J Psychiatry 1992; 149:867–876.
31. Shukla S, Cook BL, Cook S, Mukherjee C, Goodwin C, Miller MG. Mania following head trauma. Am J Psychiatry 1987; 144:93–96.
32. Clark AF, Davison K. Mania following head injury. A report of two cases and a review of the literature. Br J Psychiatry 1987; 150:841–844.
33. Miller LS, Garde IB, Moses JA, Zipursky RB, Kravitz K, Faustman WO. Head injury and mood disturbance. J Clin Psychiatry 1992; 53:171–172.
34. Burnstein A. Bipolar and pure mania disorders precipitated by head trauma. Psychosomatics 1993; 34:194–195.
35. Jorge RE, Robinson RG, Starkstein SE, Arndt SV, Forrester AW, Geisler FH. Secondary mania following traumatic brain injury. Am J Psychiatry 1993; 150(6):916–921.

36. Greenberg DB, Brown GL. Mania resulting from brain stem tumor. J Nerv Ment Dis 1985; 173:434–436.
37. Mark M, Modai I, Aisenberg D, Heilbronn Y, Elizur A. Bipolar disorder associated with an acoustic neurinoma. Hosp Commun Psychiatry 1991; 42:1258–1260.
38. Sweet R. Case of craniopharyngioma in late life. J Neuropsychiatry 1990; 2:464–465.
39. Rundell JR, Wise MG. Causes of organic mood disorder. J Neuropsychiatry 1989; 1:398–399.
40. Khouzam HR, Emery PE, Reaves B. Secondary mania in late life. J Am Geriatr Soc 1994; 42:85–87.
41. Lyketsos CG, Hanson AL, Fishman M, Rosenblatt A, McHugh PR, Treisman GJ. Manic syndrome early and late in the course of HIV. Am J Psychiatry 1993; 150(2):326–327.
42. Jacobs LA, Bloom HG, Behrman FZ. Mania and a gait disorder due to cobalamin deficiency. J Am Geriatr Soc 1990; 38:473–474.
43. Lee S, Chow CC, Wing YK, Leung CM, Chiu H, Chen C. Mania secondary to thyrotoxicosis. Br J Psychiatry 1991; 159:712–713.
44. Ur E, Turner TH, Goodwin TJ, Grossman A, Besser GM. Mania in association with hydrocortisone replacement for Addison's disease. Postgrad Med 1992; 68: 41–43.
45. Fujikawa T, Yamawaki S, Touhouda Y. Incidence of silent cerebral infarction in patients with major depression. Stroke 1995; 24:1631–1634.
46. Kobayashi S, Okada K, Yamashita K. Incidence of silent lacunar lesions in normal adults and its relation to cerebral blood flow and risk factors. Stroke 1991; 22: 1379–1383.
47. Migliorelli R, Starkstein SE, Teson A, de Quiros G, Vazquez S, Leiguardia RG. SPECT findings in patients with primary mania. J Neuropsychiatry 1993; 5(3): 379–383.
48. McDonald WM, Krishnan KRR, Doraiswamy PM, Blazer DG. Occurrence of subcortical hyperintensities in elderly subjects with mania. Psychiatry Res Neuroimag 1991; 40:211–220.
49. Aylward EH, Roberts-Twillie JV, Barta PE, et al. Basal ganglia volumes and white matter hyperintensities in patients with bipolar disorder. Am J Psychiatry 1994; 151(5):687–693.
50. Black DW, Winokur G, Hulbert J, Nasrallah A. Predictors of immediate response in the treatment of mania: the importance of comorbidity. Biol Psychiatry 1988; 24:191–198.

12

Developmental Aspects of Comorbidity in Mania

GABRIELLE A. CARLSON
State University of New York at Stony Brook
Stony Brook, New York

I. CRITERIA SHIFTS AND IMPLICATIONS FOR DIAGNOSIS OF MANIA IN CHILDREN AND ADOLESCENTS

Until recently, manic-depressive psychosis/illness has been considered rare in childhood. Kraepelin noted, "In rare cases (4 out of 903—0.4%), the first beginnings can be traced back even before the 10th year" (1). These were not cases he saw as children, and it is unclear from his brief quote whether or not they were episodes of mania or depression since he did not make the distinction. However, years later, Lish et al. (2) reported that of the 15% of bipolar members of the National Depressive Manic Depressive Association who responded, 84 (17%) "first exhibited signs of the illness" prior to age 10, 42% between the ages of 10 and 19. Signs of illness were most commonly either depression/hopelessness (33%) or mania/hyperactivity (32%). Two studies of clinical samples (3,4) reported that 16% of consecutive medication clinic referrals and 10 prebubertal children hospitalized over a 17-month period, respectively, met DSM-III-R criteria for mania.

Children meeting current criteria for mania, then, do not seem to be all that rare. The reasons for our "recognizing" these cases have to do with criteria changes, reformulations of comorbidity, and attitude shifts. This chapter, therefore, will first describe the evolution and criteria changes relevant to the diagnosis and differential diagnosis of bipolar disorder, and then examine the impact of comorbidity on phenomenological and outcome data on bipolar disorder from children, adolescents, and adults.

In the beginning, Kraepelin (1) observed:

> we distinguish first of all manic states with the essential morbid symptoms of flight of ideas, exalted mood, and pressure of activity, and melancholia or depressive states with sad or anxious moodiness and also sluggishness of thought and action. . . . But besides them we observe also clinical "mixed forms" in which the phenomena of mania and melancholia are combined with each other, . . . composed of the same morbid symptoms as these, but cannot without coercion be classified either with the one or with the other.

Kraepelin, of course, was concerned mainly with distinguishing episodic, nondeteriorating psychosis from dementia praecox. He did not concern himself with the differential diagnosis of other disorders that we now recognize in children, nor with operationalizing criteria. Thus, duration of "attacks" and level of impairment, intrinsic to our "counting" an episode of mania or hypomania, were not defined.

The last 20 years of refining our nosology to increase diagnostic reliability has had direct and indirect impact on what we define as bipolar. Direct impact has been through changes in mood disorder criteria; indirect impact has been via changes in the criteria of disorders that have traditionally been part of the differential diagnosis of mania.

While symptom wording has changed little, the definition of an "episode" has varied. In DSM-III (5), a manic episode had to last a week (unless it resulted in hospitalization). In DSM-III-R (6), this was changed to a "distinct period" with a nonspecified duration. In DSM-IV (7), the week's duration was reimposed because it was felt that the nonspecified duration had broadened the definition too far (8). Goodwin and Jamison (9) note that cycle length may vary from less than 48 hr to many years. They do not, however, address how or whether to distinguish a "cycle" from mood lability.

> Related to ultrarapid cycling is the phenomenon of mood instability, in which moods shift sharply within the same day or even hour. Although this phenomenon is a common feature of stage III mania [the peak of a severe manic episode], *it can also be encountered outside of the context of typical bipolar illness* [italics mine]. This form of rapid mood lability is probably heterogeneous diagnostically. Some patients meet criteria for borderline disorder, others for complex partial seizure, and still others for cyclothymia (p. 81).

There are, then, several diagnostic areas in which mood lability is a part, e.g., milder mood states (cyclothymia and hypomania). They, too, have also evolved considerably. In DSM-III, the criteria for hypomania defined a more euphoric (inappropriate laughing, punning, or joking; extreme gregariousness;

overoptimism) and productive (sharpened thinking, increased productivity) state than current criteria. In DSM-IV, furthermore, duration (4 days) of symptoms *observable by others as a distinct change* is demanded. These criteria are likely to be more stringent than prior iterations. On the other hand, cyclothymia no longer consists of hypomanic *episodes* and depressive symptoms, but rather hypomanic symptoms (perhaps only elevated or irritable mood) and depressive symptoms (perhaps only sad mood) without other symptoms or duration of symptoms (except for an overall duration of 1 year) specified.

Goodwin and Jamison (9) also point out that organic personality syndrome, as delineated in DSM-III-R, may account for severe mood lability. This "persistent personality disturbance" was characterized by (1) affective instability, e.g., marked shifts from normal mood to depression, irritability, or anxiety; (2) recurrent outbursts of aggression or rage that are grossly out of proportion to any precipitating psychosocial stressors; (3) marked impairment of social judgment, e.g., sexual indiscretions; (4) marked apathy and indifference; (5) suspiciousness or paranoid ideation; (6) evidence from history, physical examination, or laboratory tests of organic factors judged to be etiologically related; (7) *diagnosis not given to a child or adolescent if the clinical picture is limited to the features that characterize attention deficit hyperactivity disorder* (ADHD). No study of child/adolescent mood disorder has used this diagnosis, in part because the assessment methods in studies of mood disorders used structured interviews that did not comprehensively evaluate "organic factors." In DSM-IV, "organic personality" is mood disorder due to the "general medical condition," and characterized by either depressed mood or elated or irritable mood. It is likely that a broad range of "general medical conditions" operate in some children, from the known and obvious (e.g., fetal alcohol syndrome), to the less well understood or not yet diagnosed. Children with developmental disabilities may well fall within this rubric. As in secondary mania in adults (10), treatment may be more difficult. Unfortunately, the unreliability and variable diagnostic significance of "organic" has made this area difficult to document and study.

Changes in ADHD criteria have had an indirect impact on delineating childhood mania. In redesigning the ADHD criteria, input from DSM-IV field trials (11) was solicited. Two "classic" ADHD criteria were almost dropped because they were not felt to be discriminating from other externalizing disorders of childhood. These were: "is often distracted by extraneous stimuli, and often talks excessively." A third, "often engages in physically dangerous activities without considering possible consequences," which describes impulsivity, was eliminated. However, clinicians will recognize it as one of the most frequently complained about symptoms in children with ADHD, endorsed by parents for 77% of children with ADHD (12), and probably one of the most dangerous (13). If the only place to "count" its significance is as a criterion for mania ("excessive involvement in pleasurable activities that have a high potential for dangerous consequences"), one can see how easy it might be to confuse a child with ADHD (hyperactive, hyperverbal, distractible, impulsive) with a manic child. Add to that the fact that oppositional defiant and/or conduct disorder (ODD/CD), which takes precedence when they co-occur, accompanies ADHD, at least 30–68% of the time (12), and deciding when one is dealing with severe, co-morbid ADHD, versus mania, versus both is likely to be difficult (14,15). Conduct disorder items of cruelty to people and animals, stealing, fire setting, and property destruction are not where the confusion is likely to occur. It is the symptoms of ODD, "often loses temper, often argues with adults, often deliberately annoys, often angry, often easily annoyed," that are virtually indistinguishable from the irritability and annoying intrusiveness of mania. Unfortunately, rates of oppositional defiant disorder are often not examined or separately identified in mood disorder studies.

Finally, the relationship of mood symptoms to psychosis has undergone substantial change in the evolution of our nosology. The most significant change for young people has been recognizing that mood incongruent psychotic symptoms may occur in mood disorders as well as schizophrenia (see Ref. 14 for review) and in the comparable conceptual shift of paranoid schizophrenia (16,17). In DSM-II (18), paranoid schizophrenia was characterized by

> the presence of persecutory or grandiose delusions often associated with hallucinations. Excessive religiosity is sometimes seen. The patient's attitude is frequently hostile and aggressive, and his behavior tends to be consistent with his delusions. In general, the disorder does not manifest the gross personality disorganization of the hebephrenic and catatonic types (p. 34).

With DSM-III (5), paranoid schizophrenia became the type "dominated" by persecutory, grandiose, or jealousy delusions, and/or hallucinations (p. 191). Subsequent DSMs restricted paranoid schizophrenia to "preoccupation with one or more systematized delusions or with frequent auditory hallucinations related to a single theme" and basically without negative symptoms. Grandiose, paranoid, and religious delusions/hallucinations and irritable aggression were considered mania criteria. This evolution likely explains observations of Werry et al. (19), who used DSM-III criteria to reexamine and follow up adolescents hospitalized between 1971 and 1988. Only 57% of adolescent bipolars and 63% of schizophrenics were diagnosed accurately at first hospitalization because the concepts and rules had changed.

II. EPIDEMIOLOGY OF MANIA AND MANIC SYMPTOMS

Like depression, the frequency of mania depends on whether it is defined as a symptom, syndrome, or disorder. Two community studies illustrate that point. Carlson and Kashani (20) interviewed 150 14–16-year-olds randomly selected from a Midwest high school, using the Diagnostic Interview for Children and Adolescents (DICA) (21) and DSM-III (5) criteria. They found that 4% of teenagers endorsed the screening symptom on the DICA: "Have you ever gone through a period during which you became unusually excited?" Ten percent said they had periods during which their moods went up and down quickly; 4% met symptom *and* duration criteria (i.e., hypomania) but only 0.6% had these symptoms *for a week's duration with impairment* with symptoms confirmed by a parent. Lewinsohn et al. (22) interviewed 1709 adolescents aged 14–18 using the Schedule for Affective Disorders for School-Age Children (23) *with the adolescent only* (i.e., there was no other informant to verify the presence of manic symptoms. In this study 5.7% of subjects reported a single symptom of mania, "a distinct period of elevated, expansive or irritable mood" ("core positive symptom"); less than 1% met DSM-III-R (6) criteria for bipolar disorder. Of these, two-thirds were hypomanic and depressed.

Lewinsohn's findings are similar to those reported in the Epidemiological Catchment Area Study (24). Overall rates for 1 weeks's duration of euphoria or irritability during one's lifetime was 4.5% in 18–29-year-olds. Lifetime prevalence of bipolar I disorder in 18–29-year-olds was 1.1%, and for bipolar II, 0.7%. For the general population, the lifetime prevalence varied from 0.6 to 1.6% (see Table 1). Prevalence of subsyndromal disorders like cyclothymia varies much more widely given the differences in definition and has been cited as low as 0.4% in a community sample of adults to as high as 6% in college students (25). While rates of bipolar disorder depend on how and from whom the symptoms are elicited and how strictly it is defined, it appears that about 1 out of 20 teenagers/young adults report significant euphoria/irritability.

What is the significance of such manic symptoms? Interestingly, in both the Carlson and Kashani (20) and the Lewinsohn (22) studies, young people with manic symptoms had higher rates of other psychopathology and were functioning significantly more poorly than the sample without manic symptoms. In the Carlson and Kashani study (20), of the 20 adolescents who had several manic symptoms, 60% met criteria for lifetime major depression, 50% met DSM-III criteria for at least one anxiety disorder, 50% met criteria for oppositional disorder, and 40% met criteria for conduct disorder. Lewinsohn et al. (22) found similar disorders in their "core positive" group: 48.5% had major depression, 32% had at least one anxiety disorder, 18.6% had a disruptive behavior disorder, and 23.7% had a substance use disorder. Lower behavior disorder rates may be because the DSM-III-R criteria used in Lewinsohn's study are more stringent, and parents were not interviewed to determine the presence of externalizing disorders. In addition, the subjects in the Carlson and Kashani study had more manic symptoms than just euphoria/irritability. In either case, whether "irritable, elated, or expansive mood" is a symptom unique to mania, a symptom that identifies bipolar spectrum disorders (26), or a symptom that selects serious

Table 1 Epidemiology of Bipolar Disorder

Study	Bipolar I	Bipolar II	Males	Females
ECA—total lifetime prevalence (48)	0.8	0.5	0.7 + 0.4	0.9 + 0.5
Age 18–29	1.1	0.7		
Age 30–44	1.4	0.6		
Age 45–64	0.3	0.2		
Age 65+	0.1	0.1		
ECA—1 month (77)	0.4		0.3	0.4
Age 18–24	0.6		0.4	0.8
Age 25–44	0.6		0.5	0.6
Age 45–64	0.2		0.2	0.2
Age 65+	0.0		0.0	0.0
New Haven (lifetime) (78)	0.8	0.8		
Amish—lifetime (79)	0.46			
National Comorbidity Study—lifetime (80)			1.6	1.7
Puerto Rico—lifetime (81)			0.7	0.4
Edmonton, Alberta (Canada) (41)—lifetime	0.6		0.7	0.4
Age 18–24	0.4		0.5	0.3
Age 25–34	1.0		0.5	0.4
Age 35–44	0.7		0.3	0.6
Age 45–54	0.5		0.1	0.0
Age 55–64	0.2		0.3	0.2
Age 65+	—		0.0	0.0
Columbia, Missouri (14–16-year-olds)—lifetime (20)	0.6			
Oregon Adolescent Depression Project (ages 14–18)—lifetime (22)	0.94–0.99			

psychopathology in general, it is not trivial and bespeaks substantial comorbidity and impairment.

III. SYMPTOM PICTURE AND THE RELATIONSHIP BETWEEN PSYCHOPATHOLOGY AND AGE

The bipolar spectrum may encompass hyperthymia, a temperament that may or may not be related to bipolar disorder (27), cyclothymia, bipolar II disorder (i.e., clinical depression with hypomania), classic mania and depression, and possibly schizoaffective mania (14). Mania has been dichotomized by the prominence of euphoria versus irritability. Irritable, dysphoric, or "mixed" mania (i.e., simultaneous symptoms of depression and mania with irritability rather than euphoria as the mood component) is more severe (i.e., there is more affect dysregulation, poorer outcome, and more comorbidity), and it appears to be more treatment refractory (28). However, as noted below, there is significant overlap between dysphoric mania and comorbid mania. Thus, the presence or absence of comorbidity is another way of classifying mania (29–31).

A. Comorbidity/Mixed Episodes

Both frequency and type of comorbidity seem to vary with age. Carlson (32) first noted that one of the differences between very-early-onset bipolar disorder (under age 9) and peripubertal-onset bipolar disorder was a high rate of preexisting other psychopathology in the younger group. Recently, Kovacs and Pollock (33) found that 26 of 134 prospectively followed, depressed 9–13-year-olds developed an episode of mania or hypomania. Only 11.5% were without preexisting other serious psychiatric disorders, however. All of the sample of Wozniak et al. (34) described earlier were comorbid. Both inpatient (4) and research (35) samples were highly comorbid but rates of "pure" disorder were not specifically described. In a community sample of patients first hospitalized with psychosis, Carlson et al. (36) found that only 14.3% of patients between ages 15 and 20 had "pure" mania. Rates of specific co-occurring disorders from these studies are reported in Table 2. Rates of externalizing disorders are particularly high.

Whereas oppositional defiant/conduct disorder and anxiety disorders complicate mania in youths, in adults, the major complications came from alcohol and/or substance abuse. In the NIMH Collaborative Study, 79% of bipolar patients had alcoholism preceding their mood disorder; 29% had drug abuse first. Lower rates of both occurred after the bipolar disorder (37). In a sample of patients hospitalized with a first episode of psychosis, half (51.7%) of the 60 manic patients had another disorder (31). Of these, 18.3% had medical disorders, the

Table 2 Lifetime Comorbidity in Youth-Onset Mania/Hypomania (%)

	Kovacs and Pollack, 1995 teen	Wozniak et al., 1995 child	Fristad et al., 1995 child	Geller et al., 1995 child	Geller et al., 1995 teen	Carlson et al., 1995 ages 15–20
"n"	26	43	10	9	17	17
ADHD		98	30	88.9	29.4	
ODD		88		?	?	50
CD	54	37	80	22.2 "severe"	17.6 "severe"	
spec. ed.	?			?	?	35.7
anxiety	?	56		?66.6	?35	
depression	100	86		22.2	47.1	50
no comorb.	11.5	0	?10	0	?	14.3

remainder were psychiatric, most alcohol (26.7%) and drug (16.7%) abuse or dependence disorders. Although, in this sample, rates of anxiety disorders were less than 10%, other groups have found higher rates of anxiety disorders in manic patients (38,39).

Comorbidity is obvious in nonclinical samples as well. The comorbidity with substance abuse was 60.7% in the Epidemiologic Catchment Area (ECA) Study (40). A similar study in Edmonton, Canada, reported lifetime rates of alcohol abuse of 45%, substance abuse 34.3%, antisocial personality 18%, and phobias 54% (41).

To explore the relationship between age, adolescent behavior problems, and mania in a nonreferred sample, I used data from the Wave 1 ECA tapes (unweighted) to examine rates of conduct disorder symptoms elicited by the Diagnostic Interview Schedule (42) for persons with bipolar I (BPI) disorder. Table 3 presents impressively higher rates of conduct problems before age 15 in the 18–29-year-olds compared to the older patients with BPI disorders. While not as high as rates seen in people diagnosed with antisocial personality (for whom conduct disorder symptoms before age 15 are a requirement) (43), rates are nearly as high. Serious rule violations (truancy, school suspension, runaway behavior, getting drunk before age 15, lying) are of greater significance com-

Table 3 Comorbidity of Conduct Disorder Symptoms in Bipolar Subjects (ECA data)

	Ages 18–29			30+			Odds ratio[a] (conf. intervals)
sample size	52	4,296		80	13,806		
	BPI	Non-BP	x2[b]	BPI	Non-BP	x2[b]	
truant	40.4	15.1	25.3	13	5.2	11.4	3.4 (2.2–5.1)
suspended/expelled	48.1	15.3	41.8	12.5	4.2	13.6	3.4 (2.5–5.6)
bad grades	21.2	9	9.1	15	7.0	7.7	2.4 (2.2–2.7)
in trouble in school	32.7	12.8	17.9	15	5.4	14	3.1 (2.0–4.7)
arrested	19.2	4.8	22.5	6.25	1.8	8.9	4.1 (2.3–7.3)
runaway	21.2	3.6	43.1	10	1.5	37.2	6.7 (4.0–1.1)
lying	48.1	17.1	34.2	23.8	8.0	26.3	3.7 (2.5–5.3)
drunk <15	34.6	11.9	24.8	8.8	2.2	15.7	4.1 (2.6–6.5)
stealing	48.1	22.4	19.3	21.3	11	8.4	2.4 (1.6–3.5)
vandal	17.3	6.6	9.4	10	2.1	23.4	3.9 (2.4–6.7)
fights	15.4	9.2	ns	13.8	5.1	7.7	2.3 (1.4–3.8)

[a]Comparison of all BP subjects with all non-BP subjects controlling for age and sex. All are significant.

[b]All Chi squares are statistically significant.

pared to nonbipolars than the more "typical" conduct disorder (CD) symptoms such as stealing, vandalism, and fighting. There is a significant disparity in rates of all CD symptoms in 18–29-year-old bipolars versus nonbipolars not seen in the next age group. However, even when controlling for sex and age, bipolar subjects have higher odds ratios for every symptom compared to nonbipolar subjects. Most significantly, the childhood behavior problems occur much more frequently in adult bipolar subjects with substance abuse than bipolar subjects without (44) suggesting that childhood comorbidity is directly related to adult comorbidity. It should be clear from these data that when people who meet criteria for mania are questioned with a structured interview, they frequently meet criteria for other psychiatric disorders. In young people, ODD/CD is most frequently observed; this graduates to its older counterpart, substance abuse, in adults. CD symptoms in bipolar youths are significant at all ages. Anxiety disorders, too, occur with mania in all age groups, but at lower rates.

Several reports note that mixed episodes and/or rapid cycling are the most common bipolar subtypes with "classic" euphoria being seen a small minority of adolescents (35,45). Related to the observation of differentially high rates of "mixed" manic episodes in adolescents is the additional observation by Strakowski et al. (30) that 83.3% of those with mixed episodes were comorbid, versus 42.2% rates of comorbidity in those with nonmixed states. Rates of comorbidity, usually substance and alcohol abuse, also appear to be higher in first episodes of mania in young adults (46), though alcohol abuse, too, seems to diminish with time (47). *If comorbidity is common to both youths and adults, then what appears to be differentially uncommon in children and adolescents is uncomplicated, noncomorbid bipolar disorder.*

IV. IMPLICATIONS OF COMORBIDITY FOR AGE OF ONSET

Recent epidemiological studies report mean age of onset to be 18–20 years (41,48) for bipolar I disorder and 22 years for bipolar II disorder (48). Fogarty et al. (41) found that less than 5% reported symptoms before age 10. While data from several studies including the ECA study suggest a "cohort effect" for mania (the age of onset of mania is getting younger in successive generations) (49,50), in the Old-Order Amish, a stable society where substance abuse is virtually absent and rates of behavior disorders are lower, there is no decline in age of onset (51) in successive cohorts. Robins and Price (42), also using the ECA data, have reported that the presence of childhood CD symptoms lowers the age of onset of virtually all psychiatric disorders, and mania, from 1 to 2 years suggesting that this comorbidity may play a role in lowering age of onset for a number of psychiatric disorders in contemporary society.

A. Familiality

In addition to an apparent increase in the rate, there is a clear association between early age of onset and degree of familiality of disorder such that families with the greatest genetic loading appear to have offspring who tend to develop mood disorder at an earlier age. Strober et al. (52) found the highest lifetime rates of mood disorder in first-degree relatives of adolescent-onset bipolar youths who had preadolescent psychopathology (44.1%); adolescent-onset bipolars without prepubertal psychopathology had rates in first-degree relatives of 23.5%, similar to rates reported in other studies of early-onset bipolar patients (53). By contrast, rates in first-degree relatives of "late onset" bipolar patients (age of onset definitions variable) averaged 14.4% (53). In the Amish sample, moreover, relatives of probands with an earlier age of onset were also at increased risk for developing mood disorder (51). Among the hypotheses offered in explanation is the possibility of expansion of trinucleotide repeats, which has been observed to explain the phenomenon of genetic "anticipation" (the progressively earlier age at onset and increasing severity of illness in succeeding generations) in several genetic disorders like myotonic dystrophy and fragile X syndrome (54). However, it is also possible that declining age of onset represents the results of a greater genetic loading combined with the impact of substantial parental mental illness on offspring (55).

V. OUTCOME

Goodwin and Jamison (9) found one-third of bipolar patients to have some social incapacitation including high rates of enduring symptoms and a high level of psychosocial impairment even when episodes have remitted (56). In the most recent study delineating functioning (57), only 27% of hospitalized manics had good overall functioning at 2 years, 41% at 4.5 years. Of those doing well at 2 years, 29% worsened. Of those doing poorly, 59% improved somewhat. Unfortunately, many patients are not substantially improved even with vigorous psychopharmacological treatment (58,59). Gitlin et al. (58) attribute this poor response to "real world" clinical samples, but an examination of recent controlled trials (see below) is not substantially more encouraging.

With regard to psychosocial function in youths, the sample described by Werry et al. (19) (follow-up of 1–16 years; mean 6.2 years) is comprehensively described. Of the 23 youths who were diagnosed as bipolar at follow-up, with an average age of 20, 51% were living "independently," 48% were either working or in school full time, and 45% had had more than two episodes. With respect to treatment, 17% were taking neuroleptics, 66% mood stabilizers, and 17% were taking no medications.

Three longitudinal follow-up studies of early-onset bipolar patients (60–62) have contrasted adolescents with adults. Coryell and Norton (61) found that over 8.4 years, adolescent and adult bipolars spent 12.6% and 9.4%, respectively, in hospital. Of the 28 adolescent bipolar symptom onset patients studied (60), 60% had good social outcomes (though they might have had recurrences) similar to older onset patients. Their mean episode frequency per year of 0.38 was also similar to that of older-onset patients. McGlashan's (62) findings concurred.

What is the impact of comorbidity and/or mixed episodes on outcome in bipolar disorder? The study by Black et al. (29) specifically compares complicated (comorbid) mania to uncomplicated and finds the former patients have significantly worse treatment response at the end of hospitalization. Keller et al. (63) report that the highest probability for remaining ill for 1 year was in the mixed/rapid cycling subtype of bipolar patients, and in secondary subtype (comorbid) bipolar depressions. In adolescents, Strober et al. (52) identified a subgroup (20%) of adolescent bipolar patients with preadolescent psychopathology, usually externalizing disorders. These teenagers had a more chronic course, a more affective-disorder-loaded family history, and worse lithium response than bipolar adolescents without such premorbid psychopathology.

The relationship between comorbidity and outcome is demonstrated in a preliminary examination of data from half of the sample of the Suffolk County Mental Health Project (64) described earlier. Carlson et al. (36) found that of 17 patients (aged 15–20) who met DSM-III-R (6) criteria for mania as diagnosed at a consensus conference using structured interview and all available data including school records, 12 had externalizing/educational problems antedating their mood disorder; of 11 who had 2-year follow-up data, seven developed or had concurrent drug and/or alcohol abuse prior to their mood disorder onset. Functioning of the 11 subjects at 2-year follow-up was significantly worse than that of the five manic youths without such problems (2.09 vs. 3.4, $t = 2.17$, $p < 0.004$).

A. Suicide

In adults, the likelihood of suicide in bipolar patients is substantial, with rates ranging from 9 to 60% (9, pp. 228–231). The relationship with other psychopathology may be as high as 71% (65). In youths, a particularly malignant course was observed in 12 bipolar young adults (nine males, three females) who had been psychiatrically hospitalized in adolescence (66). One-third never graduated from high school, and all had had poor work histories, suggesting severe disorder, comorbidity, or both. Psychological autopsy studies have indicated high rates of comorbidity, usually between mood disorder and either substance abuse, CD, or personality disorders (67,68). It is unclear how many of the mood disorder youths were bipolar; Brent and his group found that 22% of their subjects met criteria for bipolar I or II (67). Shaffer's study did not replicate this (68). Given the high rate of conversion of major depressive disorders to bipolar disorder when the onset is in adolescence, however, it is likely that, had some of these young people lived, a manic episode would have eventuated sooner or later.

B. Medication Response

Medication response of adult bipolar patients has varied considerably over the past 40 years. A summary of placebo-controlled studies (not to mention open trials) from 1954 to 1971 of 116 patients yielded an overall response rate of 78% (9, p. 614). On the other hand, Bowden et al. (69), summarizing four recent trials (1987–1994), with, arguably, more sophisticated design, reported response rates of 41–52%. More pessimistically, if one counts those who could not complete the trial because of the severity of their symptoms, the response rate was closer to 34%. Several explanations have been offered to explain this decline in response rate. One argument (70) states that the patients who originally responded to lithium continue to do so. There is no rebound after discontinuation, though with continued follow-up, there is relapse. They state further: "A prompt rebound of intense manic or psychotic symptoms on discontinuation has frequently been observed during the past decade, indicating that these recently treated patients benefit mainly from a non-specific reduction of overactivity by lithium rather than from true mood stabilization."

Other explanations of lithium nonresponse are summarized in Table 4. Unfortunately, many of the poor-response criteria characterize young people who meet criteria for mania. Grof's (70) final indictment is that the current diagnostic approach "with its emphasis on standardization rather than validity of diagnosis, encourages a brief assessment with a counting of symptoms rather than a comprehensive analysis of each case."

Anticonvulsants have provided a treatment alternative to lithium. Controlled trials of carbamazepine from 1979 to 1989 show an overall response rate of 71% (9, p. 621). This was frequently administered in conjunction with other medications, however. Like valproic acid or divalproex sodium, it is said to be more effective in some of the patients (rapid-cycling patients, mixed-episode patients) who are less responsive to lithium. The most recent trials of the anticonvulsant divalproex sodium, in which efficacy was compared with that of lithium, produced comparable response rates. Acute antimanic responses have ranged from 48% (71) to 69% (72). Again, however, the seriousness of the pathology in patients studied often caused high dropout rates from the open trials before patients were even randomized (69). Taking into account such problems lowered the response rate of divalproex from 49% to 34%. That was still better than the 13% placebo response similarly derived, however.

There are no comparable studies of medication response in children and ado-

Table 4 Responders Versus Nonresponders to Lithium (With Specific Relevance to Children and Adolescents)

Good responders	Poor responders
Euphoric mania	Dysphoric, mixed mania
Grandiosity	Paranoia
Mania with mood-congruent psychosis	Mania with mood incongruent psychosis
Absense of "neurotic" personality traits	Anxious, obsessive-compulsive traits
No comorbidity	Co-occurring behavior disorders and/or substance/alcohol abuse
Mania/depression/euthymia	Rapid cycling without euthymia
Acute onset of retarded depression	Slow onset/chronic depression
Family history of mania	Family history of schizophrenia or alcoholism
Preserved family/social network	Many psychosocial stressors
	Hypothyroidism
	Folate deficiency

Source: Abou-Saleh, 1993; Solomon et al., 1995.

lescents with bipolar disorder. Summary of a variety of open, anecdotal, and small-number controlled trials of lithium from 1969 to 1988 reveal a response rate of 82% (73). In many cases, however, reports were likely published precisely because the child responded to lithium. There have been no controlled or even open small series studies of carbamazepine. One open study of valproate (74) and one of divalproex (75) have been published. In these 28 patients, most of whom were being concurrently treated with other medications as well, the addition of this anticonvulsant enhanced response. In the former study, six of the patients had "mixed" episodes; all but one of these had concurrent ADHD. Since comorbidity complicates treatment response of most illnesses, there is no reason why this should be different for bipolar disorder in children and adolescents. The particular significance for young people is that uncomplicated disorder is so rare.

VI. CONCLUSIONS

The criteria changes used to diagnose mania, and thus bipolar disorder, have broadened in the past 20 years such that this disorder appears to be more common in youths than heretofore. Classically defined, "pure," uncomplicated bipolar disorder is still rare in youths compared to adults. Conversely, in both young people and adults, changes in the definition and ascertainment have increased rates of mania comorbidity, especially with behavior disorders. In children, this includes co-occurring ADHD and oppositional ODD/CD. In adults, this has subsumed alcohol and substance abuse disorders. However, bipolar adults, young and old, have higher rates of behavior problems in childhood, too. For children and adolescents, meeting criteria for mania (even having only chronic symptoms of "elated, irritable mood") predicts considerable disability. The younger the onset, the more obvious the disability. The less obvious change from the premorbid state, the more chronic the course.

The outcome and treatment refractoriness of these comorbid children is troubling and not unlike that of comorbid ADHD/ODD/CD youths (76). Treatment implications of this have not been confronted. In addition, while there is much interest in the genetic underpinnings of bipolar disorder, family studies should account for behavioral comorbidity in relatives with bipolar disorder to determine the distinctiveness of this subtype.

ACKNOWLEDGMENT

The assistance of Evelyn Bromet, Ph.D., Joseph Schwartz, Ph.D., and Lina Jandorf, M.A., was invaluable in preparing this manuscript. Data from the Suffolk County Mental Health Project was gathered as part of MH 44801.

REFERENCES

1. Kraepelin E. Manic Depressive Insanity and Paranoia. Edinburgh: E&S Livingstone, 1921.
2. Lish JD, Dime-Meenan S, Whybrow PC, Price RA, Hirschfeld RM. The National Depressive and Manic-Depressive Association (DMDA) survey of bipolar members. J Affect Disord 1994; 31:281–294.
3. Wozniak J, Biederman J, Mundy E, Mennin D, Faraone SV. A pilot family study of childhood-onset mania. J Am Acad Child Adolesc Psychiatry 1995; 34:1577–1584.
4. Fristad MA, Weller RA, Weller EB. The mania rating scale (MRS): further reliability and validity studies with children. Ann Clin Psychiatry 1995; 7:127–132.
5. American Psychiatric Association. Diagnostic and Statistical Manual for Psychiatric Disorders II, III, III-R, IV. Washington, DC: APA Press, 1980.
6. American Psychiatric Association. Diagnostic and Statistical Manual for Psychiatric Disorders III-R. Washington, DC: APA Press, 1987.
7. American Psychiatric Association. Diagnostic and Statistical Manual for Psychiatric Disorders-IV. Washington, DC: APA Press, 1994.
8. Dunner DL. Differential diagnosis of bipolar disorder. J Clin Psychopharmacol 1992; 12(Suppl 1):7S–12S.
9. Goodwin FK, Jamison KR. Manic Depressive Illness. New York: Oxford University Press, 1990.

10. Heila H, Turpeinen P, Erkinjuntti T. Case study: mania associated with multiple sclerosis. J Am Acad Child Adolesc Psychiatry 1995; 34:1591–1595.
11. Lahey BB, Applegate B, McBurnett K, Biederman J, Greenhill L, Hynd GW, Barkley RA, Newcorn J, Jensen P, Richters J, Garfinkel B, Kerdyk L, Frick PJ, Ollendick T, Perez D, Hart EL, Waldman I, Shaffer D. DSM IV field trials for attention deficit hyperactivity disorder in children and adolescents. Am J Psychiatry 1994; 151:1673–1685.
12. Biederman J, Newcorn J, Sprich S. Comorbidity of attention deficit hyperactivity disorder with conduct, depressive, anxiety, and other disorders. Am J Psychiatry 1991; 148:564–577.
13. Barkley RA, Guevremont DC, Anastopoloulos AD, DuPaul GJ, Shelton TL. Driving-related risks and outcomes of attention deficit hyperactivity disorder in adolescents and young adults: a 3- to 5-year follow-up survey. Pediatrics 1993; 92:212–218.
14. Carlson GA. Annotation: Child and adolescent mania—diagnostic considerations. J Child Psychol Psychiatry 1990; 31:331–341.
15. Carlson GA. Identifying prepubertal mania. J Am Acad Child Adolesc Psychiatry 1995; 34:750–753.
16. Parker G, O'Donnell M, Walter S. Changes in the diagnosis of functional psychoses associated with the introduction of lithium. Br J Psychiatry 1985; 146:382.
17. Taylor MA, Abrams R. The phenomenology of mania. Arch Gen Psychiatry 1973; 29:520–522.
18. American Psychiatric Association. Diagnostic and Statistical Manual for Psychiatric Disorders-II. Washington, DC: APA Press, 1968.
19. Werry JS, McClellan JM, Chard L. Childhood and adolescent schizophrenic, bipolar and schizo-affective disorders: a clinical and outcome study. J Am Acad Child Adolesc Psychiatry 1991; 30:457–465.
20. Carlson GA, Kashani JH. Manic symptoms in non-referred adolescent population. J Affect Disord 1988; 15:219–226.
21. Herjanic B, Reich W. Development of a structured psychiatric interview for children: agreement between child and parent on individual symptoms. J Abnorm Child Psychol 1982; 10:307–324.
22. Lewinsohn PM, Klein DN, Seeley JR. Bipolar disorder in a community sample of older adolescents: prevalence, phenomenology, comorbidity and course. J Am Acad Child Adolesc Psychiatry 1995; 34:454–463.
23. Orvaschel H, Puig-Antich J, Chambers W, Tabrizi MA, Johnson R. Retrospective assessment of child psychopathology with the kiddie-SADS-E. J Am Acad Child Psychiatry 1982; 21:392–397.
24. Robins LN, Reiger DA, eds. Psychiatric Disorders in America. New York: The Free Press, 1991.
25. Howland RH, Thase ME. A Comprehensive review of cyclothymic disorder. J Nerv Ment Dis 1993; 181:485–493.
26. Akiskal HS. Mood disorders: clinical features. In: Kaplan HI, Sadock BJ, eds. Comprehensive Textbook of Psychiatry. Baltimore: Williams & Wilkins, 1995: 1123–1152.
27. Akiskal HS. Developmental pathways to bipolarity: are juvenile-onset depressions prebipolar? J Am Acad Child Adolesc Psychiatry 1995; 34:754–763.

28. McElroy SL, Keck PE, Jr, Pope HG, Jr, Hudson JI, Faedda GL, Swann AC. Clinical and research implications of the diagnosis of dysphonic or mixed mania or hypomania. Am J Psychiatry 1992; 149:1633–1644.
29. Black DW, Winokur G, Bell S, Nasrallah A, Hulbert J. Complicated mania—comorbidity and immediate outcome in the treatment of mania. Arch Gen Psychiatry 1988; 45:232–236.
30. Strakowski SM, Tohen M, Stoll AL, Faedda GL, Goodwin DC. Comorbidity in mania at first hospitalization. Am J Psychiatry 1992; 149:554–556.
31. Strakowski SM, Tohen M, Stoll AL, Faedda GL, Mayer PV, Kolbrener ML, Goodwin DC. Comorbidity in psychosis at first hospitalization. Am J Psychiatry 1993; 150:752–757.
32. Carlson GA. Bipolar affective disorders in childhood and adolescence. In: Cantwell DP, Carlson GA, eds. Affective Disorders in Childhood and Adolescence—An Update. New York: Spectrum Publications, 1983:61–84.
33. Kovacs M, Pollock M. Bipolar disorder and conduct disorder in childhood and adolescence. J Am Acad Child Adolesc Psychiatry 1995; 34:715–723.
34. Wozniak J, Biederman J, Kiely K, Ablon JS, Faraone SV, Munda E, Mennin D. Mania-like symptoms suggestive of childhood-onset bipolar disorder in clinically referred children. J Am Acad Child Adolesc Psychiatry 1995; 34:867–876.
35. Geller B, Sun K, Zimerman B, Luby J, Frazier J, Williams M. Complex and rapid-cycling in bipolar children and adolescents: a preliminary study. J Affect Disord 1995; 34:259–268.
36. Carlson GA, Fennig S, Bromet ET. The confusion between bipolar disorder and schizophrenia in youth: where does it stand in the 1990's? J Am Acad Child Adolesc Psychiatry 1994; 33:453–460.
37. Andreasen NC, Grove WM, Coryell WH, Endicott J, Clayton PJ. Bipolar versus unipolar and primary versus secondary affective disorder; which diagnosis takes precedence? J Affect Disord 1988; 15:69–80.
38. Savino M, Perugi G, Simonini E, Soriani A, Cassano GB, Akiskal HS. Affective comorbidity in panic disorder: is there a bipolar connection? J Affect Disord 1993; 28:155–163.
39. Young LT, Cooke RG, Robb JC, Levitt AJ, Jaffe RT. Anxious and non-anxious bipolar disorder. J Affect Disord 1993; 29:49–52.
40. Regier DA, Farmer ME, Rae DS, Locke BZ, Keith SJ, Judd LL, Goodwin FK. Comorbidity of mental health disorders with alcohol and other drug abuse. JAMA 1990; 264:2511–2518.
41. Fogarty F, Russell JM, Newman SC, Bland RC. Mania. Acta Psychiatr Scand 1994; 376(Suppl):16–23.
42. Robins LN, Price RK. Adult disorders predicted by childhood conduct problems: results from the NIMH Epidemiologic Catchment Area project. Psychiatry 1991; 54:116–132.
43. Robins LN, Tipp J, Przybeck T. Antisocial personality. In: Robins LN, Rieger DA, eds. Psychiatric Disorders in America. New York: The Free Press, 1991:258–290.
44. Carlson GA, Bromet EJ, Jandorf L. Conduct disorder and mania, what does it mean in adults? J Affective Disorders 48:199–205, 1988.
45. Himmelhoch JM, Garfinkel ME. Sources of lithium resistance in mixed mania. Psychopharmacol Bull 1986; 22:613–620.

46. Keck PE, Jr, McElroy SL, Strakowski SM, West SA, Hawkins JM, Huber TJ, Newman RM, DePriest M. Outcome and comorbidity in first-compared with multiple episode mania. J Nerv Ment Dis 1995; 183:320–324.
47. Winokur G, Coryell W, Akiskal HS, Maser JD, Keller MB, Endicott J, Mueller T. Alcoholism in manic-depressive (bipolar) Illness: familial illness, course of illness, and the primary-secondary distinction. Am J Psychiatry 1995; 152:365–372.
48. Weissman MM, Bruce ML, Leaf PJ. Affective disorders. In: Robins LN, Regier DA, eds. Psychiatric Disorders in America. New York: The Free Press, 1991: 53–80.
49. Gershon ES, Hamovit JH, Guroff JJ, Numberger JI. Birth-cohort changes in manic and depressive disorders in relatives of bipolar and schizoaffective patients. Arch Gen Psychiatry 1987; 44:314–319.
50. Lasch K, Weissman M, Wickramaratne P, Bruce ML. Birth-cohort changes in the rates of mania. Psychiatry Res 1990; 33:31–37.
51. Pauls DL, Morton LA, Egeland JA. Risks of affective illness among first-degree relatives of bipolar I Old-Order Amish probands. Arch Gen Psychiatry 1992; 49: 703–708.
52. Strober M, Morrell W, Burroughs J, Lampert C, Danforth H, Freeman R. A family study of bipolar I in adolescence: early-onset of symptoms linked to increased familial loading and lithium resistance. J Affect Disord 1988; 15:255–268.
53. Strober M. Relevance of early age-of-onset in genetics studies of bipolar affective disorder. J Am Acad Child Adolesc Psychiatry 1992; 31:606–610.
54. McInnis MG, McMahon FJ, Chase GA, Simpson SG, Ross CA, DePaulo JR Jr. Anticipation in bipolar affective disorder. Am J Hum Genet 1993; 53:3850–3900.
55. Downey G, Coyne JC. Children of depressed parents; an integrative review. Psychol Bull 1990; 108:50–76.
56. Coryell W, Scheftner W, Keller M, Endicott J, Maser J, Klerman GL. The enduring psychosocial consequences of mania and depression. Am J Psychiatry 1993; 150: 720–727.
57. Goldberg JF, Harrow M, Grossman SS. Course and outcome in bipolar affective disorder: a longitudinal follow-up study. Am J Psychiatry 1995; 152:379–384.
58. Gitlin MJ, Swendsen J, Heller TL, Hammen C. Relapse and impairment in bipolar disorder. Am J Psychiatry 1995; 152:1635–1640.
59. Winokur G, Coryell W, Keller J, Endicott J, Akiskal H. A prospective follow-up patients with bipolar and primary unipolar affective disorder. Arch Gen Psychiatry 1993; 50:457–465.
60. Carlson GA, Davenport YB, Jamison KR. A comparison of outcome in adolescent and late onset bipolar manic depressive illness. Am J Psychiatry 1977; 134:919–922.
61. Coryell W, Norten SG. Mania during adolescence. J Nerv Ment Dis 1980; 168: 611–613.
62. McGlashan TM. Adolescent vs adult onset mania. Am J Psychiatry 1988; 145: 221–224.
63. Keller MB, Lavori PW, Coryell W, Andreasen NC, Endicott J, Clayton PJ, Klerman GL, Hirschfeld RM. The differential outcome of pure manic, mixed/cycling and pure depressive episodes in patients with bipolar illness. JAMA 1988; 255: 3138–3142.

64. Bromet EJ, Schwartz JE, Fennig S, Geller L, Jandorf L, Kovasznay B, Lavelle J, Miller A, Pato C, Ram R, Rich C. The epidemiology of psychoses: the Suffolk County Mental Health Project. Schizophren Bull 1992; 18:255.
65. Isometsa ET, Henriksson MM, Aro HM, Lonnqvist JK. Suicide in bipolar disorder in Finland. Am J Psychiatry 1994; 151:1020–1024.
66. Welner A, Welner Z, Fishman R. Psychiatric adolescent inpatients 8 to 10 year follow-up. Arch Gen Psychiatry 1979; 36:698–700.
67. Brent DA, Perper JA, Goldstein CE, Kolko DJ, Allan MJ, Allman CJ, Zelenak JP. Risk factors for adolescent suicide. Arch Gen Psychiatry 1988; 45:581–588.
68. Shaffer D, Gould MS, Fishir P, Trautman P, Moreau D, Kleinman M, Flory M. Psychiatric diagnosis in child and adolescent suicide. Arch Gen Psychiatry 1996; 53:339–348.
69. Bowden CL, Calabrese JR, Wallin BA, Swann AC, McElroy SL, Risch SC, Hirschfeld MA. Who enters therapeutic trials? Psychopharmacol Bull 1995; 31:103–109.
70. Grof P, Alda M, Grof E, Fox D, Cameron P. The challenge of predicting response to stabilizing lithium treatment. Br J Psychiatry 1993; 163(Suppl 21):16–19.
71. Bowden CL, Brugger AM, Swann AC, Calabrese JR, Janicak PG, Petty F, Dilsaver SC, Davis JM, Rush AJ, Small JG. Efficacy of divalproex vs lithium and placebo in the treatment of mania. JAMA 1994; 271:918–924.
72. Freeman TW, Clothier JL, Pazzaglier P, Lesem MD, Swann AC. A double-blind comparison of valproate and lithium in the treatment of acute mania. Am J Psychiatry 1992; 149:108–111.
73. Faedda GL, Baldessarini MD, Suppes T, Tondo L, Becker I, Lipshitz DS. Pediatric onset bipolar disorder: a neglected clinical and public health problem. Harvard Rev Psychiatry 1995; 3:171–195.
74. West SA, Keck PE Jr, McElroy SL, Strakowki SM, Minnery KL, McConville BJ. Open trial of valproate in the treatment of adolescent mania. J Child Adolesc Psychopharmacol 1994; 4:263–267.
75. Papatheodorou G, Kutcher SP, Katic M, Szalai JP. The efficacy and safety of divalproex sodium in the treatment of acute mania in adolescents and young adults: an open clinical trial. J Clin Psychopharmacol 1995; 15:110–116.
76. Hechtman L, Offord DR. Long-term outcome of disruptive behavior disorders. Child Adolesc Psychiatr Clin North Am 1994; 3:379–403.
77. Regier DA, Boyd JH, Burke JD Jr. One month prevalence of mental disorders in the United States. Arch Gen Psychiatry 1988; 45:977–986.
78. Weissman MM, Myers JK. Affective disorders in a U.S. urban community: the use of Research Diagnostic Criteria in an epidemiological survey. Arch Gen Psychiatry 1978; 35:1304–1311.
79. Egeland JA, Hostetter AM. Amish study, I: affective disorders among the Amish, 1976–1980. Am J Psychiatry 1983; 140:56–61.
80. Kessler RC, McGonagle KA, Zhao S. Lifetime and 12 month prevalence of DSM III R psychiatric disorders among persons aged 15–54 in the United States: results from the National Comorbidity Survey. Arch Gen Psychiatry 1994; 51:8–19.
81. Canino GJ, Bird HR, Shrout PE. Prevalence of specific psychiatric disorders in Puerto Rico. Arch Gen Psychiatry 1987; 44:727–735.

Index

Acamprosate, alcohol and, 45
Acoustic neurinoma, bipolar disorder in old age, 254
Addiction and mental health treatment settings, substance abuse and depression rates in, 28
Adjustment disorder with depressed mood, depression of medically ill and, 63
Adolescents (*see* Children)
Adrenocortical hormones, 70
Age and personality disorder comobidity, 137, 141
AIDS patients, manic syndromes and, 255
Alcohol, bipolar disorder and, 198, 199, 203
Alcohol and depression
  abuse, 30
  biological markers, 33–34
  men versus women, 28
  pharmacological treatment of, 44–46
  psychosocial factors, 31
Alcoholics Anonymous (AA), 49
Alcohol-related disorders, bipolar disorder in old age and, 250–251
Anticonvulsant therapy, substance abuse and, 205–207
Antidepressants
  cancer and, 86
  cerebrovascular disease and, 79
  dementia and, 80–81
  for depression of medically ill, 74–75, 76
  diabetes mellitus and, 82
  drug interactions and, 77
  epilepsy and, 79–80
  heterocyclic for depression of medically ill, 75–76
  HIV and, 85
  Parkinson's disease and, 81
  pharmacokinetics of, 77
  tricyclic, 75
Antisocial personality disorder, mania and, 242–243
Assertive community treatment model for substance abuse, 40
Assessment of substance abuse, 35–39
Attention deficit hyperactivity disorder (ADHD)
  bipolar disorder and Axis I disorders, 231, 234
  criteria for, 265–266
Atypical antidepressants for depression of medically ill, 76
Axis II personality disorders (*see also* Bipolar disorder and

Axis II personality disorders):
co-occurence of mania and, 242–244
prevalence of, 241–242
Axis I mania disorders (*see* Bipolar disorder and Axis I mania disorders)

Beck Depression Inventory (BDI), 81
Biological factors of substance abuse, 32
Bipolar depression
comorbidity of, 1–20, 25–26
prevalence of, 2–3
Bipolar disorder (*see also* Children and bipolar disorder; Medical illness and bipolar disorder; Old age, bipolar disorder in; Substance abuse and bipolar disorder):
in depression of medically ill, 63
psychiatric comorbidity and, 230
Bipolar disorder and Axis II personality disorders, 241–245
diagnostic difficulties, 244
medications for, 244–245
Bipolar disorder and Axis I mania disorders, 229–236
attention deficit hyperactivity disorder and, 234
bulimia nervosa and, 233
diagnostic difficulties, 234–235
impulse control disorders and, 233
mania and, 230–231
multiple comorbidity, 234
obsessive-compulsive disorder and, 232–233
medications, 235–236
panic disorder and, 231–232
medications, 235–236
prevalence rate of, 231–232
Bipolar disorder and major depressive disorder (MDD), 3–6 (*see also* Major depressive disorder (MDD)):
comorbidity effects on course and severity, 11–14
effects of earlier disorders, 6–11
genetic influences, 17
with other disorders, 3–6
prevention of, 19
Bipolar mania, 220
Bipolar spectrum disorders, 201
Borderline personality disorder, mania and, 243
Brain stem tumors, bipolar disorder in old age, 254
Bromocriptine, 83
Bulimia nervosa, 231
depression and, 233
Bupropion
for alcohol and depression, 44
for depression of medically ill, 75, 76
for nicotine dependence, 35, 48

Caffeinated beverages, 32
Cancer, 85–86
antidepressants and, 86
depression of medically ill, 85–86
dexamethasone suppression test and, 70–71
drug interactions and, 86
medical illness in old age and, 158
pancreatic, 66
SSRIs and, 86
Carbamazepine, 205
Cardiovascular disease, depression of medically ill and, 83–84
Center for Epidemiologic Studies Depression (CES-D), 158

Central nervous system disorders, secondary mania and, 216, 217
Cerebrovascular disease
  bipolar disorder in old age, 250–251, 253
  medically ill depression, 79
Children and bipolar disorder
  comorbidity for age of onset, 271–272
  epidemiology of mania and manic symptoms, 266–268
  mania diagnosis, 263–266
  outcome, 272–275
    medication response, 274–275
    suicide, 273–274
  psychopathology and age, 268–271
    comorbidity/mixed episodes, 269–271
Children and depression, 179–194
  epidemiological studies of, 180–189
    anxiety disorders, 185, 188
    attention deficit/hyperactivity disorder (ADHD), 186, 188
    conduct and/or oppositional defiant disorders, 184, 188
    prevalence of depressive disorders, 182–183, 188
    substance-related disorders, 187, 188
  reasons for comorbidity, 189–194
Cigarette smoking (*see* Nicotine and depression)
Cluster A personality disorders, depression and, 131–133
Cluster B personality disorders, depression and, 133–135
Cluster C personality disorders, depression and, 135–137
Cocaine and depression, 28–29
[Cocaine and depression]
  biological markers, 34
  bipolar disorders and, 17, 198–199
  pharmacological treatment of, 46–47
  psychosocial factors, 31
Cognitive behavior therapy, for substance abuse and bipolar disorder patients, 208
Cognitive impairment in elderly manic patients, 253–254
Collaborative Study on the Genetics of Alcoholism (COGA), 38
Comorbidity
  bipolar disorder in children, 269–272
  definition of, 128
  Diagnostic and Statistical Manual of Mental Disorders (*DSM*) and, 57
  effects on bipolar disorders and major depressive disorders, 11–14
  effects on medical illness in old age, 164–166
  in mania, 230
  personality disorders and depression, 146–148
Comorbidity with depression, definition of, 179
Complicated mania, 230, 250, 256–257
  medical comorbidity, 220
Conduct disorder symptoms, 270
Construct validity, diagnosis, 59
Coronary artery disease (CAD), depression in old age and, 158
Corticotropin-releasing factor (CRF), 70
Craniopharyngioma, 254
Cushing's syndrome, 83

Dementia
  bipolar disorder in old age, 253–254
  depression of medically ill, 80–81
  electroconvulsive therapy and, 81
Dementia praecox, 229, 264
Depression (*see also* Medical illness in old age and depression; Medically ill, depression in; Personality disorders and depression; Substance abuse and depression):
  diagnosis failure in medically ill, 62
  rates of medical illness in old age, 158–159
  screening for medically ill, 66–67
Depressive comorbidity, definition of, 179
Depressive personality disorder, 142–143
Descriptive-based diagnosis, 58
Descriptive differential, depression of medically ill, 59–64
Descriptive validity
  diagnostic validity, 59
  grief and, 61
Desipramine, substance abuse and depression, 45, 46–47
Dexamethasone suppression test (DST) and cancer, 70–71
Diabetes mellitus (DM), endocrine disorders and, 81–82
Diagnostic classification, for depression of medically ill, 58
Diagnostic issues
  bipolar disorder and Axis I disorders, 234–235
  bipolar disorder and Axis II disorders, 244
  medically ill depression, 61–62
  substance abuse and bipolar disorder, 201–202
Diagnostic validity, depression of medically ill, 58–59
Differential diagnosis
  depression of medically ill, 59
  substance abuse, 35–39
Digoxin, 84
Disulfiram, alcohol and, 44–45
Dopamine (DA), 68
Drug interactions
  antidepressants, 77
  cancer, 86
  in epilepsy, 79–80
  Parkinson's Disease (PD), 81
DSM (*Diagnostic and Statistical Manual of Mental Disorders*), comorbidity and, 57
DSM-III (*Diagnostic and Statistical Manual of Mental Disorders*), 58
  personality disorders and depression, 57
  prevalence studies in family samples, 129
  prevalence studies in patient samples, 129–131
DSM-III-R (*Diagnostic and Statistical Manual of Mental Disorders*), Axis I disorder, 129–131
DSM-IV (*Diagnostic and Statistical Manual of Mental Disorders*), 58
  Axis I disorder, 129–131
  diagnostic validity of depression in, 58–59
  major depressive disorder (MDD) in, 60, 107
  personality disorders and depression, 107
  substance abuse, 36, 37
Dual-diagnosis treatment, substance abuse, 40
Dysthymia, 107

Electroconvulsive therapy (ECT), 69
in cerebrovascular disease, 79
in dementia, 81
in epilepsy, 80
medically ill depression, 78
Endocrine disorders
depression and, 65
diabetes mellitus and, 81–82
Epidemiologic Catchment Area (ECA) Study, 231, 249
mania and manic symptoms, 267
substance abuse and bipolar disorder, 197, 198
substance abuse and depression, 28
Epilepsy, depression in medically ill and, 79–80
Etiology-based diagnosis, 61
in depression of medically ill, 58
Exclusive diagnostic strategy, 61–62

Face validity
as diagnostic validity, 58–59
grief and, 60–61
First-episode mania in old age, 252
Fluoxetine, alcohol and, 45–46
Formes frustes depressions, children, 180

Genetic influences, bipolar disorders and major depressive disorders, 17
Grief, and depression of medically ill, 60–61

Hamilton Depression Rating Scale (HAM-D), 158
Head trauma
bipolar disorder in old age, 254
secondary mania and, 215–217
Health care utilization, medical illness in old age and, 163
Health effects, of medical illness in old age and depression, 162–166
Heroin, 34
Heterocyclic antidepressants, 75–76
HIV, 84–85
antidepressants for, 85
Hyperprolactinemia, depression of medically ill, 83
Hypothalamic-pituitary-adrenal (HPA), 69, 70–71, 73
Hypothalamic-pituitary-thyroid (HPT)
hypothyroidism, 71–72
TRH, 71–72
Hypothyroidism, 64, 65–66
grades of, 72
hypothalamic-pituitary-thyroid (HPT), 71–72

Imipramine
for alcohol and depression, 45
for depression of medically ill, 75–76
Immune system, and depression of medically ill, 72–73, 74
Impulse control disorders, depression and, 231, 233
Inclusive diagnostic strategies, 61–62
Infectious diseases
disorders associated with depression, 65
secondary mania and, 216, 218
Integrated treatment model for substance abuse, 40–41
Iproniazid, 76

"Kindling," substance abuse and bipolar disorder and, 204

Late onset of first-episode mania in old age, 252

Lifetime disorders, studying old age for, 249
Lithium
  for bipolar disorder in children, 274–275
  for substance abuse and bipolar disorder, 204–205, 206

Major depressive disorder (MDD) (*see also* Bipolar disorder and major depressive disorder (MDD)):
  in depression of medically ill, 59–60
  in *DSM-IV*, 107
Mania
  Axis I disorders and, 230–231
  Axis II disorders and, 242–244
  bipolar disorder in old age and, 253–254
  borderline personality disorder and, 243
  in children
    diagnosis for, 263–266
    epidemiology for, 266–268
Manic episode, definition of, 264
Manic-only symptoms, cerebrovascular lesions in old age and, 253
Manic symptoms in children, 266–268
Manic syndromes, AIDS patients and, 254–255
McLean First-Episode Mania Project, 234
Medical illness and bipolar disorder, 213–224
  medical comorbidity, 219–222
  overview, 213–214
  secondary mania and, 214–219
Medical illness in old age and depression, 157–175
[Medical illness in old age and depression]
  comorbidity effects of, 164–166
  depression identification of, 166–173
    diagnostic criteria, 168–169
    exclusive symptoms, 169–173
    inclusive symptoms, 169–173
    medical illness effect, 168
    patient self-report of symptoms, 166–167
    substitutive symptoms, 169–173
  depression rates of, 158–159
  health care utilization of, 163
  health effects of, 162–166
  mortality of, 163–164
  overview of, 157–158
  as reactive depression, 160–161
  risk factors of, 158–160
  treatment of, 173–174
Medically ill, depression in, 57–87
  cancer and, 85–86
  cardiovascular disease and, 83–84
  Cushing's syndrome and, 83
  descriptive differential and, 59–64
    adjustment disorder with depressed mood, 63
    bipolar disorders, 63
    grief, 60–61
    major depressive disorder, 59–60
    psychological factors affecting medical condition, 63–64
    symptoms resembling depression, 61–63
  diagnostic classification of, 58
  diagnostic strategies and, 61–62
  diagnostic validity of, 58–59
  differential diagnosis of, 59
  disorders associated with, 65
  endocrine disorders and

[Medically ill, depression in]
diabetes mellitus, 81–82
thyroid disorders, 82
etiological differential and
mood disorder due to general medical condition, 64–66
substance-induced mood disorder, 66
HIV and, 84–85
hyperprolactinemia and, 83
immune system, 72–73, 74
multiple sclerosis (MS), 80
natural killer cell activity (NKA), 72, 73
neurobiological issues, 68–74
neurochemistry of depression, 68–69
neuroendocrinology of depression, 69–72
hypothalamic-pituitary-adrenal (HPA), 69, 70–71, 73
hypothalamic-pituitary-thyroid (HPT), 69, 71–72
neuroimmunology of depression, 72–73
neurological disorders, 79–81
cerebrovascular disease, 79
dementia, 80–81
depression screening, 66–67
epilepsy, 79–80
Parkinson's Disease, 81
psychosocial therapies, 78–79
somatic therapies, 74–78
antidepressants, 74–75
atypical antidepressants, 76–77
electroconvulsive therapy, 78
heterocyclic antidepressants, 75–76
monoamine oxidase inhibitors, 76
psychostimulants, 77
[Medically ill, depression in]
selective serotonin reuptake inhibitors, 76–77
treatment, 74–79
Medical morbidity, medical illness in old age and depression, 162–163
Medication response, bipolar disorder in children, 274–275
Medications (*see also* Antidepressants; Pharmacotherapy):
associated with depression, 67
OCD and panic disorder, 235–236
substance abuse treatment, 48–49
Memory impairment in old age manic patients, 254
Men, alcohol abuse and, 28
Mesolimbic dopamine pathway, 32
Metabolic disorders
disorders associated with depression, 65
secondary mania and, 216, 218
Migraine, 220
Mirtazapine, 76–77
Moclobemide, 48, 76
Monoamine oxidase inhibitors (MAOIs), 76
Monoamines, depression and, 68–69
Montgomery-Asberg Depression Rating Scale (MADRS), 67
Mood disorder due to general medical condition (MDDGMC), 64–66
Mood disorders, 107
Mood symptoms in children, psychosis and, 266
Morphine, 34
Mortality, medical illness in old age and depression, 163–164

Motivational enhancement therapy (MET), substance abuse and, 41–42
Motivational Interviewing (Miller and Rollnick), 41
Motivation and substance abuse, 27
  dual-diagnosis treatment approach, 41
  stages of, 36–37, 41
Multiple comorbidity, bipolar disorder and Axis I disorders, 234
Multiple-episode mania in old age, 252
Multiple sclerosis (MS)
  depression of medically ill, 80
  medical comorbidity, 220
  pseudobulbar phenomena, 62

Naltrexone, for alcohol and depression, 44, 45
National Comorbidity Survey (NCS)
  bipolar disorders and Axis I disorders, 230
  bipolar disorders in old age, 249
  substance abuse and bipolar disorder, 197
  substance abuse and depression, 28
National Depressive Manic Depressive Association, 263
Natural killer cell activity (NKA), depression of medically ill, 72, 73
Nefazadone, for alcohol and depression, 44
Neoplastic disease, disorder associated with depression, 65
Neurobiological issues of depression in medically ill, 68–74
  neurochemistry of, 69
[Neurobiological issues of depression in medically ill]
  neuroendocrinology of, 69–72
  neuroimmunology of, 72–73
Neurological abnormalities, secondary mania and, 216, 217–218
Neurological disorders
  associated with depression, 65
  in depression of medically ill, 79–81
Neuronal sensitization or "kindling," substance abuse and bipolar disorder and, 204
Nicotine and depression, 29, 30
  biological markers, 34–35
  pharmacological treatment of, 47–48
Norepinephrine (NE), 68
Nutritional disorders associated with depression, 65

Obsessive-compulsive disorder (OCD), 231, 232–233
  panic disorder and medications and, 235–236
Old age (*see also* Medical illness in old age and depression):
  advantages of studying, 249
Old age, bipolar disorder in, 249–259
  comorbidity and outcome, 256–258
  demographic data, 251
  neuroimaging, 255–256
    silent cerebral infarctions (SCIs), 255
    subcortical hyperintensities (SCHs), 256
  neurological disorders of, 250–256

[Old age, bipolar disorder in]
cerebrovascular lesions and, 253
dementia, 253–254
mania, 253–254
other neurological conditions, 254–255
overview of, 249–250
treatment outcome, 257–259
Opiates and depression
biological markers of, 34
pharmacological treatment of, 47
Organic personality syndrome, 265

Pain, depression and, 65
Pancreatic cancer, disorder associated with depression, 66
Panic disorder and depression, 231–232
Parkinson's Disease (PD), antidepressants and, 81
Personality disorders (*see also* Axis II personality disorders):
classification, 141–144
definition of in DSM-IV, 106, 128
dysthymia and, 124–127
Personality disorders and depression, 105–148
age and, 137, 141
cluster A personality disorders, 131–133
cluster B personality disorders, 133–135
cluster C personality disorders, 135–137
comorbidity models, 146–148
prevalence of, 108–123
studies in patient samples, 129–131
[Personality disorders and depression]
studies using family samples, 129
sex and, 141
trait-state problem and, 144–146
Personality traits, 106, 107
Pharmacokinetics of antidepressants, 77
Pharmacotherapy
for substance abuse and bipolar disorder, 204–207 (*see also* Antidepressants; Medications)
Predictive diagnostic validity, 59
Prevention, bipolar disorder and major depressive disorder (MDD), 19
Pseudobulbar phenomena, in multiple sclerosis, 62
Psychiatric comorbidity, bipolar disorder and, 230
Psychological factors affecting medical condition (PFAMC), in depression of medically ill, 63–64
Psychopathology and age, in bipolar disorder in children, 268–271
comorbidity/mixed episodes, 269–271
Psychosis and mood symptoms in children, 266
Psychosocial factors of substance abuse, 30–31
Psychosocial therapies, for depression of medically ill, 78–79
Psychostimulants, for depression of medically ill, 77

Psychotherapeutic treatments, for substance abuse and bipolar disorder, 207–208

Radiological procedures, depression and, 65
Reactive depression
  medical illness in old age as, 160–161
  in medically ill, 65
Relapse prevention therapy for substance abuse, 43
Research Diagnostic Criteria for mania, 256
Reserpine, depression and, 68
Rheumatological disease, disorders associated with depression, 65
Risk factors, medical illness in old age and depression, 158–160

Screening tools
  for depression, 67
  for substance abuse disorder, 36
Secondary mania, 250
  medical illness and bipolar disorder and, 214–219
Selective serotonin reuptake inhibitors (SSRIs)
  alcohol and depression and, 46
  cancer and, 86
  depression of medically ill, 76–77
"Self-medication theory," of substance abuse, 31
Serotonin (5-HT)
  alcohol dependence and, 33
  depression and, 68–69
Sertraline, alcohol abuse and, 44, 46
Sex and personality disorders comorbidity, 141
Side effects, tricyclic antidepressants (TCAs), 75–76
Silent cerebral infarctions (SCIs), bipolar disorder in old age and, 255
Smoking cessation, depression and, 29
Social factors, substance abuse, 31
Stimulant use, bipolar disorders and, 17
Structured Clinical Interview for DSM (SCID), 38
  substance abuse and bipolar disorder and, 202
Study on the Psychobiology of Depression, 28
Subcortical hyperintensities (SCHs), bipolar disorder in old age and, 256
Substance abuse and bipolar disorder, 197–208
  clinical course of, 202–204
  diagnostic issues, 201–202
  neuronal sensitization or "kindling," 204
  pharmacotherapy, 204–207
    anticonvulsant therapy, 205–207
    lithium, 204–205, 206
  prevalence of, 198–201
  psychotherapeutic treatments, 207–208
Substance abuse and depression, 27–49
  assessment of, 36
  biological factors, 32
  biological markers, 32–35
    alcohol dependence, 33–34
    cocaine dependence, 34
    opiate dependence, 34
  differential diagnosis of, 35–39
  in *DSM-IV*, 36
  epidemiology of, 28–30
  medications and, 48–49

[Substance abuse and depression]
pharmacological treatment of, 44–48
alcohol, 44–46
cocaine, 46–47
nicotine, 47–48
opiates, 47
psychosocial factors, 30–31
treatment, 39–44
assertive community treatment model, 40
community reinforcement approach (CRA), 42–43
integrated treatment model, 40–41
motivation-based dual-diagnosis treatment approach, 41
phases, 39
relapse prevention therapy, 43
12-step recovery programs, 43–44
types, 27
Substance-induced mood disorder (SIMD), 66
Substitutive diagnostic strategy, 61–62
Suicide
bipolar disorder in children, 273–274
smokers and, 29
substance abuse and, 35
Surgery complications, in secondary mania, 253
Surgical procedures, depression and, 65
Symptoms resembling depression in medically ill, 61–63
Thyroid disorders, depression of medically ill and, 71–72, 82
Tourette's disorder, 220–221, 233
Trait-state problem, in personality disorders and depression, 144–146
Treatment
for bipolar disorder in old age, 257–259
medically ill depression, 74–79
substance abuse and depression, 39–44
pharmacological, 44–48
TRH, hypothalamic-pituitary-thyroid (HPT) and, 71–72
Tricyclic antidepressants (TCAs), 75
Triiodothyronine (T_3), 71
12-step recovery programs for substance abuse, 43

Uncomplicated form of mania in old age, 257
Unipolar depression, 1–20
prevalence of, 2–3
University of Cincinnati Mania First-Episode Project, 230, 234
University of Iowa Psychiatric Hospital, 256

Valproate, substance abuse and, 205–207
Venlafaxine, 84

Warfarin, 84
Women, alcohol abuse and, 28

Youth-onset mania/hypomania, 269

About the Editor

MAURICIO TOHEN is Global Medical Advisor, Lilly Research Laboratories, Indianapolis, Indiana. Additionally, he is an Associate Clinical Professor of Psychiatry, Harvard Medical School, Boston, Massachusetts. The author, coauthor, or coeditor of over 200 articles, abstracts, and book chapters, he is a Fellow of the American Psychiatric Association and a member of the American College of Psychiatrists. Dr. Tohen received the M.D. degree (1976) from the National University of Mexico, Mexico City, and the M.P.H. (1984) and Dr.P.H. (1988) degrees from Harvard University, Cambridge, Massachusetts.